Assessment and Management of Central Auditory Processing Disorders in the Educational Setting

From Science to Practice

A Singular Audiology Text

Jeffrey L. Danhauer, Ph.D.
Audiology Editor

Assessment and Management of Central Auditory Processing Disorders in the Educational Setting

From Science to Practice

Teri James Bellis, M.A., CCC-A

SINGULAR PUBLISHING GROUP, INC.
SAN DIEGO · LONDON

Singular Publishing Group, Inc.
401 West "A" Street, Suite 325
San Diego, California 92101-7904

Singular Publishing Ltd.
19 Compton Terrace
London, N1 2UN, UK

e-mail: singpub@mail.cerfnet.com
Website: http://www.singpub.com

© 1996 by Singular Publishing Group, Inc.

Second Printing May 1997

Illustrated by Timothy P. Bellis

Typeset in 10/12 Cheltenham by So Cal Graphics
Printed in the United States of America by McNaughton & Gunn

Library of Congress Cataloging-in-Publication Data

Bellis, Teri James.
 Assessment and management of central auditory processing disorders in
 the educational setting : from science to practice / Teri James Bellis.
  p.   cm.
 Includes bibliographical references and index.
 ISBN 1-56593-628-0
 1. Word deafness.   I. Title.
RC394.W63B45   1996
617.8—dc20   96–3917
                                                      CIP

Contents

Foreword

Auditory processing has become an important and well-known facet of communication disorders. According to a recent ASHA Task Force document, the now common term CAPD (central auditory processing disorders) refers to an observed deficiency in one or more of the following auditory behaviors: sound localization and lateralization, auditory discrimination, auditory pattern recognition, temporal aspects of audition (resolution, masking, integration, ordering), auditory performance decrements with competing acoustic signals, and auditory performance decrements with degraded acoustic signals. Abnormal results on various auditory evoked potential measurement can also define an auditory processing deficit.

Although auditory processing and its related dysfunctions have become better known, defined, and understood, education about this problem is lacking at all levels. *Assessment and Management of Central Auditory Processing Disorders in the Educational Setting: From Science to Practice* should help resolve this problem. The author Teri Bellis, is relatively new on the auditory processing scene, but brings with her considerable practical experience from a variety of clinical settings. In addition to her varied and audiological background, Teri brings a high level of enthusiasm to the complex area of brain function and hearing.

Within these pages the reader will find information not only about current assessment trends of CAPD, but also about novel management approaches. The book focuses on the educational setting, but many of the principles can be applied to a variety of settings. The book also discusses practical applications and relates them back to the science from which they evolved. This last aspect is critical and is a point far too often overlooked. In a field as complex and challenging as auditory processing, it is important that we embrace its basic science and use it to guide us through much unknown territory.

Assessment and Management of Central Auditory Processing Disorders in the Educational Setting is not an exhaustive review nor an in-depth account of assessment or management of CAPD. Rather, it is a practical, easy access and handy approach to CAPD. It also can serve as a good introduction to the field of auditory processing. Certainly it should be used with a variety of other resources to gain a well-rounded foundation in this area of study. The book is nicely organized to promote optimal learning. In each chapter there is a list of learning objectives, a summary, and review questions, and in the text key words and phrases are placed in italic and/or bold to direct the reader. The writing is understandable and easy to read. The reader will surely find this to be an approachable, informative resource for understanding CAPD.

Frank E. Musiek, Ph.D.

Preface

Few topics within the fields of audiology and speech-language pathology have resulted in more misinformation, confusion, and general frustration as the topic of Central Auditory Processing Disorders (CAPD). For years, controversy has existed concerning methods of assessment, methods and effectiveness of remediation/rehabilitation and, for some, even whether CAPD exists. For those of us in the educational arena, the frustration is intensified as we are called upon frequently by parents, teachers, and associated colleagues to assist in cases of children who are exhibiting academic difficulties. Often as a last ditch effort when all else has failed, we are asked to determine if the child in question exhibits characteristics of CAPD. The fact that we, ourselves, have little or no specialized training in the science of auditory processing combined with the paucity of practical information regarding specific diagnostic and rehabilitative tools available for use in the educational setting merely augments our own frustration and discomfort with the issue. Yet the referrals and requests keep pouring in.

The purpose of this book is to assist the professional in the educational setting in gaining the knowledge base necessary for understanding the mechanism of auditory processing. In addition, these writings will serve as a resource for practical application of scientific theory. It should be noted that the intent of this book is not to take the place of specialized training. It is not possible to provide the reader with a complete, in-depth treatment of all of the complexities of this subject within the scope of one book. However, it is possible to give the reader a basic understanding of the issues involved and to direct the reader toward areas of further study. Therefore, this book is designed to assist the reader in addressing the challenges of CAPD in the educational setting from a scientifically based perspective, and then applying that knowledge in a practical sense to his or her daily job duties, thus eliminating some of the mystique and confusion that surrounds this complex topic.

The book is divided into three parts. Each chapter concludes with questions for review to assist the reader in the learning process. Part One discusses the science of auditory processing, focusing specifically upon anatomy and physiology of the central auditory nervous system and effects of pathology. In addition, the neurophysiological bases of specific auditory processes (dichotic listening, temporal processing, and binaural interaction), and neuromaturation and neuroplasticity of the auditory system are covered. A complete presentation of the aforementioned material is not the intent of the author. However, with a core knowledge of the scientific aspects of CAPD, the reader may achieve a level of understanding necessary for appropriate assessment and recommendations for rehabilitation. Therefore, Part One serves as an overview of basic science so that the clinician may better understand the "Whys" as well as the "Hows."

Part Two focuses on specific assessment and management tools. Included in this section are recommendations for a multidisciplinary approach to screening for CAPD, methods of determining whether a comprehensive CAP evaluation is indicated, choosing the test battery, overview of current assessment tools, interpreting the test battery, and making recommendations for deficit-specific management based upon test outcomes combined with what is known about brain function.

We consider Part Three to be our "Nuts 'n' Bolts" section. This section includes recommendations for development of a service delivery program within the educational setting. Attention will be given to a variety of subjects including methods of educating educators, parents, and colleagues through inservice training, child study processes, and concise report writing. In addition, although recommendations for rehabilitation are based upon neurophysiological function, very little data exist regarding actual efficacy of specific remediation techniques. One possible explanation for this is the widening gulf between science and practice. In general, it seems that scientists rarely present the practical, remediation-based application of science. By the same token, practitioners rarely present the scientific bases for their remediation practices. It appears likely that the data regarding which remediation activities are most efficient will eventually come from those practitioners engaged in the assessment and rehabilitative process. Therefore, the final chapter of this book looks at methods in which we, as practitioners in the educational setting, can utilize appropriate scientific methodology in our daily settings with an eye toward data collection regarding efficacy of assessment and remediation strategies, thus helping to bridge the gap between science and practice. If unfamiliar with scientific methodology, the reader may wish to read the final chapter of this book first, and then begin at the beginning, in order to facilitate understanding of the earlier chapters, as well as to complete the loop from science to practice and back to science again.

Those of us in the educational setting have been hoping for the "easy answer" to the CAPD question. It will perhaps dishearten some readers to realize that such an answer does not exist. In fact, as more is learned about the function of the central auditory nervous system, it is likely that the entire CAP arena will move toward the more complex. Therefore, it is essential that the clinician engage in continuing education activities and make all attempts to keep up with the literature. The author has no doubt that what is recommended in ten years is likely to be very different from the recommendations made today. All of the answers are not in yet, and they may never be. However, it is our fondest hope that this book will assist the clinician "in the trenches" to become familiar with the current knowledge about CAPD in order to better serve the children with whom we work every day.

The author wishes to acknowledge the invaluable assistance of the following individuals: Frank Musiek, Ph.D., whose professional guidance and technical assistance provided the catalyst for this book; Jeffrey Danhauer, Ph.D., whose editorial assistance and timely suggestions were greatly appreciated at every step along the way; Tim Bellis for his brilliant illustrations and helpful comments; Jeff Simmons, whose generous contribution of time and effort helped to lighten the load; and, last but never least, Jeanane Ferre, Ph.D., for her unconditional professional and personal support.

This book is dedicated to Tim, Jennifer, Christopher, and the littlest Bellis—as yet unnamed—each of whom made the greatest sacrifice of all to see this dream realized.

PART
ONE

The Science of Central Auditory Processing

CHAPTER

Neuroanatomy and Neurophysiology of the Auditory System

It is essential for the clinician involved in the assessment of central auditory processes to have a basic understanding of the anatomical and physiological bases underlying those processes. Without knowledge of the functioning of the central auditory nervous system (CANS), the full clinical value of central tests may go untapped.

This chapter provides an overview of the anatomy and physiology of the CANS. Although it is not within the scope of this book to give the reader a complete review of this subject, the topics discussed herein will provide a basic understanding of the function of the CANS as well as direction for further study. There are numerous sources available in which more detailed analyses of neuroanatomy and neurophysiology can be found. The reader is directed to the References at the end of this book for further resources.

Learning Objectives

After studying this chapter, the reader should be able to

1. Define technical terms related to planes of brain section and directional reference
2. Identify primary lobes of the brain and discuss the general function of each lobe
3. Discuss the general mechanism of synaptic transmission
4. Identify primary central auditory nervous system brainstem structures and discuss their functions
5. Identify primary central auditory nervous system cortical structures and discuss their functions
6. Discuss the structure and function of the corpus callosum, particularly as it relates to auditory function
7. Discuss current theory relating to the function of the central auditory nervous system efferent pathways and the olivo-cochlear bundle
8. Discuss general effects of pathology on various levels of the central auditory nervous system.

Terminology

Specific terminology is used in neuroscience to indicate the direction and position of various structures with relation to other structures in the brain. In this section, we will discuss terminology related to *planes of brain section* and *directional reference.*

The human brain can be sectioned into three primary planes: *sagittal, coronal,* and *horizontal.* The term sagittal refers to a cut in which the brain is divided into right and left sides. A midsagittal section is one in which the brain is divided at midline, or center, thus separating the brain into two equal halves (Figure 1–1a). A coronal section divides the brain into front (anterior) and back (posterior) sections (Figure 1–1b), whereas a horizontal section divides the brain into upper (superior) and lower (inferior) portions (Figure 1–1c). Another important term relating to planes of section is *transverse.* A transverse cut is one which is diagonal to the horizontal plane (Figure 1–1d). Because of the curvature of the brainstem and other structures, transverse sections are often necessary to view internal landmarks of these structures adequately.

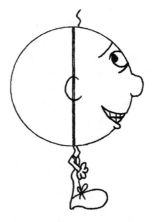

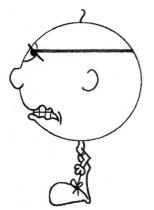

a. sagittal and midsagittal section

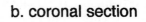

b. coronal section

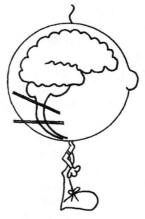

c. horizontal section

d. transverse section

Figure 1-1.   Planes of brain section.

Neuroscience also utilizes terminology relating to directionality in the brain as well as location of a structure in relation to other structures. The term *rostral* refers to locations toward the head and away from the tail, whereas *caudal* indicates the opposite: toward the tail and away from the head. For example, in gross terms, the brainstem is caudal to the cerebrum, but rostral to the spinal cord. Finally, the term *lateral* indicates a structure away from the midline, and *medial* refers to a structure toward the midline. For example, the cochlea is lateral to the VIIIth nerve, but medial to the tympanic membrane.

Although there are other common terms relating to neuroanatomy, these are the primary ones that will be used throughout this chapter.

Gross Anatomy of the Brain

The adult human brain weighs approximately 2 lb and represents 2% of total body weight. The cerebrum, which consists of the two cerebral hemispheres, makes up the largest portion of the brain. The surface of the brain is referred to as the *cortex* and consists of gray (unmyelinated) matter. The cortical surface is convoluted, forming ridges (*gyri*) and valleys (*sulci*), which serve as landmarks for important primary structures. The number and size of gyri and sulci vary greatly from individual to individual; therefore, they serve only as rough frames of reference.

The two cerebral hemispheres are separated by the *longitudinal fissure* (Figure 1–2). Each cerebral hemisphere is essentially a mirror image of the other although, as will be discussed later in this chapter, there exist some significant asymmetries in terms of size and length of cerebral landmarks.

Each cerebral hemisphere consists of four primary lobes named for the bones of the skull that they underlie: the *frontal, parietal, temporal* and, most posterior, *occipital* (Figure 1–3). The frontal lobe lies anterior to the central sulcus and superior to the lateral (or Sylvian) fissure. This lobe contains the primary motor cortex in which motor activity for the entire human body is represented.

The parietal lobe is located between the frontal and occipital lobes and above the temporal lobe. It is primarily concerned with perception and elaboration of somatic sensation and integration of multimodality or crossed modality information. The temporal lobe is located inferior to the frontal and parietal lobes and anterior to the occipital lobe. The Sylvian (lateral) fissure marks the superior boundary of this lobe. The temporal lobe is the site of the primary auditory cortex, auditory association areas, and auditory language associational cortex (Wernicke's or Brodmann area 22). This lobe will be discussed further later in this chapter. Only a small portion of the occipi-

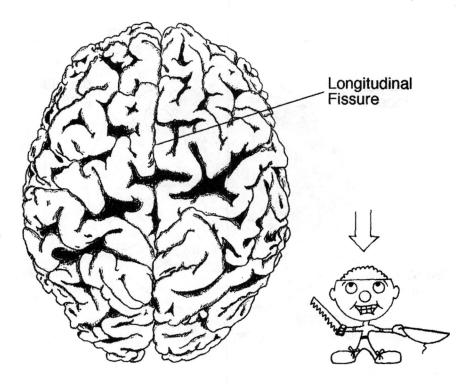

Figure 1-2. Superior view of brain showing cerebral hemispheres separated by longitudinal fissure.

tal lobe can be seen on the lateral surface of the brain. The majority of this lobe lies along the medial surface of the cerebral hemisphere. This lobe contains the primary and secondary visual cortices.

Upon midsagittal sectioning of the brain, further structures can be viewed (Figure 1–4). Most notable for our purposes is the *corpus callosum*. Present only in mammals, the corpus callosum is the largest fiber tract in the primate brain. Heavily myelinated (white matter), it is located at the base of the longitudinal fissure and connects most cortical areas of the two cerebral hemispheres. Because of its importance in central auditory processing, the corpus callosum will be discussed further later in this chapter.

Other structures of the brain seen in the midsagittal view include the *cerebellum*, which is located below the occipital lobe and posterior to the brainstem and which is concerned primarily with coordination of

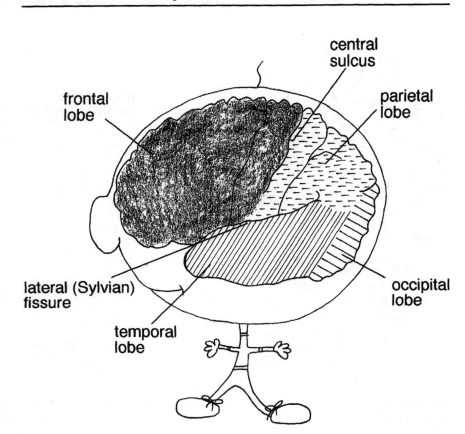

Figure 1-3. Lateral view of brain showing primary lobes, central sulcus, and lateral (Sylvian) fissure.

motor activities and maintenance of equilibrium; the *diencephalon*, which consists of both the *thalamus*, concerned with relay of sensorimotor information to the cortex and some speech and language functions, and the *hypothalamus*, which regulates various autonomic functions such as body heat production, hormone production, and reproduction, among others; the *pineal body*, which appears to contribute to circadian rhythm and sexual reproduction cycles; and the *hypophysis (pituitary gland)*—called the "master gland" of the body—which secretes hormones that regulate a variety of functions including metabolism, sexual drive, pain, emotion, temperature, and electrolyte control.

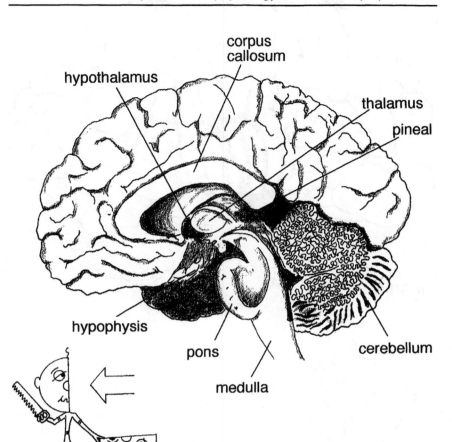

Figure 1–4. Midsagittal section of brain.

These are only a few of the important structures of the brain, and the reader is referred to the References at the end of this book for further, more detailed study.

Two additional cerebral structures are worthy of mention: the *insula* and the *limbic system*. The *insular cortex*, also known as the *isle of Reil*, is located within the lateral fissure and cannot be viewed from the surface without spreading or removing portions of the frontal, parietal, and temporal lobes (Figure 1–5). As will be discussed later, the insula has important implications in audition.

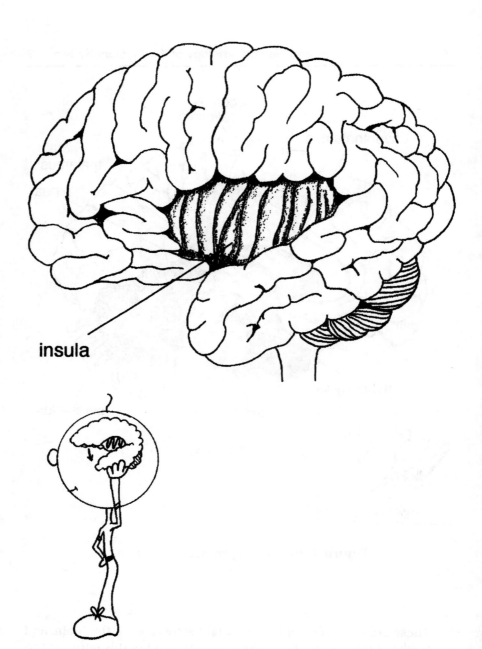

insula

Figure 1-5. Lateral view of brain with temporal lobe displaced to expose insula.

The limbic system is located along the most medial margins of the frontal, parietal, and temporal lobes. The structures within this system provide emotional drive to a variety of functions necessary for survival, including instinctual reflexes, aggression, defensive behaviors (including the "fight or flight" response), mating, and other primitive functions.

The *brainstem*, which will be considered in depth later in this chapter, consists of three structures: the *midbrain, pons,* and *medulla oblongata.* In addition, some sources consider the structures of the diencephalon (thalamus and hypothalamus) to be part of the brainstem (Bhatnagar & Andy, 1995).

There are four *ventricles* (or cavities) within the brain that function to circulate cerebrospinal fluid: two *lateral ventricles*, one *third ventricle*, and one *fourth* ventricle. The body of the lateral ventricle is formed by the corpus callosum and the floor is formed by the superior surface of the thalamus. The lateral ventricle extends from the frontal lobe (anterior horn) to the occipital lobe (posterior horn). The third ventricle is located between the two thalami and connects superiorly to the lateral ventricle through Monro's foramen and inferiorly to the fourth ventricle of the brainstem through the cerebral aqueduct. The floor of the third ventricle is formed by the nuclei of the hypothalamus. The floor of the fourth ventricle is located in the brainstem at the level of the pons and medulla. The fourth ventricle contains openings through which cerebrospinal fluid can access the subarachnoid space surrounding the central nervous system.

The *basal ganglia* are subcortical (gray matter) structures which help to regulate muscle tone and motor functions (Figure 1–6). The primary structures of the basal ganglia are the *caudate, putamen,* and *globus pallidus.* The putamen and globus padillus lie between the *internal capsule* and the *external capsule,* which are pathways composed of white matter. The internal capsule is of particular interest as it is the pathway through which auditory information is transmitted from the brainstem to the auditory cortex. The external capsule contains fibers that carry auditory (as well as somatic and possibly visual) information from the internal capsule to the insula. Within the external capsule lies a thin strip of gray matter, the *claustrum,* which also seems to be highly responsive to acoustic stimulation.

The brain is protected within the head by the *meninges* (three fibrous tissue membranes that surround the central nervous system), the cerebrospinal fluid, and the bones of the skull.

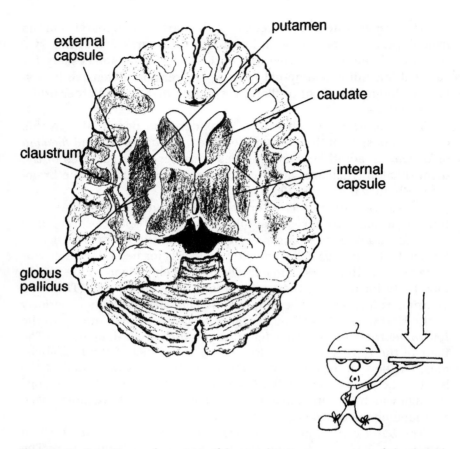

Figure 1-6. Coronal section of brain showing structures of the basal ganglia, internal and external capsules, and claustrum.

Basis of Neural Transmission

Nerve cells communicate through nerve impulses that are mediated by *neurotransmitters*, chemical substances that are released at the synapse and cause specific events to take place. The *synapse* is the point at which nerve cells interact. There are two primary effects of neurotransmitters: *excitatory* and *inhibitory*.

Excitatory neurotransmitters lower the postsynaptic cell's membrane potential or threshold, thus allowing the cell to fire and propogate the nerve impulse. Inhibitory neurotransmitters work in the opposite way: They raise the threshold of the postsynaptic cell, making it less likely to fire. Both excitatory and inhibitory neurotransmitters are critical to appropriate functioning of the nervous system. Speed of transmission is related to diameter of the nerve cell and amount of myelination, among other factors.

Although a complete discussion of neurochemistry is not within the scope of this chapter, it should be noted that the chemical composition at the synapse site is affected by a variety of drugs. Therefore, pharmacologic intervention holds great promise for the treatment of many auditory and vestibular complaints, either by increasing excitability of the postsynaptic neurons or by encouraging inhibition (Musiek & Hoffman, 1990; Sahley, Kalish, Musiek, & Hoffman, 1991).

Brainstem Auditory Pathways

The anterior surface of the brainstem can be seen in Figure 1–7. The most caudal portion of the brainstem is the *medulla*. Proceeding in a caudal to rostral direction, the next portion is the pons, and the most rostral portion is termed the *midbrain*. In order to view the posterior surface of the brainstem, the cerebellum must first be removed. The posterior surface of the brainstem is shown in Figure 1–8. Although a few structures essential to auditory function can be seen on the surface of the brainstem, many cannot, and require transverse sectioning of the brainstem in order to be viewed adequately. Several brainstem structures comprise the ascending auditory pathway. These include the *cochlear nuclei, superior olivary complex, lateral lemniscus, inferior colliculus,* and *medial geniculate body* (Figure 1–9).

Cochlear Nuclei—Pons

The most caudal structures in the CANS are the cochlear nuclei (CN). There are three main nuclei: the *anterior ventral, posterior ventral,* and *dorsal.* The CN are located on the posterolateral surface of the pontomedullary junction where the pons, medulla, and cerebellum meet. This area is also known as the *cerebellopontine angle* and is a common site of tumors.

The cells within the CN complex are tonotopically arranged. That is to say, there is a one-to-one relationship between tonotopic organization of the hair cells within the cochlea and tonotopic organization

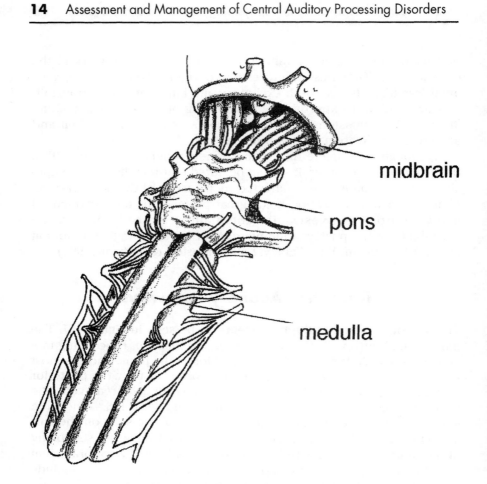

midbrain

pons

medulla

Figure 1-7.   Anterior view of brainstem.

of the cells within the CN. This cochlear representation is repeated throughout the ascending auditory pathways (Kiang, 1975).

The CN project to more rostral structures by way of three main tracts: the *dorsal acoustic stria, intermediate stria,* and the *ventral stria.* Although the majority of auditory fibers from the CN cross the midline and project contralaterally, many of the fibers remain ipsilateral. The fibers of the dorsal stria project to the contralateral superior olivary complex, lateral lemniscus, and inferior colliculus. Fibers of the intermediate stria communicate with the contralateral lateral lemniscus and inferior colliculus. The ventral stria, by far the largest fiber tract, projects to the contralateral superior olivary complex. All of the cells that cross midline form the *nucleus of the trapezoid body.*

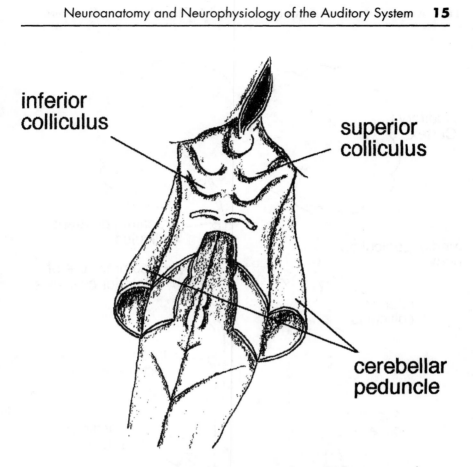

inferior
colliculus

superior
colliculus

cerebellar
peduncle

Figure 1–8.   Posterior view of brainstem with cerebellum removed.

Those fibers from the CN that remain ipsilateral project to either the ipsilateral superior olivary complex or lateral lemniscus. The fact that the CN are located on the posterolateral surface of the brainstem makes it particularly susceptible to pathological effects of tumors such as acoustic neuromas.

Superior Olivary Complex—Pons

The superior olivary complex (SOC) is medial to the cochlear nucleus in the caudal pons, thus it cannot be viewed on the surface of the brainstem. It receives information from both ipsilateral and contralat-

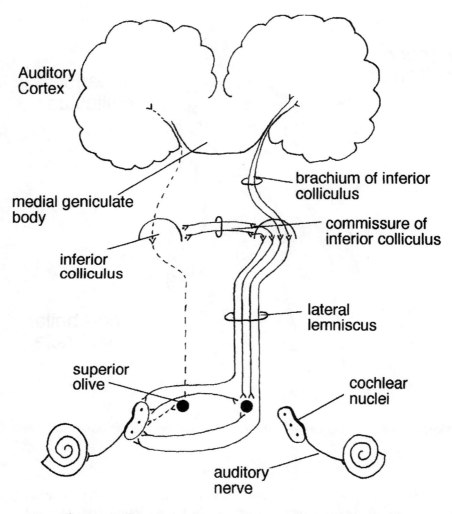

Figure 1-9. Ascending brainstem auditory pathways.

eral cochlear nuclei. A distinctive feature of the SOC is the presence of "binaural cells" that are sensitive to time and intensity cues. Since input from the ipsilateral ear reaches the SOC milliseconds sooner than input from the contralateral ear, the SOC is implicated in successful localization, lateralization, and binaural integration.

Lateral Lemniscus—Pons

Composed of both ascending and descending fibers, the lateral lemniscus (LL) is the primary ascending auditory pathway. It extends from the SOC to the inferior colliculus in the midbrain. Like the SOC, the LL cannot be seen from the surface of the brainstem. It contains cell bodies (nuclei) along its length that receive crossed and uncrossed projections from more caudal auditory structures, thus continuing bilateral representation of auditory stimuli.

Inferior Colliculus—Midbrain

The inferior colliculus (IC) is located on the posterior surface of the brainstem and is easily viewed following removal of the cerebellum. It is considered to be the "way station" for auditory information, as both ICs are connected by commissural fibers. As a result, the IC is another structure that has profound implications in the ability to localize a sound source and other binaural processes. Part of the auditory information received by the IC is projected to the *superior colliculus, reticular formation,* and *cerebellum* for coordination of eye, head, and body movements in reflexive localization toward a sound source. Through the *brachium of the IC,* auditory information is sent to the ipsilateral medial geniculate body.

Medial Geniculate Body—Midbrain

The medial geniculate body (MGB) is located on the inferior surface of the thalamus, medial to the auditory cortex. It serves as the thalamic relay station for transmission of auditory information. The MGB receives information primarily from the ipsilateral brachium of the IC and projects to the internal capsule where fibers transmit information to the auditory cortex via the external capsule and insula.

The Cerebrum

Primary and Associative Auditory Cortex

The primary auditory cortex, *Heschl's gyrus,* is located approximately two thirds of the way posteriorly on the upper surface of the temporal lobe. This upper surface is also referred to as the *supratemporal plane*. Heschl's gyrus cannot be observed on the lateral surface of the cortex; instead, the temporal lobe must be removed or displaced inferiorly in order to expose the supratemporal plane (Figure 1–10). The primary auditory cortex is the site of auditory sensation and perception and receives projections from the medial geniculate body via the internal capsule, insula, and external capsule. The primary auditory cortex is known to retain the tonotopic organization of the cochlea.

The *planum temporal* extends along the cortical surface from the most posterior portion of Heschl's gyrus back along the lateral (Sylvian) fissure to its end point. The *supramarginal gyrus* curves around the most posterior aspect of the lateral fissure. This area, along with the *angular gyrus* (located immediately posterior to the supramarginal gyrus) is the approximate region of Wernicke's area, the auditory associational cortex (Figure 1–11). *Wernicke's area* is thought to be concerned with recognition of linguistic stimuli and comprehension of spoken language as well as contributing to language

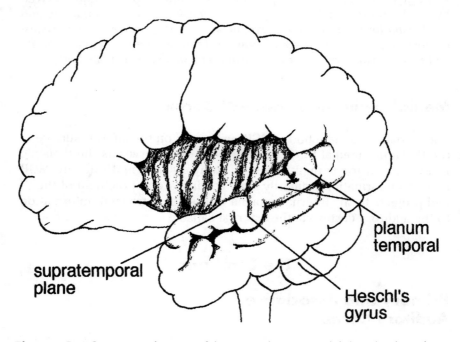

Figure 1–10. Lateral view of brain with temporal lobe displaced to expose Heschl's gyrus.

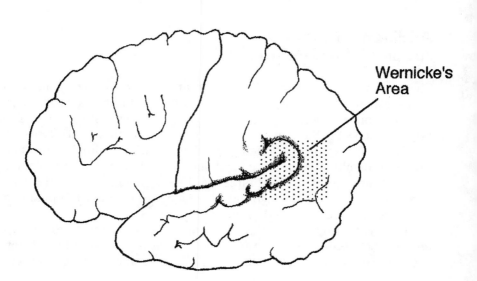

Wernicke's
Area

Figure 1-11.   Lateral view of brain.

formulation. The primary and associational auditory cortices are connected by an extensive axonal bundle.

Asymmetries of Auditory Areas of the Cerebrum

Geschwind and Levitsky (1968) initially discovered that the planum temporal was larger on the left side than the right in the majority of their subjects studied. The implications of this finding are significant when theories of hemispheric dominance for language are considered. In addition, Musiek and Reeves (1990) reported a relationship between the length of the Sylvian fissure and the length of the planum temporal, with both structures significantly longer on the left side in all specimens studied. The length of Heschl's gyrus was also found to be longer on the left side. It is possible that these cerebral asymmetries contribute to left hemisphere dominance for functions involving binaural listening and as a basis for greater language development potential for the left side (Musiek & Reeves, 1990).

Additional Auditory Areas of the Cerebrum

The inferior portion of the parietal and frontal lobes are also responsive to acoustic stimulation. In addition, as mentioned previously, the insula has a large number of fibers that are responsive to acoustic stimulation. The posterior aspect of the insula is immediately adjacent to Heschl's gyrus.

There are two primary pathways through which auditory information is transmitted from the medial geniculate bodies in the thalamus to the auditory cortex. The first is via the internal capsule to Heschl's gyrus. The second is through the internal capsule, under the putamen to the external capsule, and to the insula.

Finally, Wernicke's area in the temporal lobe connects to *Broca's area* in the frontal lobe via the *arcuate fasciculus*, a large fiber tract. Broca's area is considered to be responsible for motor speech output.

The Corpus Callosum

The primary auditory cortical areas in both hemispheres are not connected directly to each other. Instead, they are connected only through their association cortices which are, in turn, connected to each other via the corpus callosum. As mentioned previously, the corpus callosum is the largest commissural fiber bundle and connects the two cerebral hemispheres.

The corpus callosum consists of five main parts: the *anterior commissure, rostrum, genu, body,* and *splenium* (Figure 1–12). It appears that different portions of the corpus callosum contain fibers specific to different functions. For example, the occipital lobe projects solely through the splenium of the corpus callosum. Research indicates that the auditory segment of the corpus callosum is confined to its posterior portion. Baran, Musiek, and Reeves (1986) found that, although anterior sectioning of the corpus callosum resulted in essentially no change in central auditory function, posterior commissurotomy significantly altered auditory function. Specifically, the splenium and most posterior portion of the trunk, or the posterior one-fourth of the corpus callosum, appears to carry the majority of auditory fibers (Sugishita et al., 1995). Damage anywhere along the transcallosal auditory pathway can significantly affect interhemispheric exchange of auditory information. In addition, because the corpus callosum has contact with such a large part of the brain, lesions of the cortex, which is very thin, may also affect fibers of the corpus callosum.

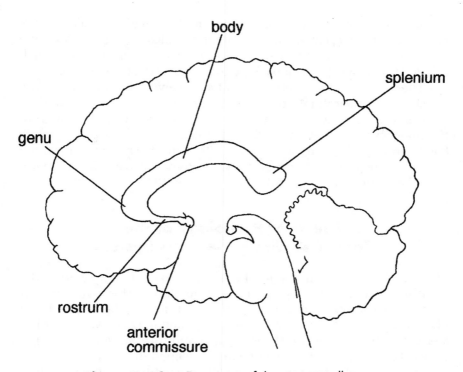

Figure 1-12. Five parts of the corpus callosum.

The corpus callosum is primarily responsible for the communication and integration of information from the two cerebral hemispheres. In the case of auditory function, the left hemisphere is dominant for language and rapid sequencing of auditory stimuli as well as for analysis. The right hemisphere is dominant for music perception and other acoustic contour recognition and perception of the gestalt. In order for an individual to perform certain auditory tasks—such as dichotic listening, which will be discussed in Chapter 2—the two cerebral hemispheres must be able to communicate. Lesions affecting the corpus callosum will significantly affect the individual's ability to perform these auditory tasks.

Efferent Auditory Pathways

To date, little is known about the efferent auditory pathways. It is known that an efferent system runs from the auditory cortex to the cochlea and parallels the afferent system. Information available indicates that the efferent auditory system includes both excitatory and inhibitory activity, and has significant implications in functions such as detection of a signal in a background of noise (Noback, 1985).

The *olivocochlear bundle* (OCB) has received the majority of the focus of the research into the efferent auditory pathways. As its name implies, the OCB extends from the superior olivary complex (SOC) to the fibers beneath the hair cells of the cochlea. The OCB apparently has inhibitory effects upon the hair cells themselves as well as on the acoustic reflex. In addition, it has been hypothesized that the OCB may play a role in auditory attention (Musiek, 1986).

Effects of Pathology of the Central Auditory Nervous System

The CANS extends from the level of the low brainstem upward to the auditory cortex. Pathology along any portion of this pathway can result in a variety of auditory symptoms that may be isolated and identified by diagnostic tests of auditory function. Knowledge of the anatomy and physiology of the normal auditory nervous system is critical to prediction of effects of pathology upon the CANS.

In this section, the term *lesion* will be used to denote any pathological condition. A lesion may be structural, as in the case of a tumor or infarct, or it may be neurochemical or idiopathic (no known etiology). **Used in this sense, the term lesion indicates site-of-dysfunction, be it structural or otherwise.**

Cerebral Hemisphere Lesions

The location and extent of the lesion within the cerebral hemisphere will largely determine the effects of the lesion. For example, a lesion confined to the left frontal lobe (Broca's area) will primarily result in a difficulty in speech execution while comprehension of spoken language will remain largely intact (Broca's aphasia). Likewise, a lesion of the temporal-occipital-parietal junction around the area of the supramarginal and angular gyri (Wernicke's area) will result in difficulty in comprehension of spoken language (Wernicke's aphasia). The most common destructive lesion of the language areas is a middle cerebral artery stroke, which results in a mixed aphasia with characteristics of both Broca's and Wernicke's aphasia (Bhatnagar & Andy, 1995).

Lesions of the primary auditory cortex typically produce a contralateral behavioral deficit that can be seen during dichotic presentation of auditory stimuli (simultaneous presentation of different stimuli to both ears). For example, a lesion in the right temporal lobe affecting the primary auditory cortex will typically result in a left ear deficit upon dichotic stimulation. The reader is referred to Chapter 2 for a more complete discussion of dichotic listening. In addition, lesions of the temporal lobe have been documented to cause impairment of sound localization in the auditory field contralateral to the temporal lobe lesion (Sanchez-Longo & Forster, 1958). Bilateral involvement of the primary auditory cortex is extremely rare and can be associated with cortical or "central" deafness.

In a study in which temporal ablation procedures were performed on 10 Japanese macaques, Heffner and Heffner (1986) further delineated the effects of unilateral and bilateral lesions of the temporal lobe. The animals, having been trained to discriminate between two types of coos, underwent systematic temporal lobe ablation in which the entire primary and secondary auditory areas were removed, resulting in severe to total degeneration of subcortical structures such as the medial geniculate body of the thalamus.

Results of this study indicated that unilateral right temporal lobe ablation did not affect the animals' ability to discriminate the coos. Unilateral ablation of the left temporal lobe resulted in an initial impairment in the animals' ability to discriminate the coos; however, this ability improved, and the animals were performing at preoperative levels within 5 to 15 sessions. Finally, bilateral temporal lobe ablation resulted in hearing loss that improved somewhat over time (unilateral temporal lesions typically do not affect hearing acuity) as well as a permanent deficit in discriminatory ability. The authors suggested that their findings indicate that **the perception of vocalizations is primarily mediated by the left hemisphere, although other cortical areas (specifically, the right temporal lobe) can assume this function in the case of left hemispheric damage.**

Brainstem Lesions

Lesions of the brainstem can be divided primarily into two categories: *intra-axial* and *extra-axial*. An intra-axial lesion arises from within the brainstem itself whereas an extra-axial lesion (the more common type) originates from outside but immediately adjacent to the brainstem. A common intra-axial lesion is the *pontine glioma*, a tumor that arises within the pons. This type of lesion is likely to result in bilateral auditory effects due to the large number of decussating (crossing) auditory fibers found in the pontine level of the brainstem.

The most common extra-axial tumor is the *acoustic schwannoma,* which usually arises from the vestibular division of the VIIIth cranial nerve. This type of tumor generally produces unilateral auditory effects (acuity and auditory brainstem response test results) in the ear ipsilateral to the lesion; however, depending upon the size of the lesion and the level at which it occurs in the brainstem, results on psychophysical auditory tests, such as tests of central auditory processing, may be unilateral or bilateral. Knowledge of brainstem anatomy and physiology is essential in order to be able to predict auditory and other sensory system effects of brainstem lesions.

Other disorders that can affect the auditory structures of the brainstem and result in auditory symptoms include degenerative diseases such as multiple sclerosis and olivopontocerebellar degeneration. Musiek, Weider, and Mueller (1982) have reported a case in which Charcot-Marie-Tooth disease resulted in severe hearing loss. In addition, Drulovic, Ribaric-Jankes, Kostic, and Sternic (1994) reported two cases in which sudden, unilateral hearing loss was the initial and sole symptom of multiple sclerosis involving the pontine level of the brainstem.

Lesions of the Corpus Callosum

Lesions of the posterior portion of the corpus callosum will result in deficits related to interhemispheric transfer of auditory information. Since the left hemisphere is considered to be dominant for language and the right hemisphere is considered to be dominant for functions such as gestalt perception and recognition of acoustic contour, the two hemispheres must be able to interact in order for normal processing to take place. **Surgical sectioning of the posterior portion of the corpus callosum (posterior commissurotomy) results in left ear deficit on dichotic tasks** (Musiek, Reeves, & Baran, 1985) **combined with bilateral deficit on tasks requiring linguistic labeling of patterned tonal stimuli.** This is probably because recognition of the tonal pattern is reliant upon the right hemisphere whereas linguistic labeling is primarily a left hemisphere function (Musiek, Pinheiro, & Wilson, 1980). Virtually any activity that requires interhemispheric transfer of information will be affected by commissurotomy. For more information regarding auditory effects of commissurotomy, the reader is referred to Chapter 2.

Interestingly, agenesis (congenital absence) of the corpus callosum, a rare condition, does not result in the same type of deficits observed in the surgically split-brain patient. Although further research in needed in this area, it has been hypothesized that, in these cases, each hemisphere develops its secondary functions to the point where it is able to function independently. Another theory is that intact portions of the corpus callosum, specifically anterior portions, may take on the functions usually mediated by the posterior portion (Musiek, 1986).

Finally, it should be noted that, due to the extreme thinness of the cortex (approximately ¼ inch thick), lesions thought to be confined to the cortex may well affect fibers of the corpus callosum, which lie immediately beneath the cortex. **Because damage anywhere along the fiber can result in dysfunction of the entire fiber, cortical lesions may also result in callosal dysfunction** (Musiek, 1986).

Effects of Lesions of the Efferent Auditory System

As little is known about the efferent auditory system, lesion effects are difficult to predict. However, if the efferent system serves inhibitory functions, as is hypothesized, behaviors such as difficulty hearing in noise may well be due, at least in part, to pathology affecting the efferent system.

A summary of the effects of lesions of the central auditory pathways is presented in Table 1–1.

Summary

Familiarity with the anatomy and physiology of the central auditory nervous system is critical for appropriate assessment of central auditory processing. The human brain consists of two cerebral hemispheres separated by the longitudinal fissure. The cerebrum can be divided into four primary lobes, each with specific functions: the frontal, parietal, occipital, and temporal lobes. The brainstem consists of three major divisions: the pons, medulla oblongata, and midbrain. The ascending central auditory nervous system extends from the low brainstem to Heschl's gyrus, the primary auditory cortex, and contains several levels at which decussation of auditory fibers occurs. Cochlear tonotopic representation of auditory input is repeated

Table 1–1

Effects of Lesions of the Central Auditory Pathways

Site of Lesion	Effect(s) on Auditory Behavior
Unilateral Temporal Lobe	Contralateral deficit on dichotic listening tasks; impairment of localization in contralateral auditory field
Bilateral Temporal Lobe	Possible cortical or "central" deafness
Brainstem	Behavioral indicators may be unilateral or bilateral depending on locus and size of lesion; may cause deficits in both acuity and processing
Corpus Callosum	Bilateral deficits on any task that requires interhemispheric integration; left ear deficit on dichotic speech tasks
Efferent Auditory System	Possible difficulty hearing in noise due to disruption of inhibitory function

throughout the CANS. The efferent central auditory system parallels the ascending system and is thought to be instrumental in the detection of auditory signals in noise and auditory attention, as well as in performing other inhibitory and excitatory activities.

The effects of pathological conditions upon auditory processing depends on the level of the CANS affected and the extent of the lesion. Unilateral lesions of the primary auditory cortex typically result in contralateral ear deficits upon dichotic stimulation. Lesions involving corpus callosal fibers interfere with the interhemispheric transfer of acoustic information. The effects of brainstem lesions are largely dependent upon the level of brainstem affected and whether the lesion is intra- or extra-axial.

Review Questions

(Answers to all review questions are provided in the Appendix.)

1. Define the following terms related to planes of reference and directional orientation within the brain:

    sagittal   coronal
    horizontal   transverse

anterior   posterior
rostral   caudal
lateral   medial

2. Using the following diagram, identify and discuss the anatomical significance of the following cerebral landmarks and lobes:

longitudinal fissure   central sulcus
lateral (Sylvian) fissure   frontal lobe
parietal lobe   temporal lobe
occipital lobe

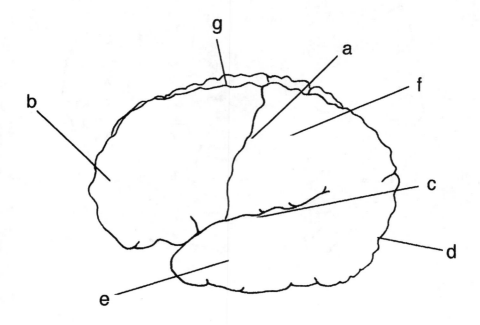

3. Discuss the general function of the following structures:

limbic system   ventricles
meninges

4. Using the following diagram, identify the following structures:

caudate   globus padillus
putamen   internal capsule
external capsule   claustrum

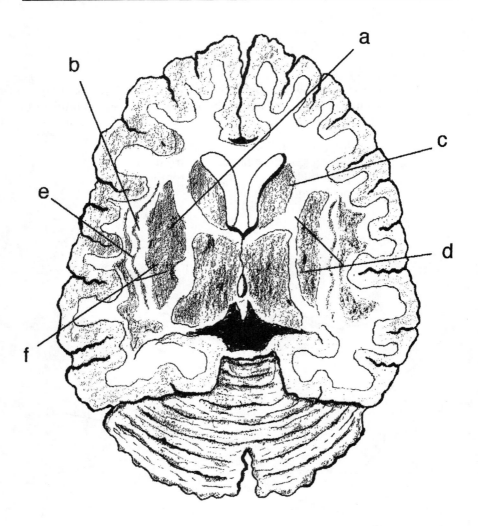

5. Discuss the two primary effects of neurotransmitters.
6. Identify the three divisions of the brainstem.
7. Discuss the function of the following significant auditory brainstem structures:

cochlear nucleus   superior olivary complex
lateral lemniscus   inferior colliculus
medial geniculate body

8. Discuss the significance related to auditory function of the following cerebral structures:

supratemporal plane	Heschl's gyrus
planum temporal	supramarginal gyrus
angular gyrus	insula
arcuate fasciculus	

9. Using the diagram below, identify the five main parts of the corpus callosum.

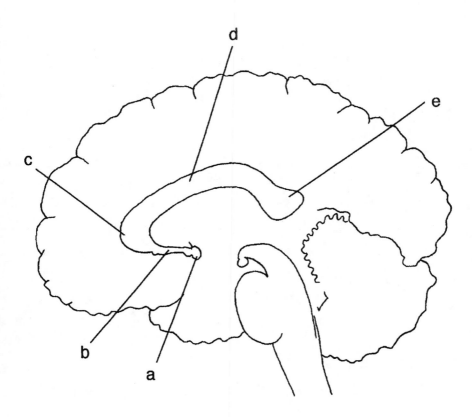

10. Discuss the function of the corpus callosum as it relates to audition.

11. Discuss the probable significance of the efferent auditory system.

12. Identify the primary types of brainstem lesions and give an example of each.

13. Discuss probable auditory effects of pathology involving the following structures:

VIIIth nerve   brainstem
right temporal lobe   left temporal lobe
both temporal lobes   corpus callosum
efferent auditory system

CHAPTER

Dichotic Listening, Temporal Processing, and Binaural Interaction

The act of hearing does not end with the mere detection of an acoustic stimulus. Rather, several neurophysiological and cognitive mechanisms and processes are necessary for the accurate decoding of auditory input. As seen in the previous chapter, the CANS is a highly complex, redundant system, and optimal functioning of the CANS is critical to the recognition and discrimination of even the most simple, nonverbal acoustic stimuli as well as of highly complex stimuli such as spoken language.

Much of what is considered to be central auditory processing is preconscious; that is, it occurs without the listener being aware of it. However, even the simplest auditory event is further influenced by higher level cognitive factors such as memory, attention, and learning. What is ultimately experienced by the listener is referred to as an *auditory perceptual event* (American Speech-Language-Hearing Association [ASHA], 1995). For purposes of this text, we will use the term auditory processing to refer specifically to those processes that occur within the CANS in response to acoustic stimuli. The term auditory perception will denote the listener's conscious experience of the auditory stimulus, which is influenced by the higher level neurocognitive, non-modality-specific factors mentioned previously. However, it should be noted that, although analysis of an acoustic signal relies initially upon detection and processing within the CANS, the higher level neurocognitive and behavioral factors greatly influence the listener's ultimate ability to recognize, decode, and interpret the acoustic signal.

The ASHA Task Force on Central Auditory Processing (ASHA, 1995) suggested the following definition of central auditory processing: Central Auditory Processes are the *auditory system* mechanisms and processes responsible for the following behavioral phenomena:

- Sound localization and lateralization
- Auditory discrimination
- Auditory pattern recognition
- Temporal aspects of audition, including:

    temporal resolution

    temporal masking

    temporal integration

    temporal ordering

- Auditory performance decrements with competing acoustic signals
- Auditory performance decrements with degraded acoustic signals.

The reader should note that the above definition concerns itself specifically with the auditory system. **Memory, learning, attention, long-term phonological representation, and other higher level neurocognitive processes are considered in the definition only as they relate to the processing of acoustic signals.**

With these distinctions and definitions in mind, this chapter will explore the mechanisms of and pathological effects on three central auditory functions: dichotic listening, temporal processing, and binaural interaction. Only by having a thorough understanding of how these processing tasks are accomplished by the CANS can the clinician appropriately interpret tests of central auditory processing that tap these processes.

The reader should be aware that, while certain studies are reviewed in this chapter in order to illustrate relevant concepts, this chapter is not intended to be a comprehensive treatment of the literature. Therefore, many relevant studies in the areas of dichotic listening, temporal processing, and binaural interaction are not mentioned herein.

Learning Objectives

After reading this chapter, the reader should be able to

1. Discuss hemispheric specialization and cerebral dominance
2. Discuss possible anatomic and physiologic bases of dichotic listening
3. Discuss the mechanism of temporal processing
4. Identify types of auditory tasks that rely on temporal processing
5. Identify the physiological structures most crucial to binaural interaction
6. Identify types of auditory tasks that rely on binaural interaction
7. Discuss the effects of various pathological conditions on dichotic listening, temporal processing, and binaural interaction.

Dichotic Listening

The term *dichotic* **refers to auditory stimuli that are presented to both ears simultaneously, with the stimulus presented to each ear being different.** This is contrasted with use of the terms *diotic* or *binaural*, which denote that the same, identical stimulus is presented to both ears simultaneously. Broadbent (1954) was the first to utilize a technique of presenting competing sets of digits to both ears simultaneously. Kimura (1961a) is generally credited with the introduction of dichotic speech tests into the field of central auditory assessment by adapting Broadbent's technique for assessing hemispheric asymmetry and unilateral lesion effects, and her research has served as the basis for much of the current theory regarding dichotic listening. Kimura used a test in which triads of digits were presented dichotically to patients who had undergone unilateral temporal lobectomies. She found that unilateral temporal lobectomy resulted in impairment of digit recognition in the ear contralateral to the excision, but only during dichotic stimulation. Monotic (noncompeting) presentation of digit triads to patients having undergone right temporal lobectomy indicated no deficit in either ear. However, damage to the left temporal lobe resulted in bilaterally depressed scores upon monotic presentation of digits, supporting the hypothesis that, while both temporal lobes are active in auditory processing, the left temporal lobe is particularly important in the auditory perception of verbal stimuli.

In a related study, Kimura (1961b) studied a group of patients with various epilepsy-related lesions of the brain. She noted that, in all cases, the ear contralateral to the dominant hemisphere for speech was more efficient than the ipsilateral ear, regardless of handedness or site of lesion.

These findings led Kimura to postulate a theory of dichotic listening. As discussed in Chapter 1, auditory input is represented both ipsilaterally and contralaterally throughout the CANS. Kimura theorized that **the contralateral pathways are stronger and more numerous than are the ipsilateral pathways** (Figure 2–1). When monotic or non-

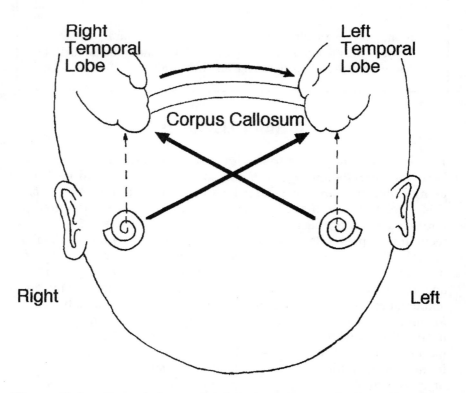

Figure 2–1.   Kimura's theory of dichotic listening. Bold lines represent contralateral, dominant pathways; dotted lines represent ipsilateral pathways.

competing stimuli are introduced, either pathway is capable of transmitting the appropriate neural signal. However, **when dichotic (competing) auditory stimuli are presented, the ipsilateral pathways are suppressed by the stronger contralateral pathways.** Therefore, if a lesion exists in one hemisphere, a deficit would be expected in the ear contralateral to the lesion when acoustic stimuli are presented dichotically. Aiello et al. (1995) reported that electrophysiological measures from a patient with corpus callosum agenesis indicated more efficient transmission of monaural auditory stimuli through the ipsilateral pathways. The authors concluded that this finding provided objective support for Kimura's theory of dichotic listening.

In addition, a variety of researchers in the early 1960s documented the existence of a *cerebral dominance effect* in dichotic listening, indicating a preexisting ear asymmetry in normal right-handed listeners in which the scores for the right ear are consistently higher than the scores for the left ear for dichotically presented digits (Bryden, 1963; Dirks, 1964; Kimura, 1961a; Satz, Achenback, Pattishall, & Fennell, 1965). This phenomenon has come to be known as the *Right Ear Advantage (REA)* and, in normal listeners, it is usually apparent only upon dichotic stimulation or other tasks that significantly challenge the auditory system (Kimura, 1961a). These findings have been considered as further evidence of the left hemisphere's dominance for speech perception.

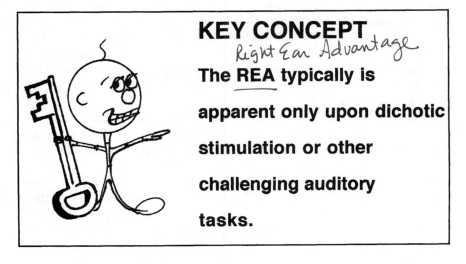

KEY CONCEPT

Right Ear Advantage

The REA typically is apparent only upon dichotic stimulation or other challenging auditory tasks.

It should be noted that other researchers have posited theories regarding the mechanism of dichotic listening as it relates to speech perception (Sidtis, 1982; Speaks, Gray, Miller, & Rubens, 1975); however, Kimura's model continues to be the one that is most widely accepted.

Effects of Temporal Lobe Lesions on Dichotic Listening

In a study of 28 left aphasic and 20 right nonaphasic lesioned adults, Sparks, Goodglass, and Nickel (1970) confirmed previous researchers' findings regarding temporal lobe lesions. They used double digits and familiar words (animal names) presented dichotically and concluded that, for subjects with right temporal lobe lesions, left ear suppression/extinction occurs due to the contralateral effect previously discussed. Likewise, for subjects with left temporal lobe lesions, right ear suppression/extinction occurs due to the contralateral effect. In addition, the authors explained that right ear extinction does not occur with right temporal lobe lesions because the primary contralateral pathway to the left hemisphere remains intact; however, ipsilateral left ear extinction can and does occur with left hemisphere lesions due to the fact that the stimulus to the left ear must arrive at the right hemisphere, then cross to the left hemisphere by way of the corpus callosum. **Lesions affecting either the auditory areas of the left temporal lobe or the fibers of the corpus callosum would therefore interrupt the successful arrival of information at the speech-dominant left hemisphere** (Figure 2–2). The findings of Grote, Pierre-Louis, Smith, Roberts, and Varney (1995) supported this contention. In a study of 49 patients with seizures, the authors reported that, whereas right ear impairment on dichotic listening tasks was always associated with left hemisphere lesions, left ear extinction occurred with lesions of either hemisphere.

The authors also hypothesized that a reverse effect may be noted when using nonverbal stimuli due to the dominance of the right hemisphere for this type of acoustic stimuli (i.e., right ear extinction of nonverbal dichotic stimuli in cases of right temporal lobe lesions). Damasio and Damasio (1979), studying patients with well-defined, focal lesions, postulated further that seemingly "paradoxic" ear extinction (i.e., extinction of dichotically presented stimuli in the ear ipsilateral to the lesion) only occurs with deep suprasylvian lesions involving the pathway from the medial geniculate body to the cortex (geniculocortical pathway). Focal occipital and frontal lesions do not produce ear effects simply because no auditory areas are affected.

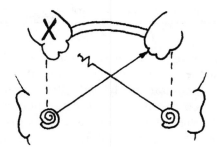

A

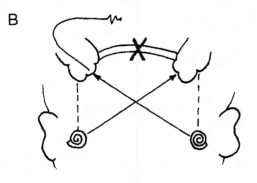

B

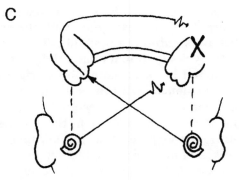

C

Figure 2–2. Effects of lesions of the CANS on dichotic listening showing pattern of interruption for (a) right temporal lobe lesion, (b) corpus callosum lesion, and (c) left temporal lobe lesion.

Finally, Berlin, Lowe-Bell, Jannetta, and Kline (1972) studied four temporal lobe lesioned patients using consonant-vowel (CV) nonsense syllables presented simultaneously and with interaural lags of 15, 30, 60, and 90 msec. Their results also indicated depressed scores in the ear contralateral to the site of lesion, as well as ipsilateral ear extinction with lesions deep enough to interfere with the right-to-left interhemispheric transfer of information. In addition, the authors reported that **those subjects with posterior temporal lobe lesions exhibited greater auditory deficit**, which is consistent with placement of the primary and associative auditory areas in the more posterior aspect of the temporal lobe. In normal listeners, acoustic stimuli received at the right ear are generally reported more accurately, as shown by previous researchers, and the lagging message is better perceived when lags of 30–90 msec are utilized.

Effects of Corpus Callosal Lesions on Dichotic Listening

Milner, Taylor, and Sperry (1968) studied seven "split brain" patients (patients who had undergone complete sectioning of the corpus callosum) and compared their results on a test of dichotically presented digit triads with normal listeners and cases of temporal lobectomies in which Heschl's gyrus was completely excised. Findings with normal listeners and temporal lobectomies agreed with the results of other studies: **Normal listeners exhibited a slight REA on dichotic tasks, left temporal lobectomy resulted in a bilateral deficit, and right temporal lobectomy resulted in an accentuation of right ear superiority/contralateral left ear deficit. With the split brain patients, significant left ear suppression or extinction resulted**, even though monotic presentation of the digits to the left ear in these patients remained unaffected. The authors concluded that the left ipsilateral pathway can be utilized in cases of monaural stimulation; however, during the more challenging task of dichotic listening, the contralateral pathway is dominant.

In a similar study utilizing dichotically presented single digits and words, Sparks and Geschwind (1968) reported 100% left ear extinction in patients with complete commissurotomies. When the listeners were instructed to attend closely to the left ear, performance for that ear improved but remained significantly depressed.

The authors also presented the verbal stimuli to the left ear along with contralateral white noise and babble masking to the right ear.

They found that right masking did not affect left ear performance significantly. The introduction of a distorted stimulus to the right ear impacted left ear performance on dichotic tasks, depending on the degree of distortion. As the degree of right ear distortion decreased, the degree of left ear extinction increased. The authors concluded that the likelihood of left ear extinction in split brain patients increases when the stimuli delivered to both ears are very similar and that the localization and depth of the lesion significantly affects the degree of left ear suppression/extinction.

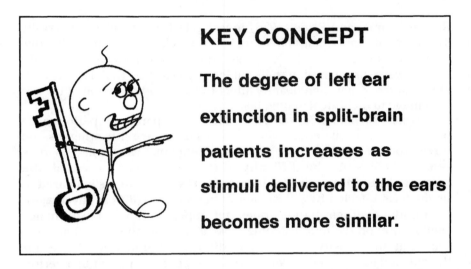

KEY CONCEPT

The degree of left ear extinction in split-brain patients increases as stimuli delivered to the ears becomes more similar.

Musiek, Reeves, and Baran (1985) investigated the effects of sectioning of the corpus callosum on a subject's performance on a variety of central tests. The subject was a patient undergoing a two-stage commissurotomy to control intractable epileptic seizures in which the posterior portion of the corpus callosum was sectioned first, followed by anterior sectioning five months later. Following posterior sectioning of the corpus callosum, left ear extinction on dichotic tasks occurred. In addition, right ear performance was enhanced. The authors suggested that this finding was due to a release from competition: Following posterior sectioning, the left hemisphere was required only to process information from the right ear. Subsequent anterior sectioning did not result in further auditory deficit.

In a related study, Baran et al. (1986) studied eight right-handed adults who underwent partial commissurotomies to control seizures. In all cases, the anterior portion of the corpus callosum was sectioned, leaving the posterior half intact. Results of the study indicated that, while complete commissurotomy results in a marked left ear deficit on dichotic tasks, anterior sectioning alone does not. These findings led the authors to conclude that **the majority of auditory fibers travel interhemispherically in the posterior portion of the corpus callosum.**

Effects of Other Pathological Conditions on Dichotic Listening

Roeser, Johns, and Price (1976) investigated the effect of bilaterally symmetrical sensorineural hearing loss on dichotic listening using digits and CV nonsense syllables as stimuli. Large ear advantages (right or left) were discovered in their subjects, suggesting that sensorineural hearing loss may significantly affect the size and direction of the ear advantage in dichotic listening tasks.

Speaks, Niccum, and Van Tasell (1985) compared the performance of listeners with bilaterally symmetrical sensorineural hearing loss on three types of dichotic tests: digits, concrete noun words, and CV nonsense syllables. **As the difficulty of the test stimuli increased, the amount of ear advantage also increased. The use of digits appeared to be the least affected by sensorineural hearing loss** (0% ear advantage).

Conductive hearing loss does not appear to affect performance significantly on dichotic listening tasks as long as the stimuli are presented at an intensity of at least 12 dB above the monotic "knee" for the affected ear(s). The *monotic knee* represents that point in a performance-intensity function at which the listener reaches a 95% accuracy level for monotic presentation of the stimuli (Niccum, Speaks, Katsuki-Nakamura, & Van Tassell, 1987).

In cases of multiple sclerosis with cerebral involvement, left ear suppression on dichotic tasks may be observed (Jacobson, Deppe, & Murray, 1983; Rubens, Froehling, Slater, & Anderson, 1985). It is possible that the existence of multiple sclerosis lesions in the deep white matter of the cerebral hemispheres results in an interruption of the auditory corpus callosal pathway, resulting in findings similar to that of split brain patients (Rubens et al., 1985).

For further information regarding dichotic listening, the reader is referred to the References at the end of this text. For information regarding methods of assessing dichotic listening, the reader is referred to Chapter 5, Overview of Central Tests and Chapter 6, Comprehensive Central Auditory Assessment. For management suggestions, the reader is referred to Chapter 8, Management of Central Auditory Processing Disorders. The effects of pathology of the CANS on dichotic listening are summarized in Table 2–1.

Temporal Processing

In this section, the term **temporal** **refers to time-related aspects of the acoustic signal**. Temporal processing is critical to a wide variety of everyday listening tasks, including speech perception and perception of music (Hirsh, 1959). For example, the perception of melody in music depends on the listener's ability to perceive the order of several musical notes or chords and to determine if the frequencies of the notes or chords are ascending or descending with respect to the adjacent chords or notes. In speech perception, temporal processing is one of the functions necessary for the discrimination of subtle cues such as voicing (e.g., voicing begins earlier in the word *dime* than in the word *time*) and the discrimination of similar words (e.g., discrimination between the words *boost* and *boots* depends in large part on discrimination of consonant duration and temporal ordering of the final two consonants of each word). These are just two examples of how the processing of time-related cues is used in everyday listening tasks.

Hirsh (1959) studied the effect of interstimulus intervals (ISI) on the perception of temporal order. Using a variety of acoustic stimuli, he determined that **an ISI of only 2 msec is required for the normal listener to perceive two sounds instead of only one; however, this**

Table 2-1
Effects of Lesions of the CANS on Dichotic Listening

Site of Lesion	Effect(s) on Dichotic Listening
Right Temporal Lobe	Left ear suppression/extinction
Left Temporal Lobe	Contralateral or bilateral suppression/extinction
Posterior Corpus Callosum	Marked left ear deficit/extinction; possible right ear enhancement
Anterior Corpus Callosum	No effect
Peripheral: Cochlear	Size and direction of ear advantage may be affected depending on task difficulty
Peripheral: Conductive	No effect at adequate presentation levels

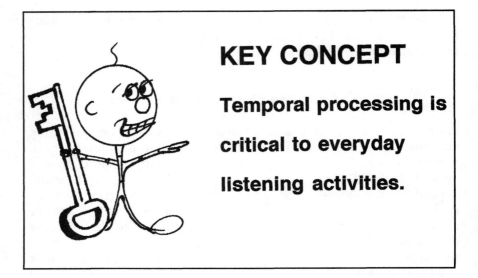

KEY CONCEPT

Temporal processing is critical to everyday listening activities.

ISI must be increased tenfold (or approximately 17 msec) for the listener to report which of the two sounds came first with 75% accuracy. In addition, the judgment of temporal order appears to be independent of the acoustical nature of the sounds (e.g., the ISI necessary for the reporting of temporal order was approximately the same regardless of whether musical notes or clicks were used and whether certain variations in the acoustic characteristics of the stimuli were made). The author did note the existence of some minor exceptions to the above rule: Although pitch had no effect, rise time and duration of click stimuli did have some minor effect on the perception of temporal order. In addition, when a burst of wide-band noise preceded a high-frequency brief tone, the ISI necessary to perceive temporal order was slightly longer, possibly due to a forward masking effect. Hirsh concluded that the judgment of temporal order does not occur at the ear, but rather represents a central auditory function and that, **in cases in which a listener requires more than 15 or 20 msec to perceive the temporal order of two consecutive stimuli, the examiner should look to possible central involvement.**

In 1961, Hirsh and Sherrick explored the effect of sense modality on the perception of temporal order. They reported that an ISI of approximately 20 msec continues to be necessary to report temporal order with 75% accuracy regardless of whether the stimuli are acoustic, visual, tactile, or a combination of modalities, despite the fact that the visual system requires a longer ISI to perceive a separation between two stimuli. Their results suggest that some type of time-organization system exists within the human brain that is independent of the peripheral and central modality-specific systems themselves.

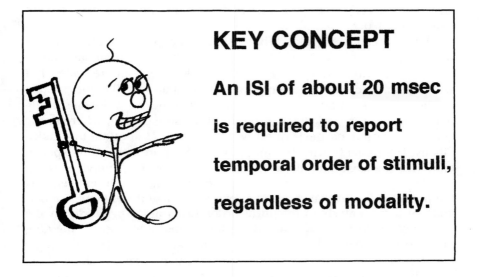

KEY CONCEPT

An ISI of about 20 msec is required to report temporal order of stimuli, regardless of modality.

Massaro (1972) posited a theory of auditory recognition in which auditory detection is distinguished from recognition and short-term memory storage. Using previous studies of forward (masking precedes stimulus) and backward (stimulus precedes masking) masking, Massaro suggested that auditory input results in the production of a preperceptual auditory image, or "echo," that preserves the characteristics of the stimulus and remains in storage for as long as 10 sec. Discrimination and recognition of the auditory input follows analysis of this preperceptual auditory image, rather than analysis of the initial input itself, which would require almost instantaneous perception—an impossible task. In addition, as contralateral masking does not appear to affect the detection of the stimulus but does interfere with recognition of the stimulus, Massaro suggested that the preperceptual auditory image is located centrally rather than peripherally. Finally, he hypothesized that, as the maximum duration of preperceptual auditory images is approximately 250 msec, **the first 100 to 250 msec of an auditory stimulus presentation are the most critical for stimulus recognition, which has significant implications for speech perception.**

Efron (1963) studied the effects of temporal lobe lesions on the perception of temporal order utilizing visual and auditory stimuli. His subjects were inpatients, 12 of whom had documented lesions of the left hemisphere (11 aphasics) and four of whom had documented lesions of the right hemisphere (no aphasics). The aphasic patients were considered to be the experimental group, the nonaphasics were used as controls.

Efron's results suggested that lesions which result in disruption of temporal order perception all lie in the left, or speech-dominant, hemisphere. The one patient who exhibited a left hemisphere lesion but was nonaphasic exhibited temporal discrimination skills comparable to the controls. In addition, the expressive aphasics in Efron's study exhibited poorer performance on auditory sequencing, whereas the receptive aphasics performed worse on visual sequencing tasks. Finally, the patients with the most difficulty in understanding speech exhibited the least difficulty with auditory sequencing, and vice versa.

Based on his results, Efron suggested that, although unconscious temporal processing takes place at every synapse throughout the nervous system, **analysis of temporal order takes place primarily in the dominant hemisphere, specifically in the temporal lobe and extending posteriorly to Wernicke's area and the angular gyrus.** The seemingly paradoxical finding that the most severe receptive aphasics exhibited the least difficulty with temporal sequencing is explained by the hypothesis that the functional deficit in speech understanding exhibited by the receptive aphasics occurs after the input is temporally sequenced. Thus, the receptive component of an expressive aphasic's difficulty may be at an earlier stage than the receptive component of a receptive aphasic, resulting in lower temporal sequencing abilities in the expressive aphasic. Efron stressed that severity of cerebral damage cannot be correlated with results on a temporal sequencing task, as variability is high.

Efron also discussed the conscious perception of time as being mediated primarily in the dominant hemisphere. He set forth the theory that the conscious perception of an event occurs when the sensory data reaches the left hemisphere. This theory helps to explain the existence of subjective time sense disturbances in patients with temporal lobe lesions. Efron also suggested that the phenomenon of déjà vu—the feeling that an individual has experienced an event previously—may occur because a lesion in the right temporal lobe delays the propagation of the sensory data to the left hemisphere. Thus, the patient "experiences" the sensory event twice: Once directly, and once through delayed transmission from the right hemisphere, giving rise to the sensation of déjà vu.

In any case, early data concerning temporal processing suggests that, while temporal cues are processed throughout the CANS, the left temporal lobe is critical to the accurate perception of temporal order.

Effects of Cerebral Pathology on Temporal Processing

Hughes (1946) discovered that, in normal listeners, **as the temporal duration of a brief tone decreases below 200 msec, the intensity required for threshold progressively increases.** This has been referred to as *temporal integration* or *summation*. Results of studies investigating the effect of cerebral pathology on temporal integration have been somewhat variable (Cranford, 1984). In a study of a patient with bilateral temporal lobe lesions, Jerger, Lovering, and Wertz (1972) reported elevated temporal integration functions for both ears. Cranford, Stream, Rye, and Slade (1982) discovered that thresholds for brief tones may be elevated in the case of temporal lobe lesions but that, given a sufficient period of time following cerebral insult, the threshold functions may return to normal. However, the authors noted a significant increase in frequency difference limens (smallest detectable difference) for signals shorter than 50 msec in the ears contralateral to the temporal lobe lesions. They suggested that a cortical lesion may result in a dissociation between detection and discrimination of brief tones, indicating that the peripheral system is primarily responsible for detection of an auditory stimulus whereas the central system is the primary mediator for temporal analysis. The authors concluded that standard temporal integration tests may have little or no value in identifying cerebral lesions; however, frequency difference limens utilizing brief tones may have some utility.

Thompson and Abel (1992a, 1992b) studied the effects of anatomical site of lesion on the processing of intensity, duration, and frequency cues. Using a two-alternative, forced choice procedure, the authors obtained difference limens for the above three acoustic parameters from a subject group that included peripheral (cochlear) lesions, acoustic nerve lesions, and cortical lesions. Their findings indicated that the group with left temporal lesions exhibited the greatest deficits in processing all three acoustic parameters, and that the degree of deficit in duration processing was significantly correlated with consonant discrimination skills. Therefore, the authors concluded, tests of temporal processing may be a good predictor of speech perception ability at the central level.

Carmon and Nachshon (1971) studied 26 patients with right hemisphere lesions, 21 patients with left hemisphere lesions, and 42 controls without lesions and compared their performance on a task of temporal sequencing of auditory as well as visual stimuli. Although none of the subjects was overtly aphasic, the authors required a motor (pointing) response in case those patients with left hemisphere lesions had subtle difficulties with verbalization. The authors found that those patients with left hemisphere lesions demonstrated decreased performance on all sequencing tasks, whereas the patients with right hemisphere lesions did not differ significantly from the control group. They concluded that, **although temporal perception does not depend on speech, speech perception may well depend, at least in part, on the sequential analysis of temporal order.** This study also supported previous evidence that temporal perception is mediated by the left hemisphere.

Swisher and Hirsh (1972) studied the effects of cerebral pathology on the ability to order two temporally successive stimuli. Using visual and auditory stimuli, the authors found that subjects with left hemisphere lesions and fluent aphasia required the longest ISI to report the order of the two stimuli, especially when the stimuli were auditory in nature. Subjects with right hemisphere lesions and no aphasia did not differ significantly from controls when both auditory stimuli were delivered to the same ear; however, they did require a longer ISI than controls to make temporal judgments when the stimuli were delivered to opposite ears. The authors concluded that the left hemisphere is particularly important for temporal ordering of events occurring at one place and that the right hemisphere also plays a part in the analysis of temporal order of tonal stimuli when one of the stimuli arrives at the left ear.

Lackner and Teuber (1973) utilized dichotic click stimuli varying in interaural ISI and asked subjects to hold up two fingers when two clicks were heard and one finger when the clicks fused and only one stimulus was heard. This activity was repeated in a bracketing paradigm in order to determine the subjects' threshold for click fusion/separation. The authors found that subjects with penetrative lesions of the posterior left hemisphere required a longer ISI in order to perceive a separation. Patients with right hemisphere penetrative lesions did not differ in ability to perform the task from the normal control group.

In an ablation study using cats, Colavita, Szeligo, and Zimmer (1974) found that the ability to attend to a full pattern is successful only when the insular-temporal cortex is intact. Surgical ablation of the insular-temporal cortex in cats resulted in inability to order three stimuli, but did not affect the ability to order two stimuli. The authors suggested that the postablative deficit noted in their study may not be due to the inability to sequence temporally per se, but rather to a reduction in attention span so that triads of stimuli can no longer be processed. The authors concluded that, due to the predisposed tendency to attend to the full pattern in temporally ordering three or more consecutive stimuli, breaking down a complex message into its component parts may not be a useful strategy for individuals with brain damage.

Efron and his colleagues (Efron, 1985; Efron & Crandall, 1983; Efron, Crandall, Koss, Divenyi, & Yund, 1983; Efron, Dennis, & Yund, 1977; Efron, Yund, Nichols, & Crandall, 1977) have conducted several studies to determine the effects of unilateral temporal lobe lesions on several auditory tasks, including gap detection and temporal ordering. Again, their findings suggest a clear pattern of deficit in the ears contralateral to posterior temporal lobe lesions. Interestingly, the authors also found contralateral deficits in patients with anterior temporal lobe lesions—an area previously thought to have no role in auditory processing. They suggested the possible existence of an efferent system responsible for enhancing the perception of auditory stimuli in the contralateral auditory space. Several other researchers have documented contralateral deficits in temporal ordering in cases of temporal lobe lesions (Belmont and Handler, 1971; Blaettner, Scherg, & Von Cramon, 1989; Karaseva, 1972).

Pinheiro and Ptacek (1971; Ptacek & Pinheiro, 1971) introduced a test of temporal processing involving triads of tone bursts. In each triad, two tone bursts are of the same frequency and a third is of a different frequency. The listener is required to report the order in which the bursts were heard (for example, high-high-low, low-high-low, etc.) Subjects with temporal lobe lesions demonstrate significant bilateral deficits on this test (Musiek, Gollegly, & Baran, 1984; Musiek & Pinheiro, 1987). In addition, those patients with lesions involving the interhemispheric pathways exhibit great difficulty in verbally reporting patterns that differ in intensity and frequency, whereas, when asked to hum the patterns heard (thus removing the linguistic labeling component), these same subjects exhibit scores near the normal range (Musiek et al., 1980).

In conclusion, the research indicates that **temporal lobe lesions result in significant difficulty in the temporal ordering of two successive auditory stimuli in the ear contralateral to the lesion. When a patterning test involving more than two successive auditory stimuli and linguistic labeling is involved, integrity of both hemispheres as well as the corpus callosum is necessary for normal performance.**

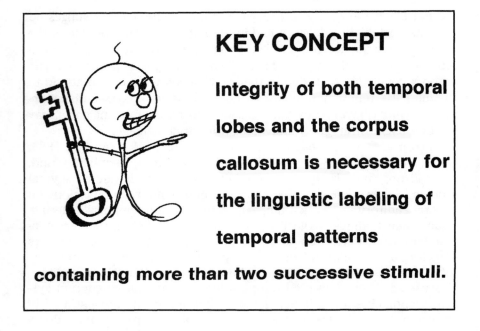

KEY CONCEPT

Integrity of both temporal lobes and the corpus callosum is necessary for the linguistic labeling of temporal patterns containing more than two successive stimuli.

In cases of lesions involving the interhemispheric pathways, removing the linguistic labeling portion of the temporal patterning test results in performance closer to that of normal listeners. Finally, although standard temporal integration tasks may not have much utility in the detection of cerebral lesions, evaluation of duration difference limens may differentiate peripheral from central pathology.

Effects of Other Pathological Conditions on Temporal Processing

The effect of brainstem lesions on subjects' ability to perform tasks of temporal ordering is variable and appears to depend upon the site of lesion and the type of task (Musiek & Pinheiro, 1987). In addition, Papsin and Abel (1988) found that subjects with VIIIth nerve pathology exhibited flat temporal integration functions, a finding that was supported by Thompson and Abel (1992b), who reported relatively little effect of stimulus duration on the ability of patients with acoustic neuromas to detect acoustic stimuli. Therefore, **it appears that tests of temporal processing may not be as sensitive to VIIIth nerve or brainstem pathology as they are to cerebral lesions.**

Likewise, cochlear lesions (peripheral hearing loss) do not appear to affect performance significantly on temporal patterning tests, provided that the stimuli are detectable (Musiek, Baran, & Pinheiro, 1990; Musiek & Pinheiro, 1987). Cranford (1984) did report that temporal integration was affected by cochlear site of lesion, resulting in a significantly less steep integration function similar to those of subjects with brainstem lesions; however, the author was unable to correlate the slope of the temporal integration function with recruitment or etiology of sensorineural hearing loss.

Finally, conductive hearing loss appears to have little effect on temporal integration (Cranford, 1984) or temporal patterning. Therefore, it appears that some tests of temporal processing may have promise for use in evaluating central auditory processing in the child and adult with hearing impairment.

For further information regarding temporal processing, the reader is referred to the References at the end of this book. Chapters 5 and 6 will provide information regarding specific tests of temporal processing, and the reader is referred to Chapter 8 for management suggestions. The effects of CANS lesions on temporal processing are reviewed in Table 2–2.

Binaural Interaction

The term *binaural interaction* or *integration* refers simply to the way in which the two ears work together. Functions that rely on binaural

Table 2–2
Effects of Lesions of the CANS on Temporal Processing

Site of Lesion	Effect(s) on Temporal Processing
Right Temporal Lobe	Contralateral deficit on two-tone ordering or gap detection; bilateral deficit on temporal patterning tasks involving more than 2 stimuli
Left Temporal Lobe	Significant contralateral and/or bilateral effects
Corpus Callosum	Bilateral deficit on temporal patterning tasks involving more than 2 stimuli
Brainstem	Variable, depending upon site of lesion and type of task
Peripheral	Little effect on temporal patterning performance

interaction include but are not limited to localization and lateralization of auditory stimuli, binaural release from masking, detection of
signals in noise, and binaural fusion (Durlach, Thompson, & Colburn,
1981; Noffsinger, Schaefer, & Martinez, 1984). As will be shown below,
it is believed that auditory structures within the brainstem are most
important for binaural interaction to occur, although the actual perception of the auditory event appears to occur in the cortex. As discussed in Chapter 1, the level of **the superior olivary complex in the
pons is the most caudal structure in the CANS to receive binaural
input, which implicates the low brainstem as being particularly critical to binaural processing.**

Localization and Lateralization

Studies of localization (determining direction of the source) and lateralization (place perception in the head) of auditory stimuli date back to
the late 1920s (Greene, 1929). Several investigators have studied the
mechanisms of localization and lateralization and the effects of various
lesions upon listeners' ability to localize and/or lateralize auditory stimuli (Abel, Bert, & McLean, 1978; Bergman, 1957; Matzker, 1959; Norlund,
1964; Pinheiro & Tobin, 1969; Sanchez-Longo & Forster, 1958; Sanchez-
Longo et al., 1957; Viehweg & Campbell, 1960; Walsh, 1957).

Bergman (1957) found that, in cases of unilateral middle ear
surgery, the ability of listeners to localize was poor if the auditory
stimulus was presented at a level below the threshold of the poorer
ear; however, localization ability rapidly improved at suprathreshold
levels and reached normal performance at 10 dB Sensation Level (SL)
(re: poorer ear threshold). Nordlund (1964), in a study of subjects
with a variety of lesions, discovered that lesions of the vestibular system had the least effect on localization ability whereas lesions of the
auditory nerve and low brainstem and unilateral deafness had the
greatest impact on the listener's ability to localize.

These two studies combined with the findings of the other researchers suggest that, **although unilateral deafness and asymmetrical
hearing sensitivity degrades localization performance, auditory nerve
and low brainstem lesions have a much greater impact upon localization and lateralization of an auditory stimulus.** In addition, localization
and lateralization ability is not easily predicted on the basis of the listener's audiometric configuration (Durlach et al., 1981). Therefore, it would
appear that, while peripheral considerations must be taken into account,

a large portion of localization and lateralization involves at least the auditory nerve and low brainstem. In addition, Sanchez-Longo and Forster (1958) and Pinheiro and Tobin (1969) showed degraded performance on tasks related to localization in subjects with temporal lobe lesions indicating that, although critical processing of localization and lateralization information occurs in the brainstem, **the actual perception of sound location occurs in the cortex** (Pickles, 1985).

Binaural Release From Masking

Licklider (1948) investigated the effects of interaural phase on the intelligibility of binaurally presented speech stimuli. He presented speech and white noise to both ears at the same time while systematically varying the phase relationship between the two ears. He found that when both speech and noise were in phase or out of phase *(homophasic condition)*, the intelligibility of the speech was lower for normal listeners than when the speech was out of phase and the noise was in phase or when the speech was in phase and the noise was out of phase *(antiphasic condition)*. In addition, speech intelligibility was found to be better for binaural antiphasic conditions than for monaural presentation alone. Conversely, speech and noise presented binaurally in a homophasic condition resulted in lower intelligibility than did monaural presentation. Therefore, he concluded that **interaural inhibition (or the decrease in binaural performance over monaural performance in some conditions) may well be linked to interaural phase.**

In a related study, Hirsh (1948) utilized a similar paradigm to investigate the effects of interaural phase, pure-tone frequency, and stimulus intensity on interaural summation and inhibition. The following six experimental conditions were utilized: (1) tone monaural/noise binaural and in phase (SNø), (2) tone monaural, noise binaural and 180° out of phase (SNπ), (3) tone and noise binaural and in phase (SøNø homophasic condition), (4) tone and noise binaural and out of phase (SπNπ homophasic condition), (5) tone binaural and in phase/noise binaural and out of phase (SøNπ antiphasic condition), and (6) tone binaural and out of phase/noise binaural and in phase (SπNø antiphasic condition). These conditions are illustrated in Figure 2–3.

Hirsh found that noise presented 180° out of phase to the two ears resulted in the listener perceiving the noise to be located at the ears, whereas noise presented in a homophasic condition resulted in a perception of the noise as being located in the middle of the head (midline).

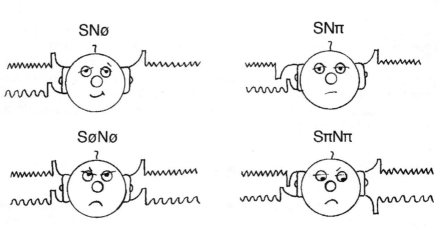

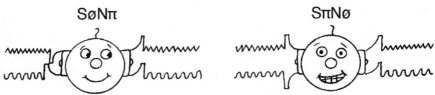

Figure 2–3. Phase conditions utilized in Hirsh's (1948) study.

Therefore, the monaural pure-tone threshold was better when the noise was in phase since the noise was perceived at midline and the tone was perceived at the ear. Similarly, binaural pure-tone thresholds were much better for the antiphasic conditions since the pure tone was heard more easily when it was located at midline and the noise was located at the ears or vice versa, a phenomenon that has come to be known as "release from masking." An additional finding was the effect of stimulus frequency on binaural summation and inhibition: as the pure-tone frequency increased, localization on the basis of phase became more difficult. Thus, **the difference in binaural thresholds between homophasic and antiphasic conditions (otherwise known as the *Masking Level Difference* or *MLD*) decreased as the stimulus frequency increased.** The author added that the fact that the monaural pure-tone thresholds masked by noise in the same ear shifted when noise was added to the opposite ear suggests that masking is not merely a peripheral phenomenon but, rather, that it must involve some degree of central interaction.

A variety of stimulus variables affects the size of the MLD. The choice of a continuous masking stimulus will result in greater release from masking—a larger MLD—than will a masking stimulus that is designed to match the cycle of the pure tone (Green, 1966). An increase in stimulus intensity has been shown to result in a decrease in the amount of release from masking in the antiphasic condition (Townsend & Goldstein, 1972). Finally, **utilization of the antiphasic condition in which the signal delivered to the two ears is out of phase and the masking noise is in phase (SπNø) will result in the largest MLDs** (Olsen, Noffsinger, & Carhart, 1976).

That the mechanism of binaural release from masking occurs at the low brainstem level is evidenced by the findings of Lynn, Gilroy, Taylor, and Leiser (1981) who found that, whereas patients with low brainstem lesions exhibited very small or nonexistent MLDs, patients with cortical lesions exhibited release from masking comparable to normal controls. In addition, lesions of the upper brainstem corresponding to Auditory Brainstem Response (ABR) Waves IV and V do not affect the size of the MLD (Noffsinger, Schaefer, & Martinez, 1984).

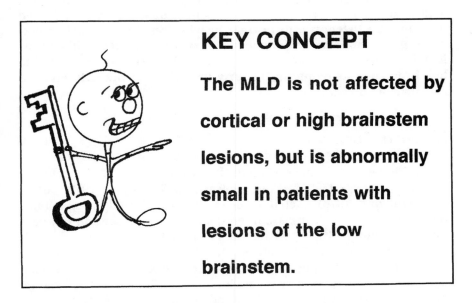

KEY CONCEPT

The MLD is not affected by cortical or high brainstem lesions, but is abnormally small in patients with lesions of the low brainstem.

Detection of Signals in Noise

The ability of a listener to detect a signal in a background of noise is critically related to the interaural relationship between the target signal and the masking signal (Durlach et al., 1981). Therefore, localization and lateralization play a crucial role in this ability.

It is generally known that two ears are better than one and that listeners with unilateral or asymmetrical hearing loss exhibit difficulty detecting signals in noise. However, this **"binaural advantage" is dependent not only upon the hearing sensitivity of the listener but also on the angle or direction of the noise as it relates to the target signal** (Nordlund & Fritzel, 1963). The binaural advantage, or improvement in masked threshold in the binaural condition over the monaural condition, is most evident when the speech and noise are separated by 90° and is essentially nonexistent when the speech and noise arise from the same angle or are separated by 180° (Dirks & Wilson, 1969; Tonning, 1971).

In essence, this dependence of the masked threshold on the angles of the signal and noise in sound field is analogous to the binaural release from masking (MLD) exhibited under headphones (Durlach et al. 1981). It is apparent from the literature that the ability to detect a signal in a background of noise can be affected by a variety of factors including peripheral hearing sensitivity, localization/lateralization ability, and binaural release from masking. **Thus, it may be inferred that, for the listener with normal hearing sensitivity, similar processing mechanisms are engaged for speech-in-noise skills as for localization/lateralization and the MLD, which would implicate the low brainstem as being particularly important in the extraction of signals from noise.**

Binaural Fusion

Several investigators have studied the mechanism of binaural fusion (Lynn & Gilroy, 1975; Matzker, 1959; Smith & Resnick, 1972; Tobin, 1985; Willeford, 1976). Each of these studies has utilized the simultaneous presentation of high-pass filtered stimuli to one ear and low-pass filtered stimuli to the opposite ear in order to assess the listener's ability to fuse the two disparate inputs into one perceptual event.

In all studies, for normal listeners, the presentation of either band pass alone resulted in poor recognition scores; however, the binaural presentation of low-pass stimuli to one ear and high-pass to the other resulted in a significant improvement in recognition performance. Matzker (1959) found that the performance of subjects with cortical lesions was comparable to normal listeners whereas subjects with brainstem lesions had difficulty with the fusion task. The findings of Smith and Resnick (1972) and Lynn and Gilroy (1975) also indicated abnormal fusion performance in subjects with brainstem pathology, suggesting that **the mechanism of binaural fusion is also mediated primarily in the brainstem.**

Effects of Cerebral Pathology on Binaural Interaction

As mentioned previously, the mechanism of binaural interaction is mediated primarily in the low brainstem. Therefore, it would be expected that cerebral pathology would have little effect upon binaural processing. Indeed, Lynn et al. (1981) found that subjects with cerebral pathology demonstrated essentially normal MLDs. However, if the perception of the auditory event occurs in the cortex, lesions of the cerebral hemispheres may result in disrupted binaural perception.

Sanchez-Longo et al. (1957) and Sanchez-Longo and Forster (1958) investigated localization ability in subjects with temporal lobe lesions. The authors found that subjects with lesions of the temporal lobe demonstrated impaired sound localization ability in the auditory field contralateral to the lesion.

Pinheiro and Tobin (1969, 1971) studied the amount of interaural intensity difference (IID) required for subjects to lateralize auditory stimuli. **Whereas normal listeners required an IID of approximately 4 dB for lateralization, subjects with central lesions required a greater IID in the ear ipsilateral to the lesion in order to lateralize auditory stimuli successfully.** Of the subjects in this study, those who exhibited neurological symptoms characteristic of temporal and/or parietal pathology demonstrated elevated IIDs, whereas those with symptoms of occipital or frontal lesions exhibited IIDs comparable to normal subjects.

Based on these findings, it would appear that the auditory cortex is instrumental in the development of the concept of auditory space as well as in the perception of the location of a sound source. Therefore, pathology affecting the auditory areas of the cortex could be expected to disrupt these perceptual behaviors.

Effects of Brainstem Pathology on Binaural Interaction

In addition to transmission of sound and reflexive action as seen in the acoustic reflex, the brainstem auditory pathways are responsible for reception and processing of binaural input (Noffsinger et al., 1984). Therefore, auditory functions involving binaural interaction are likely to be affected by brainstem lesions. The MLD paradigm represents the brainstem's ability to extract a signal from background noise and is the most sensitive behavioral procedure for assessing auditory brainstem integrity (Noffsinger et al., 1984). Specifically, lesions involving the pontomedullary junction are particularly likely to result in abnormal MLDs (Lynn et al., 1981; Noffsinger et al., 1984; Olsen & Noffsinger, 1976).

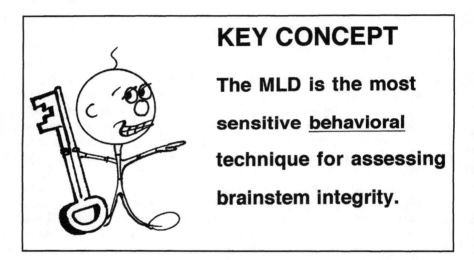

KEY CONCEPT

The MLD is the most sensitive behavioral technique for assessing brainstem integrity.

Multiple sclerosis has been shown to slow transmission time throughout the brainstem auditory pathways (Chiappa, 1980). Several researchers have studied the effects of multiple sclerosis on binaural interaction (Hendler, Squires, & Emmerich, 1990; Levine et al. 1993a, b; Noffsinger et al., 1972; Noffsinger et al., 1984; Olsen & Noffsinger, 1976; Quine, Regan, & Murray, 1983).

Olsen and Noffsinger (1976) studied a variety of subjects with cochlear and brainstem lesions using MLDs for tones and spondaic words. They reported that those subjects with multiple sclerosis exhibited reduced MLDs for both tones and speech and concluded that this finding was most likely due to a disruption of brainstem integration of binaural input.

Quine et al. (1983) conducted a study in which the interaural delay of tones presented to one ear was varied relative to a fixed 1000 Hz tone in the other ear. Subjects were required to indicate which ear received the tone first and responses were analyzed to determine the smallest interaural delay necessary for judgment, similar to temporal ordering tasks but involving both ears. The authors reported that the majority of subjects with multiple sclerosis exhibited significantly longer interaural delays than did control subjects. In addition, the authors found that this delay could be present at one, two, or all three of the frequencies tested (500, 1000, and 2000 Hz). Therefore, it appears that delays can occur for specific frequencies and not others, a finding which may be explained by the presence of local plaques of demyelination occurring at those anatomical sites responsible for the affected frequency or frequencies.

In a similar study investigating the ability of subjects with multiple sclerosis to process changes in interaural intensity, Noffsinger et al. (1972) found that 12 of 60 subjects were unable to experience a single fused midline image when tones presented to both ears were of equal intensity. Hausler and Levine (1980) reported that, of 29 patients with multiple sclerosis, 13 exhibited degraded interaural time discrimination abilities, and these findings were related to abnormalities in brainstem auditory evoked potentials.

Levine et al. (1993a, b) cautioned that, **because multiple sclerosis may cause focal lesions anywhere throughout the auditory pathways, the performance of multiple sclerosis patients on various tests of central auditory processing is likely to be quite varied depending on the site of lesion.** In their two-part study, the authors investigated the performance of subjects with multiple sclerosis on behavioral tests involving discrimination of interaural time and frequency. The findings on the behavioral tests were then compared to results of brainstem auditory evoked potential testing and magnetic resonance imaging (MRI) to determine site of lesion. The stimuli utilized were noise bursts that were either high-pass filtered (4000–2000 Hz) or low-pass filtered (20–1000 Hz). The authors' objective was to determine the just noticeable difference (jnd) in interaural time and interaural intensity required for subjects to perceive a displacement of sound from one ear to the other.

The authors' findings indicated that the majority of subjects exhibited abnormal time jnds for high-pass stimuli. Abnormal performance on any of the other tests was always associated with abnormal time jnds for high-pass stimuli. The least sensitive measures were the jnds for interaural intensity. In addition, the authors found that there were no "silent" multiple sclerosis lesions in that every subject with documented lesions of the brainstem auditory pathways exhibited some abnormality in tests that required microsecond accuracy in neural timing. Specifically, a disruption in interaural discrimination for high-frequency sounds was correlated with unilateral lesions between the cochlear nucleus (CN) and superior olivary complex (SOC). The authors suggested that **the processing of high-frequency sounds requires a greater amount of neural synchrony than does processing of low-frequency sounds and, thus, is most likely to be affected by lesions involving transmission of sound through the brainstem auditory pathways.**

In conclusion, pathological conditions involving the brainstem auditory pathways are likely to result in some disturbance of binaural interaction.

Effects of Cochlear Pathology on Binaural Interaction

Olsen and Noffsinger (1976) reported that subjects with unilateral Meniere's disease exhibited reduced MLDs for 500 Hz tones and spondaic words compared to normal controls. In addition, subjects with noise-induced cochlear hearing loss also exhibited reduced MLDs for speech, although MLDs for 500 Hz tones were within normal limits. They concluded that **binaural release from masking is affected by cochlear pathology** when spondaic word stimuli are used and that this finding may provide an explanation for why individuals with noise-induced hearing loss often report difficulty understanding speech in the presence of background noise.

Several other studies have shown that the MLD is often abnormally reduced in subjects with cochlear pathology (Hall, Tyler, & Fernandez, 1984; Jerger, Brown, & Smith, 1984; Quaranta & Cervellera, 1974; Schoeny & Carhart, 1971; Staffel, Hall, Grose, & Pillsbury, 1990). The abnormalities found in the MLD are likely to be more apparent with increasing severity of loss and interaural asymmetry in hearing sensitivity.

Regarding localization and lateralization abilities in subjects with cochlear hearing loss, it appears that cochlear lesions have a much lesser effect than lesions involving other parts of the auditory system and CANS (Nordlund, 1964; Roser, 1966; Pinheiro & Tobin, 1971). In addition, although subjects with asymmetrical hearing loss tend to do worse on these tasks, **unilateral deafness does not always destroy localization performance** (Gatehouse, 1976; Jongkees & Van der Veer,

1957; Tonning, 1973, 1975), and the degree of difficulty in performing localization and lateralization tasks is difficult to predict on the basis of the degree of hearing loss or audiometric configuration (Nordlund, 1964; Tonning, 1973). The fact that some individuals with cochlear hearing loss report significant difficulty in activities such as understanding a speaker in a noisy situation and others do not may be explained, at least in part, by this variability found in binaural interaction skills in patients with cochlear pathology.

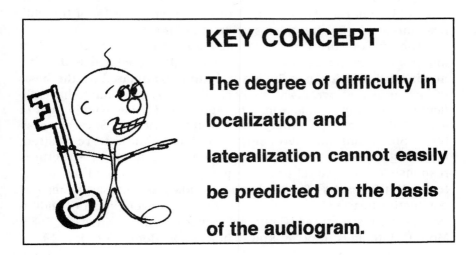

KEY CONCEPT

The degree of difficulty in localization and lateralization cannot easily be predicted on the basis of the audiogram.

Effects of Middle Ear Pathology on Binaural Interaction

Some of the most interesting research in the area of binaural interaction have concerned the effect of otitis media and other middle ear disorders on MLDs, particularly in children. **The MLD at 500 Hz is generally reduced in children as compared to adults and increases as a function of age, reaching adult values at approximately 5 to 6 years of age** (Hall & Grose, 1990). In addition, adults show a greater release from masking for time-compressed speech than do children of 8 to 9 years of age (Bornstein, 1994). Finally, children with a history of chronic otitis media have been shown to have difficulty recognizing words presented in a competing speech background (Jerger, Jerger, Alford, & Abrams, 1983).

Pillsbury, Grose, and Hall (1991) studied the MLD for 500 Hz tones in a group of children with a history of chronic otitis media with effusion (OME) and hearing loss. The children, aged 5 to 13 years of age, were tested just prior to the insertion of pressure equalizing (PE) tubes and one month following surgery. Several of the children also returned for additional testing three months post-operatively. Findings from this group were compared to a group of children with no history of otitis. The authors found that the children with a history of otitis media demonstrated significantly reduced MLDs and greater variability than did the control children. This MLD abnormality continued to be present for 64% of the children three months after the insertion of PE tubes.

The authors drew several conclusions from their study. Most importantly, **the extent of hearing disability associated with otitis media with effusion may be severely underestimated on the basis of pure-tone audiograms** as many children may continue to have difficulty extracting signals from a background of noise even in light of essentially normal postoperative hearing sensitivity. Several possible explanations for the observed deficit in MLDs were posited, including abnormal development of brainstem auditory structures responsible for binaural processing, a finding that would be consistent with the results of several animal studies in which asymmetrical conductive hearing loss resulted in abnormal development of auditory brainstem structures (Clopton & Silverman, 1978; Knudsen, 1983; Moore, Hutchings, King, & Kowalchuk, 1989; Moore & Irvine, 1981). Other possible explanations included inaccurate mapping of stimulus frequency onto cochlear place and reduced ability of the CANS to process cues for signal detection and extract the signal from the noise. Whatever the cause, it does appear from the authors' data that children with a significant history of chronic otitis media with effusion may exhibit long-term difficulty in binaural interaction, possibly due to sensory deprivation.

To explore further the relationship between abnormal MLDs and possible abnormal brainstem function in children with a history of otitis media with effusion, Hall and Grose (1993) studied a group of 14 children, aged 5 to 9, all of whom had a significant otologic history and were tested approximately one month following the insertion of PE tubes. The authors compared MLD results with results of brainstem auditory evoked potential testing. Results of this study indicated modest correlation between abnormal MLDs and interaural asymmetry for interpeak interval values. There was no correlation noted between

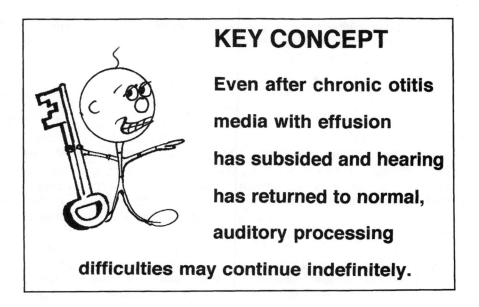

KEY CONCEPT

Even after chronic otitis media with effusion has subsided and hearing has returned to normal, auditory processing difficulties may continue indefinitely.

abnormal MLDs and absolute latency prolongation or interpeak intervals. The authors concluded that the degree of interpeak interval abnormality in one ear may be related to the degree of auditory deprivation in that ear relative to the other ear. In addition, the results suggest that reduced MLDs in children with otitis media with effusion may indeed be related to abnormal brainstem processing as opposed to more centrally located factors.

Hall, Grose, and Pillsbury (1995), in a longitudinal study of the effects of OME on MLD performance, reported that the abovementioned abnormalities in the MLD continued to be present up to two years following medical intervention. By three years post-surgery, a small proportion of children continued to exhibit reduced MLDs; however, the OME group did not differ significantly from that of the control group in terms of MLD performance. These results suggest a slow recovery of binaural function over a long period of time in children with a history of chronic otitis media with effusion.

Finally, conductive hearing loss can degrade localization and lateralization abilities significantly (Hausler, Colburn, & Marr, 1983; Nordlund, 1964; Roser, 1966), and abnormalities in binaural processing have been found to persist even after hearing thresholds are returned to normal by middle ear surgery (Hall & Derlacki, 1986, 1988; Hall, Grose, & Pillsbury, 1990; Pillsbury et al., 1991).

For further information regarding assessment and management of binaural interaction, the reader is referred to Chapters 5, 6, and 8. Table 2–3 summarizes the effects of CANS pathology on binaural interaction.

Summary

The term *central auditory processing* encompasses a variety of auditory system mechanisms. This chapter has focused on three central auditory functions: dichotic listening, temporal processing, and binaural interaction. With an understanding of the neurophysiological bases of and pathological effects on these processes, the clinician may be better able to interpret tests of central auditory processing and make appropriate recommendations for management.

Dichotic listening is the processing of auditory stimuli that are presented to both ears simultaneously, with the stimulus being different in each ear. **Theory regarding the mechanism of dichotic listening suggests that, although auditory input is represented both ipsilaterally and contralaterally throughout the CANS, the contralateral pathways are stronger than the ipsilateral pathways. Thus, when competing auditory stimuli are introduced, the weaker ipsilateral pathways are suppressed by the contralateral pathways.**

Lesions of the right temporal lobe result in contralateral (left ear) suppression or extinction of dichotically presented auditory stimuli. Left temporal lobe lesions often result in bilateral suppression, as

Table 2-3
Effects of Pathology of the CANS on Binaural Interaction

Site of Lesion	Effect(s) on Binaural Interaction
Temporal Lobe	Impairment of localization in contralateral auditory field; greater IID required in ear ipsilateral to lesion for lateralization
Low Brainstem	Deficit in all binaural interaction tasks
High Brainstem	No effect on MLD
Peripheral: Cochlear	Variable, possible deficit in localization and lateralization; reduced MLD
Peripheral: Conductive	Reduced MLD; may exhibit ongoing deficit in binaural interaction tasks

auditory information from both ears is prevented from arriving at the speech-dominant left hemisphere. Complete sectioning of the corpus callosum results in left ear extinction of dichotically presented stimuli due to the interruption in interhemispheric transfer of auditory information from the right hemisphere to the left. Individuals with cochlear hearing loss may exhibit a greater ear advantage than do normal listeners. Conductive hearing losses do not appear to affect dichotic listening significantly.

Temporal processing refers to the processing of time-related cues in the auditory signal and is critical for speech and music perception. The processing of temporal cues takes place throughout the CANS; however, the primary and associative auditory cortex appear to be particularly important for the processing of temporal order. **Although VIIIth nerve and brainstem lesions may have some effect on temporal processing, lesions of the temporal lobe and/or corpus callosum are most likely to disrupt the processing of temporal cues.**

Binaural interaction, or the way in which the two ears work together, is important for a variety of everyday listening activities including localization and lateralization of auditory stimuli, binaural release from masking, detection of signals in a background of noise, and binaural fusion. The level of the pons in the low brainstem is implicated as being particularly crucial to the processing of binaural input, although the actual perception of the auditory event occurs in the cortex. **Lesions of the low brainstem are most likely to disrupt binaural interaction. In addition, conductive hearing loss has been shown to have an effect upon binaural interaction**, possibly due to abnormal development of brainstem auditory structures following sensory deprivation. Cortical and cochlear lesions may affect binaural interaction depending on the extent of the pathology and the type of binaural interaction task.

Review Questions

1. Define the term *central auditory processes.*
2. Distinguish between *dichotic* and *diotic* listening.
3. Describe Kimura's theory of dichotic listening.
4. Define the term *Right Ear Advantage.*
5. Describe the effects of pathology of the following structures on dichotic listening:

right temporal lobe	left temporal lobe
corpus callosum	cochlea
middle ear	

6. Define *temporal processing.*
7. Identify examples of listening tasks that rely on processing of temporal cues.
8. Describe the effects of pathology of the following structures on temporal processing:

> temporal lobe   corpus callosum
> brainstem   cochlea
> middle ear

9. Define *binaural interaction.*
10. Identify examples of auditory functions that rely on binaural interaction.
11. Describe the phenomenon of binaural release from masking (Masking Level Difference) and define the following four stimulus conditions:

> SπNπ   SøNø
> SπNø   SøNπ

12. Which of the above four stimulus conditions will result in the largest MLDs in the normal listener and why?
13. Describe the effects of pathology of the following structures on binaural interaction:

> temporal lobe   midbrain
> pons   cochlea
> middle ear

14. How does multiple sclerosis affect binaural interaction?

CHAPTER

THREE

Neuromaturation and Neuroplasticity of the Auditory System

Any discussion of central auditory processing in children must take into account the effects of maturation upon auditory function. Age-dependent morphological changes within the brain will determine in large part the child's ability to perform certain auditory tasks. The clinician engaged in central auditory assessment must be familiar with normal variations in CNS development in order to select the most appropriate assessment tools, interpret test results in the context of age-appropriate normative data, and develop management plans based on the stage of neuroaudiological development. In addition, neuromaturation, or lack thereof, may remain a factor in the evaluation and remediation of a given child for several years following the initial assessment; therefore, attempts to determine the efficacy of remediation must take into consideration those improvements in auditory function that may be attributed to CNS development over time as opposed to direct results of rehabilitative techniques.

The term *functional plasticity* refers to the nervous system's ability to reorganize and adapt in response to internal and external changes. Two familiar examples of neuroplasticity are the organizational rearrangement of neural pathways after a stroke or other pathology and the functional and morphological changes that occur as a result of sensory deprivation. The ability of the CNS to adapt to internal and external changes has important implications for learning. Because neuroplasticity is greatest in the early years and diminishes with age, early exposure to sensory stimuli is critical to the normal development of CNS structures and pathways. Likewise, early identification of pathological conditions will increase the chance of (re)habilitative success.

This chapter will provide an overview of how age affects auditory function, including the normal course of development and maturation within the auditory system and implications for valid age-appropriate assessment and interpretation. In addition, current research regarding neuroplasticity of the auditory system and its implications for remediation of CAPD will be discussed.

Learning Objectives

After studying this chapter, the reader should be able to:
1. Describe the prenatal development of the auditory system
2. Describe the normal course of myelination and synapse formation in the maturing auditory system
3. Discuss auditory behavioral correlates to neuromaturation of the auditory system
4. Discuss neuroplasticity and its potential significance in remediation of central auditory processing disorders.

Prenatal Development of the Auditory System

It is not even remotely within the scope of this text to provide the reader with a comprehensive discussion of human embryological development. Indeed, what is currently known about prenatal development of the auditory and central nervous systems would fill volumes of text.

Therefore, the purpose of this section is to give the reader a brief overview of the development of the auditory system, focusing in particular on the development of central auditory structures.

Prenatal Development of the Brain

First, it is important to note that the human brain is not fully developed at birth. Although the production of neurons through cell division is completed by approximately 16 to 20 weeks after conception and no new neurons are produced after that time, **the development of new and more efficient synaptic connections continues into adulthood** (Kalil, 1989; Restak, 1986).

Development of the brain and spinal cord begins during the third week after conception (gestational age, GA) with the appearance of the *neural plate*, a hollow tube approximately 3 mm in length. As the brain of a newborn baby contains more than 100 billion neurons, the developing brain must grow at the remarkable rate of about 250,000 nerve cells per minute throughout the course of pregnancy (Ackerman, 1992).

By 4 weeks GA, the main divisions of the brain can be seen: the *forebrain*, which will give rise to the cerebral hemispheres, *midbrain, hindbrain,* and *spinal cord.* Within another week, swellings appear that mark the future site of the cerebral hemispheres and other structures, becoming identifiable by 8 weeks GA. By 18 weeks GA, the primary grooves on the surface of the hemispheres have appeared, but the surface itself remains smooth. Finally, by 28 weeks GA, the primary lobes of the brain are clearly formed as is the lateral (Sylvian) fissure. From this point, the brain continues to grow in size and complexity of synaptic pathways, reaching an average weight of 8,400 g at birth.

Cell Differentiation and Migration in the Developing Embryo

At the earliest stages of development, all cells within the human embryo have the potential to develop into any cell of the body. However, at 15 to 16 days after fertilization, differentiation begins, with cells assuming specific "identities." The cells differentiate into three cellular layers, termed *germ layers*: the *ectoderm*, which will give rise to outer skin layers, the nervous system, and sense organs; the

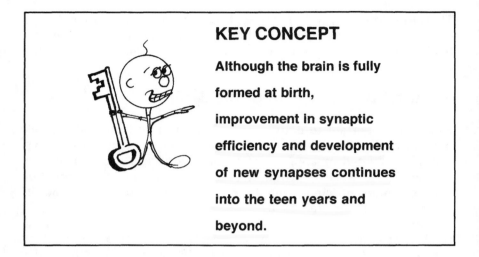

KEY CONCEPT

Although the brain is fully formed at birth, improvement in synaptic efficiency and development of new synapses continues into the teen years and beyond.

mesoderm, which is associated with skeletal, circulatory, and reproductive organs; and the *endoderm*, from which the digestive and respiratory organs will arise.

Following the appearance of the germ layers, a massive migration of cells begins wherein cells continually divide and travel to their final predetermined destinations. Upon arrival, each cell seeks out and recognizes others like itself, aggregating in groups in distinct regions and forming synapses. The exact mechanism through which this clustering and finely tuned differentiation occurs is not fully understood at this time; however, it is likely that both genetic programming and distinctive cellular secretions play a role (Restak, 1986).

Prenatal Development of the Auditory System

The outer ear, inner ear, and CANS structures arise from ectodermal tissues, which is why abnormalities of the outer ear may coincide with sensory or neural abnormalities. In contrast, the bony structures of the middle ear develop from the mesodermal germ plate. This section will focus on the prenatal development of the inner ear and CANS.

The inner ear is the first of the three anatomical divisions of the ear to appear embryologically, beginning with the appearance of the *otic placodes*—slight thickenings on the lateral aspect of the neural plate—at approximately 20 days GA. The otic placode consists of a small island of neural tissue that is similar to brain-wall ectoderm. In a short period of time, the otic placode sinks into the surrounding tissue and forms the otic pit, which subsequently deepens and forms a vesicle—the otocyst. By the end of the 5th week GA, the otocyst has divided into two lobes which will ultimately become the organs of hearing and the vestibular system. **By the end of the 5th month GA, all of the structures necessary for inner ear function are present and adultlike in structure and size.** In fact, the youngest human fetus reported to have responded to acoustic stimuli was 26 weeks GA, a period that coincides with the completion of inner ear development (Wedenberg, 1965).

This is not the case with the structures of the CANS. As previously mentioned, the human brain is not completely developed until well into the teenage years. Likewise, CANS structures, while present and functioning at birth, continue to form new synaptic connections and to increase synaptic efficiency for several years following birth.

Little is known about the prenatal development of the central auditory pathways. It is known that cells of the cochlear ganglion begin to migrate toward the brainstem during the 6th week GA and that the cochlear nerve appears abruptly at approximately 7 weeks GA, with its appearance occurring in all parts of the nerve's course simultaneously (Streeter, 1906). It is likely that the fibers of the auditory brainstem structures develop at the same time as the nerve fibers of the otic vesicle; however, there are no empirical data to determine the timing of their maturation definitively (Maue-Dickson, 1981). **That the brainstem auditory pathways are structurally complete by 30 weeks GA is evidenced by the ability to obtain brainstem auditory evoked potentials from infants as young as 10 weeks premature** (Cervette, 1984; Despland & Galambos, 1980; Galambos, Wilson, & Silva, 1994; Starr, Amlie, Martin, & Sanders, 1977). **However, the synaptic efficiency of auditory brainstem fibers continues to improve until approximately 3 years of age** (Cox, 1985; Salamy, 1984; Salamy, Mendelson, Tooley, & Chaplin, 1980). The information presented here regarding prenatal development of the auditory system is summarized in Table 3–1.

Neuromaturation of the Auditory System

It is a well-accepted fact that the normal human infant, just minutes after birth, can hear. The newborn startles to loud sound and even turns, to the degree that its immature musculature will allow, toward an off-center sound (Kelly, 1986; Wertheimer, 1961). This behavioral

Table 3-1

Overview of Prenatal Development of the Brain and Auditory System

Gestational Age	Developmental Characteristics
15-16 days	Differentiation of cells into 3 neural germ layers
3rd week	Appearance of neural plate
20 days	Appearance of otic placodes
4 weeks	Main divisions of the brain can be seen
5th week	Division of otocyst into lobes that will give rise to organs of hearing and balance
6th week	Cells of cochlear ganglion begin to migrate toward brainstem
7 weeks	Cochlear nerve appears abruptly
18 weeks	Primary grooves have appeared on brain surface
5 months	Structures of inner ear are present and adultlike in structure and size
28 weeks	Primary lobes of brain and lateral fissure are fully formed
30 weeks	Brainstem auditory pathways structurally complete; auditory brainstem response can be obtained
Birth	Brain weighs approximately 8,400 grams

orienting response, basic to hearing, has been shown to be affected by the type of stimulus used. Very brief stimuli appear to be unsuccessful in eliciting a response in newborns (Butterworth & Castillo, 1976; McGurk, Turnure, & Creighton, 1977), but high-frequency, longer duration stimuli such as rattle sounds and human speech are extremely effective in eliciting head turns (Brazelton, 1973; Muir & Clifton, 1985; Weiss, Zelazo, & Swain, 1988).

In addition, evidence suggests that the newborn exhibits definite preferences not only to certain types of sounds, but even to content of linguistic stimuli. A study was undertaken at the University of North Carolina in which pregnant mothers were asked to read a children's book (*The Cat in the Hat* by Dr. Seuss) twice every day during the last 6 months of their pregnancy. Shortly after birth, the newborn infants were attached to a device that monitored sucking activity. The infants learned immediately to alter their sucking patterns to produce a tape-recorded rendition of the mother reading the familiar book; however, taped renditions of the mother reading another children's book with similar intonation failed to elicit the sucking response (Kolata, 1984). Although it is not clear which auditory cues were most influential in the infants' preferences, **these findings suggest that the ability of infants to perceive differences in the linguistic content of auditory stimuli is present to some degree at birth, and may even be present prior to birth while still in the womb.**

Although newborn infants exhibit surprisingly sophisticated auditory abilities, there is no question that the auditory system of the infant and child is not like that of the adult. **In the infant and small child, masked thresholds are higher** (Schneider, Trehub, Morrongiello, & Thorpe, 1989), **discrimination of intensity, frequency, and temporal cues is poorer** (Hall & Grose, 1994; Irwin, Ball, Kay, Stillman, & Bosser, 1985; Jensen, Neff, & Callaghan, 1987; Wightman, Allen, Dolan, Kistler, & Jamieson, 1989), **the right ear advantage on linguistically loaded dichotic listening tasks is more pronounced** (Keith, 1984; Willeford & Burleigh 1994), and the list goes on. What accounts for these marked differences between the auditory perceptual abilities of children and adults? The answer, simply, is neuromaturation. While the auditory system of the newborn may be structurally intact from a gross anatomical and physiological perspective, the efficiency of the system continues to develop and improve for several years following birth (Aoki & Siekevitz, 1988).

Age-Dependent Morphological Changes of the Central Auditory Nervous System

There is a variety of age-dependent morphological changes that occur in the brain and influence auditory behavior, the most prominent of which is degree of myelination (Romand, 1983). Myelin is the white matter of the brain, a multilayered sheath that insulates and protects the nerve fiber. The speed of transmission of nerve impulses depends on the diameter of the nerve fiber and its degree of myelination. Some areas of the brain are heavily myelinated; others (gray matter) are unmyelinated.

The formation of myelin begins during fetal development and continues until maturity. Therefore, the time span of myelination is directly related to the development of sensorimotor and cognitive development (Lecours, 1975; Lenneberg, 1967). **Myelination proceeds in a caudal to rostral direction, with those structures of the brainstem necessary for survival completed before the first year of age whereas cortical communication areas may not be myelinated until early adulthood** (Yakovlev & Lecours, 1967). Myelination of the corpus callosum, critical for interhemispheric transfer of information, continues through adolescence (Salamy, 1978). The fact that different areas of the brain undergo myelination at different times has profound implications for auditory processing, as those processes that depend upon brainstem function will develop much earlier than will those that rely upon efficient inter- and intra-hemispheric communication.

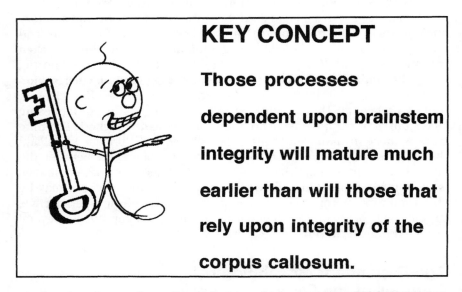

KEY CONCEPT

Those processes dependent upon brainstem integrity will mature much earlier than will those that rely upon integrity of the corpus callosum.

Another factor that affects degree of neuromaturation is *arborization* or *dendritic branching*. Dendrites are extensions of the nerve cell body that transmit information to the cell body from other, adjacent cells. As the organism develops, the dendrites branch out in various directions, thus increasing the surface area available for synapses with the axons of other nerve cells. As a result, additional connections are made for the transfer of more information.

There is some evidence to suggest that arborization and the development of new synapses continue indefinitely in some brain systems. In fact, those systems responsible for learning must retain some ability to alter neural "wiring" throughout life; otherwise, no new learning could take place (Kalil, 1989).

Electrophysiological Indicators of Auditory Neuromaturation

The caudal to rostral course of neuromaturation within the CANS may be illustrated through the use of electrophysiological measures of CANS function, in which the speed of transmission appears to be directly related to the degree of myelination (Musiek, Verkest, & Gollegly, 1988).

The Auditory Brainstem Response

The auditory brainstem response (ABR), first described by Jewitt and Williston (1971), is an electrical, far-field recording of synchronous activity in the auditory nerve and brainstem and is characterized by five to seven waveforms which occur within 10 msec following presentation of auditory stimuli (clicks or tone pips). A typical adult ABR is illustrated in Figure 3–1. The ABR is most often analyzed according to absolute wave latencies of waves I, III, and V; interwave intervals; and interaural latency differences, as well as interwave amplitude ratios in order to obtain information regarding hearing sensitivity and neurological brainstem integrity (Jacobson, 1985).

Although absolute generators of the ABR have been in dispute for a number of years, it is generally agreed that **wave I represents the action potential within the acoustic nerve and wave III arises from the region of the superior olivary complex. The generator for wave V appears to be the region of the lateral lemniscus in the mid pons** (Chiappa, 1983; Moller, Jannetta, & Moller, 1981).

Studies of the effects of age on the ABR provide us with valuable information regarding neuromaturation of the brainstem. As previous-

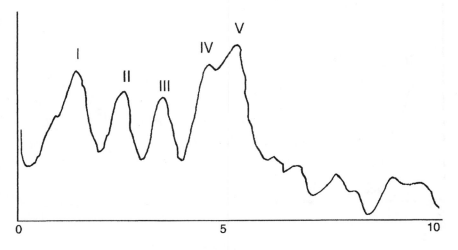

Latency (msec)

Figure 3–1. Typical Auditory Brainstem Response (ABR).

ly mentioned, waves I, III, and V of the ABR may be obtained by 30 to 32 weeks gestational age. However, absolute wave latencies, interwave intervals, and amplitude ratios continue to change as a function of age, with **waves III and V continuing to change until age 2 or 3 even though absolute latency of wave I reaches adult values by 3 months of age** (Cox, 1985; Salamy et al. 1980).

The Middle Latency Response

The middle latency response (MLR) was first described by Geisler, Frishkopf, and Rosenblith (1958). Like the ABR, the MLR can be recorded from the scalp in response to tone pips or clicks. **The MLR follows the ABR, occurring between 10 and 90 msec following stimulus onset and is characterized by waves Na, Pa, and Pb** (Figure 3–2). **Brain structures thought to be involved in the generation of the MLR include auditory-specific structures as well as structures outside the CANS.** Presumed generators include the temporal lobe and/or thalamocortical projections (Kileny, Paccioretti, & Wilson, 1987; Kraus, Ozdamar, Hier, & Stein, 1982; Ozdamar & Kraus, 1983), the reticular formation in the midbrain and thalamus (Buchwald, Hinman, Norman, Huang, & Brown, 1981; McGee, Kraus, Comperatore, & Nicol,

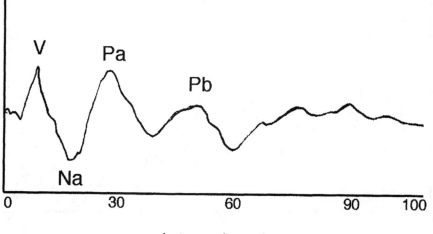

Figure 3–2. Typical Middle Latency Response (MLR). Wave V of the ABR can be visualized.

1991; Osterhammel, Shallop, & Terkildsen, 1985), the inferior colliculus in the midbrain (Caird & Klinke, 1987; Fischer, Bognar, Turjman, & Lapras, 1995; Hashimoto, Ishiyama, Yoshimoto, & Nemoto, 1981; McGee et al., 1991), and the medial geniculate body in the midbrain (Fischer et al., 1995).

Although the effects of maturation upon the MLR are not as well understood as that on the ABR, it has been shown that **MLRs obtained from infants and young children show longer latencies, poorer waveform morphology, and greater variability than those from adults** (Suzuki, Hirabayashi, & Kobayashi, 1983). In addition, while the earlier Na component of the MLR is present in 60 to 70% of children younger than 1 year of age, the later Pa component is present in only 20% of these children. In contrast, both Na and Pa components are present in nearly 100% of children 10 to 12 years of age, demonstrating a clear, caudal-to-rostral, progressive effect of neuromaturation on the MLR (Kraus, Smith, Reed, Stein, & Cartee, 1985).

The Late Evoked Potentials

The ABR and the MLR are considered to be primarily *exogenous* potentials; that is, they occur in response to external events (although subject state does have some effect upon the MLR). Portions of the late evoked potentials (LEPs), conversely, are *endogenous* potentials, occurring in response to internally generated events related to attention to the stimulus (Squires & Hecox, 1983). As such, **the generators of the LEPs are those that involve the integrative and attentional functions of the brain including the limbic system and the auditory cortex itself** (Perrault & Picton, 1984; Ritter, Simson, Vaughan, & Macht, 1982; Scherg, Vasjar, & Picton, 1989; Vaughan & Ritter, 1970).

The typical LEP consists of the N1, P2, and P3 waves which occur at 100, 200, and 300 msec poststimulus, respectively (Picton, Woods, Baribeau-Braun, & Healey, 1977) (Figure 3–3). Whereas the N1 and P2 can be elicited simply by presentation of tonal or click stimuli to an awake, passive individual, the P3 requires conscious attention to and discrimination of stimulus differences (Sutton, Braren, Zubin, & John, 1965). In addition, speech stimuli may be used to elicit potentials comparable to N1 and P2 (Rugg, 1984a, b) as can visual and somatosensory stimuli (Davis, 1939).

Although many components of the LEPs may be recorded in infants, **complete maturation of N1 and P2 does not occur until adolescence, and the P3 response reaches its shortest latency values in the early to mid teenage years** (Courchesne, 1978; Davis & Onishi, 1969; Goodin, Squires, Henderson, & Starr, 1978; Polich, Howard, & Starr, 1985).

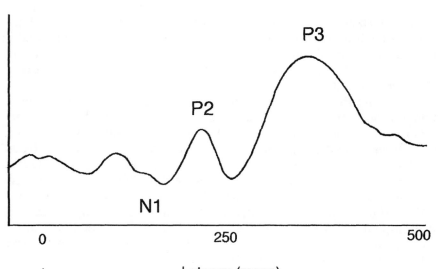

Figure 3–3. Typical Late Evoked Potentials (LEP), including P300 response to deviant stimuli.

In conclusion, examination of the available data regarding maturation of auditory electrophysiology measures reveals a **caudal-to-rostral progression of maturation with auditory brainstem potentials reaching adult values by 3 years of age, followed by middle latency potentials and, finally, late potentials, which may not reach adult values until the teen years**. These findings are consistent with those regarding myelination which indicate that, whereas some brainstem structures may complete the myelination process during the first year of life, myelination of higher level structures continues throughout adolescence and into early adulthood.

Developmental Psychoacoustics

Given the fact that neuromaturation of the CANS continues for several years following birth, it would be expected that those behavioral auditory phenomena and processes that rely upon auditory system integrity would follow a maturational course consistent with the physiological neuromaturation of the system. Indeed, when psychophysical data regarding the effect of age on the ability of children to perform certain auditory tasks are studied, this does appear to be the case. Following is a discussion of maturational effects upon the processes described in Chapter 2: dichotic listening, temporal processing, and binaural interaction.

Maturation and Dichotic Listening

The effect of age on dichotic listening may be different depending on the type of stimuli used. As discussed in Chapter 2, dichotic listening requires communication between cerebral hemispheres as well as functional integrity of both temporal lobes. A review of the literature on dichotic listening and children suggests that **the more linguistically loaded the stimuli presented are, the more pronounced the maturational effects are likely to be**.

Berlin, Hughes, Lowe-Bell, and Berlin (1973) studied the performance of normally hearing children between the ages of 5 and 13 on a test of dichotic, consonant-vowel (CV) nonsense words. Their results showed a right ear advantage (REA) that remained relatively constant throughout the age range. However, the number of incidences in which stimuli presented to both the left and the right ear were reported correctly increased significantly as a function of age. The authors suggested that this improved performance reflected an increase in the brain's ability to process two-channel stimuli as a function of age.

In contrast, when dichotically presented sentences are used, right ear scores reach adult values by 5 years of age while the left ear exhibits poor performance which improves with age, resulting in a decrease in the size of the REA with increasing age (Willeford & Burleigh, 1994). Age-related normative data from our own clinic show the same, general trend. While the REA for dichotically presented digits continues to be approximately 10% for the age range of 7 years through adult, overall test performance does improve, reaching adult values by 9 years of age. However, our normative data using dichotic sentence stimuli indicate that 7 year olds exhibit an REA on the order of nearly 40% which rapidly decreases as a function of increasing age, reaching adult values by 10 to 11 years of age. Right ear performance of the younger children using dichotic sentences is not significantly different from that of adults (Figure 3–4). It should be noted that, in our clinic, normative data for children younger than age 7 are not available due to the high variability found in these children on central tests.

A possible explanation for these findings lies in the degree of complexity of the stimuli utilized. CV nonsense syllables (as well as digits) are less linguistically complex than sentences. As such, both hemispheres may process these stimuli relatively equally (Porter & Berlin, 1975). In contrast, dichotic sentences are more heavily linguistically loaded. As discussed in Chapter 2, processing of dichotic speech stimuli

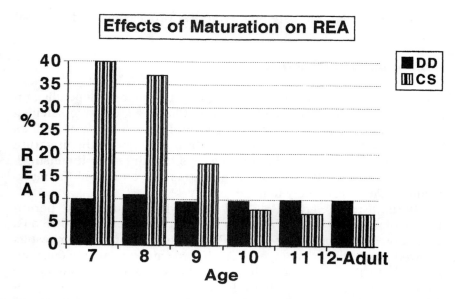

Figure 3–4. Comparison of the size of the REA for Diochotic Digits (DD) and Competing Sentences (CS) between children and adults.

requires adequate interhemispheric communication via the corpus callosum as well as integrity of both temporal lobes. **Poor left ear performance on dichotic sentence tasks in children may reflect a decreased ability of the corpus callosum to transfer complex stimuli from the right hemisphere to the left hemisphere. As the child becomes older and myelination of the corpus callosum is completed, interhemispheric transfer of information improves and left ear scores approach those found in adults** (Musiek, Gollegly, & Baran, 1984).

Maturation and Temporal Processing

Like dichotic listening, there appear to be definite effects of age on temporal processing. Werner, Marean, Halpin, Spetner, and Gillenwater (1992) studied the ability of 3-, 6-, and 12-month-old infants to perform gap-detection tasks. The infants were conditioned to respond when a gap occurred in the presentation of broadband noise, but not when the noise was continuous. In addition, the effect of masker frequency on gap detection was investigated. High-pass, continuous maskers with cutoff frequencies of 500, 2000, and 8000 Hz were added that would allow the listener to use only those frequencies below the masker cutoff to detect gaps in the broadband noise

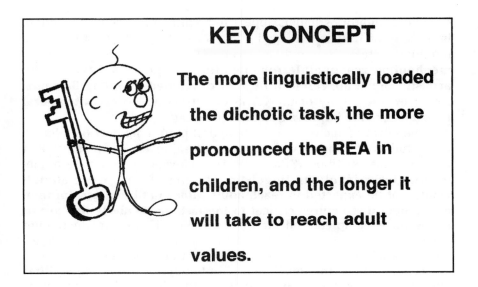

KEY CONCEPT

The more linguistically loaded the dichotic task, the more pronounced the REA in children, and the longer it will take to reach adult values.

stimulus. The authors found that, although the infants' ability to perform the gap detection task was quite poor as compared to adults, the general effect of masker frequency on gap detection was the same for infants as for adults, with improvement in gap detection as masker frequency increased. In other words, **infants performed qualitatively like adults, suggesting that the poor temporal resolution in the younger population was due to the primary effect of age**.

Studies of temporal resolution in older children have exhibited the same general finding. Irwin et al. (1985) found that gap detection ability improved in subjects from 6 years of age up until approximately 8 to 10 years of age. Morrongiello and Trehub (1987) reported a progressive increase in duration discrimination from infancy to adulthood. Wightman et al. (1989) found that, for subjects in their study, gap detection improved from age 3 to 5 years, but was not significantly different from adults by 6 years of age. However, the authors reported that the within- and across-subject variability in their population was very high, with some very young children at times performing comparably to adults. The authors suggested that memory or attention may have played a role in these findings, although a very real age effect on temporal resolution did appear to be present. Finally, Grose, Hall, and Gibbs (1993) found that the temporal resolution in their subjects improved as a function of age to 7 to 10 years of age.

As discussed in Chapter 2, temporal encoding occurs in the peripheral auditory system and is represented at various levels throughout the CANS. However, extraction and analysis of temporal cues in an auditory stimulus appear to be primarily a central function. In a study of 18 listeners aged 4 years to adult utilizing a temporal modulation task, Hall and Grose (1994) found that **the peripheral mechanism responsible for encoding temporal aspects of the acoustic signal appeared to be well developed in young listeners. However, the ability of the CANS to extract and process temporal cues appeared to improve as a function of age.**

The effect of age on tests of temporal patterning may be inferred from studies of patients with corpus callosal involvement (Musiek et al., 1980; Musiek, Kibbe, & Baran,1984). **Performance on temporal patterning tasks involving linguistic labeling of nonspeech stimuli would not be expected to reach adult values until neuromaturation of the neural structures critical to the task, particularly the corpus callosum, is complete.** Indeed, our own clinic norms, in which adult values on the Frequency Pattern and Duration Pattern tests are not attained until 11 to 12 years of age, support this hypothesis.

To summarize, **the development of temporal processing abilities appears to follow the course of neuromaturation, with skills improving as a function of age until approximately 12 years of age.** In addition, the effect of age upon temporal processing will depend on the task selected and, to some degree, on attentional factors.

Maturation and Binaural Interaction

As previously mentioned, a newborn will turn toward an off-center sound, indicating that at least a portion of those brainstem structures necessary for basic localization are developed by birth (Kelly, 1986; Wertheimer, 1961). However, stimulus frequency and stimulus duration have a significant effect on the newborn's ability to localize. High-frequency stimuli appear to be most effective in eliciting head turns in the newborn, as do stimuli at least 1 sec in duration. Stimuli less than 500 msec in duration result in nonresponsiveness (Clarkson, Clifton, & Morrongiello, 1985; Clarkson, Clifton, Swain, & Perris, 1989; Morrongiello & Clifton, 1984).

Interestingly, when infants reach approximately 6 to 8 weeks of age, they stop turning toward a sound source (Field, Muir, Pilon, Sinclair, & Dodwell, 1980; Muir, Abraham, Forbes, & Harris, 1979). Muir and Clifton (1985) suggested that this change in behavior does not reflect the infants' sudden inability to process interaural cues but, rather, the maturational shift from a subcortical to a cortical site of processing control. Whereas the head turn of a newborn toward a sound source may be almost a reflexive action, **the reappearance of the head-turning behavior at approximately 4 months of age, accompanied by visual searching, may signal the onset of conscious perception of auditory space.**

Although infants aged 4 months and older demonstrate repeatable orienting responses toward sound, the precision and accuracy of their ability to localize when the sound is presented at decreasing angles from midline continues to improve until approximately 5 years of age (Litovsky, 1991). Again, it appears that factors other than simply binaural sensitivity are at work in the developing infant. Rather, this developmental change in localization acuity may well be attributed to the integration of binaural cues with head movement and changing head size (Ashmead, Davis, Whalen, & Odom, 1991; Knudsen, Esterly, & Knudsen, 1984).

Results of studies of the effect of age on the Masking Level Difference (MLD), described in Chapter 2, have been somewhat contradictory. Nozza (1987) reported that the MLD for 500 Hz tones was significantly smaller in infants than in adult subjects. In a related study, Nozza, Wagner, and Crandall (1988) concluded that, although significant differences appear to exist between the size of the MLD for infants and adults, those of preschool children do not differ significantly from those of adults when sensation level of masking presentation is taken into account. Likewise, other studies have suggested that the MLD of 4- to 6-year-old children does not differ significantly from that of adults (Roush & Tait, 1984; Sweetow & Reddell, 1978).

In a study of 26 children aged 3.9 to 9.5 years of age, Hall and Grose (1990) found that the MLD for a pure tone presented in a wide band (300 Hz) masker progressively increased up to approximately 5 or 6 years of age. In addition, MLDs presented in narrow band (40 Hz) maskers continued to be smaller in the 6-year-old subjects than those of adults. The authors concluded that **these developmental changes observed in the MLD of children younger than 6 years of age are most likely related to central auditory processing rather than to sensitivity to interaural timing cues**.

A review of the data regarding brainstem neuromaturation supports this hypothesis. As previously discussed, the ABR reaches adult values by age 3, indicating that the brainstem structures necessary for the detection of interaural cues are essentially intact at this age. However, the higher level pathways responsible for integration and processing of binaural cues continue to mature beyond this age. Therefore, the time span of neuromaturation in the developing auditory system may be correlated with the development of localization acuity and binaural release from masking in the infant and child. **Overall, it appears that binaural interaction abilities continue to improve from infancy until at least 6 years of age.**

To conclude, auditory behaviors related to dichotic listening, temporal processing, and binaural interaction reflect a developmental course that can be explained in large part by neuromaturation of the auditory system. The implications for the clinician involved in the

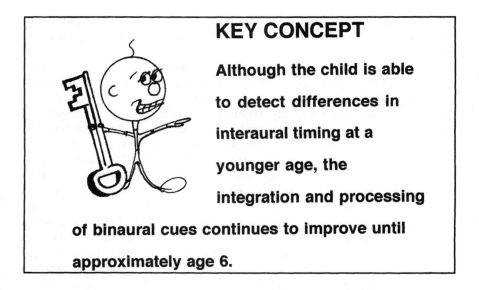

KEY CONCEPT

Although the child is able to detect differences in interaural timing at a younger age, the integration and processing of binaural cues continues to improve until approximately age 6.

assessment of central auditory processing abilities in children are obvious. **Assessment must be undertaken with an awareness of maturational effects upon the test protocols utilized, and age-related normative data must be obtained up through 11 to 12 years of age, at which time performance on the majority of central tests will have reached adult values. In addition, the assessment of children under the age of 7 years must be undertaken with caution due to the high degree of variability in performance seen on many of the commonly used tests in this younger population.** The information presented in this section is summarized in Table 3–2.

Neuroplasticity of the Auditory System

The term *neuroplasticity* refers to the nervous system's ability to undergo organizational changes in response to internal and external changes. In 1949, D.O. Hebb suggested that synaptic changes occur in response to synaptic activity in the CNS and that these synaptic changes are critical to learning and memory. While it was once thought that CNS representation of sensory events was predetermined and unchangeable, it is now understood that the CNS can and does alter its neural wiring to at least some degree throughout life. Neuromaturation, as discussed in the previous section, is one example of the nervous system's ability to form new connections as the organism grows and changes and as the tasks placed upon it become more and more challenging.

Table 3-2

Effects of Neuromaturation on Dichotic Listening, Temporal Processing, and Binaural Interaction

Process	Neuromaturational Effects
Dichotic Listening	Right ear advantage for linguistically loaded stimuli reaches adult values at 10-11 years of age
	Right ear advantage for stimuli that are lightly linguistically loaded remains relatively constant
	Overall performance improves until age 12 or 13
Temporal Processing	Temporal resolution abilities improve until age 8 to 10 years
	Performance on temporal patterning tasks reaches adult values at approximately 12 years of age
Binaural Interaction	Gross localization abilities are present at birth
	Conscious perception of auditory space occurs at age 4 months
	Precision and accuracy of localization abilities improves until approximately 5 years of age
	MLD reaches adult values at approximately 6 years of age

The majority of research conducted in the area of neuroplasticity has examined the effects of sensory deprivation upon the CNS. Studies of the effects of sensory deprivation on the visual system of cats indicate that the blocking of action potentials at any time during the critical 2-month period following birth results in abnormal development of the visual nervous system, indicating that visual stimulation is crucial to the normal development of the visual system in cats (Kalil, 1989; Kalil, Dubin, Scott, & Stark, 1986; Stryker & Harris, 1986).

The reorganization of the somatosensory cortex following peripheral nerve injury has been demonstrated in a variety of mammals. For example, sectioning the median nerve in the wrist of adult monkeys results in reorganization of the somatosensory cortex over time, with those areas of the brain responsive to the adjacent, intact digits expanding to occupy the deprived area (Merzenich & Haas, 1982). The fact that these organizational changes were observed in adult monkeys suggests that **plasticity is not simply confined to the immature or developing mammal**.

Studies of the barn owl have shown that neurological mapping of information related to spatial hearing occurs very early in life and is influenced by both auditory and visual experience (Knudsen & Knudsen, 1985; Knudsen et al., 1984). When one ear of the barn owl is plugged, a disruption in localization ability occurs (Knudsen, 1987). These effects of early auditory deprivation appear to occur in humans, as well.

It is currently accepted that an early history of chronic otitis media with effusion (OME) is associated with a higher incidence of learning difficulties, language deficits, and attention disorders (Haggard & Hughes, 1991). Pillsbury et al. (1991) have shown that children with a history of OME often exhibit abnormally reduced MLDs, and that this reduction continues even after the placement of PE tubes, resulting in a reduced ability to extract signals from noise in these children. In addition, ABR interwave intervals were found to be abnormal in the affected ear(s) of many of these children, suggesting a physiological correlate to early auditory deprivation (Hall & Grose, 1993). Furthermore, **deprivation need not occur solely during the developmental years in order to have an impact on brainstem auditory processing. Similar results have been seen in adults in whom hearing was repaired following several years of otosclerosis** (Hall & Derlacki, 1986; Hall, Grose, & Pillsbury, 1990).

The effect of sensory deprivation upon the auditory cortex may be examined through the use of electrical recording of cortical activity before and after inducing auditory deprivation in animals. Studies have demonstrated reorganization of the topographic representation of the auditory cortex following induced cochlear lesions (Irvine, Rajan, Wize, & Heil, 1991; Robertson & Irvine, 1989). It has been suggested that **the ability of the auditory cortex to reorganize continues throughout life and reflects the ability to acquire new skills and behaviors** (Kalil, 1989; Merzenich, Rencanzone, Jenkins, Allard, & Nudo, 1988).

If auditory deprivation results in morphological changes in the CANS and the nervous system retains the ability to reorganize throughout its lifetime, then it may be hypothesized that an increase in auditory stimulation may also result in morphological alterations within the CANS. Indeed, studies have shown that frequency response characteristics of single neurons can be altered by behavioral auditory conditioning (Disterhoft & Stuart, 1976; Kitzes, Farley, & Starr, 1978; Olds, Disterhoft, Segal, Kornblith, & Hirsh, 1972; Ryugo & Weinberger, 1978). In addition, Rencanzone, Schreiner, and Merzenich (1993) have shown that changes in the cortical tonotopic representations of monkeys following auditory training are correlated with improvements in discrimination ability. In other words, **auditory deprivation may result in morphological changes within the CANS that correlate with** decreased auditory processing ability, but auditory stimulation and training have been shown to facilitate improvement in auditory processing abilities. Stimulation and experience activates and strengthens neural pathways whereas unstimulated pathways atrophy (Aoki & Siekevitz, 1988; Rauschecker & Marler, 1987).

One of the mechanisms thought to be responsible for this improvement in processing abilities is **long-term potentiation (LTP). LTP is the increase in synaptic activity and efficacy following strong and repeated stimulation of a sensory system** (Bliss & Lomo, 1973; Gustafsson & Wigstrom, 1988). Although it is not clear whether all brain systems exhibit LTP in the same manner or whether the changes in synaptic activity observed are permanent, there have been reports of morphological and structural alterations within nerve cells, including increases in size and postsynaptic density, accompanying LTP (Gustafsson & Wigstrom, 1988).

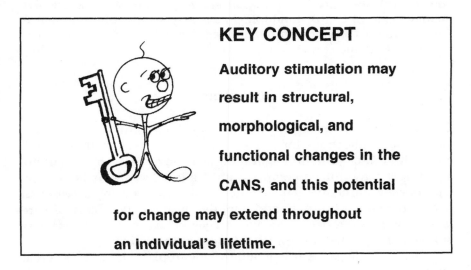

KEY CONCEPT

Auditory stimulation may result in structural, morphological, and functional changes in the CANS, and this potential for change may extend throughout an individual's lifetime.

The implications of these findings are monumental when one considers the potential for remediation of children with auditory processing disorders. **Auditory stimulation of inefficient CANS pathways may result in morphological and functional alterations, culminating in improvement in auditory processing abilities.** Jirsa (1992) demonstrated a significant decrease in P3 latency and an increase in P3 amplitude in the evoked potentials obtained from children with CAPD following an intensive therapeutic intervention program. The children in the experimental group also exhibited improvement on selected auditory tasks and positive changes in overall school performance as reported by parents and teachers. Age-matched controls of individuals with and without CAPD demonstrated no such change, suggesting that the therapeutic intervention utilized was, at least in part, responsible for the changes observed in the experimental group. It should be noted that Jirsa (1992) did not describe the specific auditory stimulation activities utilized in his study but, rather, stated that the activities focused on intensive listening exercises emphasizing auditory memory and language comprehension.

Although the results of studies regarding auditory neuroplasticity appear promising, it must be recognized that data regarding specific treatment efficacy are scarce. **Therefore, a comprehensive approach to management of CAPD including compensatory strategies and environmental modifications as well as therapeutic intervention should be undertaken. In addition, since auditory neuromaturation and neural plasticity depend upon auditory stimulation, aggressive management of CAPD should begin as early as possible** (Chermak & Musiek, 1992). For more information regarding deficit-specific management of CAPD, the reader is referred to Chapter 8.

Summary

Neuromaturation and neuroplasticity of the auditory system have important implications for the assessment and remediation of children with CAPD. **As neuromaturation of some portions of the auditory system may not be complete until age 12 years or later, age-appropriate normative data should be obtained for any assessment tools utilized clinically. In addition, due to the high degree of variability in children below the age of 7 years, many central tests may not be appropriate for use with this young population.**

Recent findings regarding auditory neuroplasticity suggest great promise for therapeutic intervention with children exhibiting CAPD. Further research is needed in the area of specific treatment efficacy; however, management of CAPD in children should be undertaken as early and aggressively as possible.

Review Questions

1. At what gestational age do the brain and spinal cord begin to develop?

2. At what gestational age are the primary lobes of the brain clearly formed?

3. Identify the anatomical structures which arise from the following three embryonic cell layers:

   ectoderm   mesoderm
   endoderm

4. By what gestational age are the structures necessary for hearing, including the brainstem auditory pathways, structurally complete?

5. Define *myelination* and discuss the course of myelination within the nervous system.

6. Define *dendritic branching*.

7. Briefly describe the following electrophysiological measures and discuss the maturation of each:

   ABR   MLR
   LEP

8. Discuss the effects of maturation on dichotic listening.

9. Differentiate the effects of maturation on linguistically loaded vs. nonlinguistically loaded dichotic listening tasks.

10. Discuss the effects of maturation on temporal processing.

11. Discuss the effects of maturation on binaural interaction.

12. By what age do children's performance on tests of central auditory function reach that of adults'?

13. Why is it important to obtain age-appropriate normative data on tests of central auditory processing?

14. Define *neuroplasticity*.

15. Discuss the effects of auditory deprivation on auditory processing.

16. Define *long-term potentiation*.

17. Discuss the implications of neuroplasticity in the remediation of children with CAPD.

PART

Assessment and Management of Central Auditory Processing Disorders

CHAPTER

FOUR

Screening

Teri James Bellis and John R. Burke

In the identification and treatment of children with central auditory processing disorders, many questions and preconceived ideas spring to the minds of administrators and special education professionals: What is the purpose of CAPD screening? How much will it cost to fund a screening program? What will occur after a child is identified through the screening process? The task of providing a plan for the development of a CAPD screening program, as well as for defending the time and cost required to implement such a plan, will often fall to the audiologist in the school setting.

The intent of this chapter is to help the reader develop a CAPD screening program using a mutidisciplinary team approach that will efficaciously identify children in need of comprehensive diagnostic central auditory processing assessment with a minimum amount of money and time investment on the part of the already taxed school system. The rationale behind the need for such a program is similar to that found for other screening programs, not the least of which is a reduction in the number of inappropriate referrals of children with learning disabilities who are erroneously suspected of CAPD. By effectively selecting the most appropriate population for comprehensive central assessment, overall costs are reduced, and efficiency of identification and rehabilitation is improved.

Learning Objectives

After studying this chapter, the reader should be able to

1. Discuss the rationale for a CAPD screening program
2. Develop a CAPD screening program for implementation in the educational setting
3. Discuss categories and types of test tools that may be used in the screening process
4. Determine the need for referral for comprehensive central auditory evaluation

---

Rationale for Central Auditory Processing Disorders Screening

Lessler (1972) stated that the purpose of screening is to acquire preliminary information about an individual's characteristics, particularly those which may impact significantly his or her health, education, or well-being. In addition, the author emphasized that the screening process should be economical in terms of money, time, and resources, because screening, by definition, likely will deal with large numbers of persons.

The justification for a CAPD screening program should comply with the above-stated factors, and should take into account concerns regarding the need, cost, design, and outcomes of the program. To this end, we will attempt to deal with some of the questions that may be posed by administrators and others in the special education profession regarding the need for and cost of a CAPD screening program. In this manner, it is hoped that clinicians may be able to justify the screening program's development, implementation, and maintenance.

Do central auditory processing disorders exist? Are tests available that can diagnose the disorder and provide information to assist in the remediation process? Are effective intervention strategies available? Although these questions may seem irrelevant to some, the fact is that many professionals in the educational setting have, over the course of time, come to disallow the existence or effective treatment of CAPD. Citing a lack of valid diagnostic tools and effective therapeutic interventions, these professionals prefer either to ignore the existence of CAPD as a whole or to label it as a kind of learning disorder that is best addressed through the use of a generic list of compensatory strategies appropriate for all affected children. Therefore, a CAPD screening program, as the first step in the overall diagnosis of CAPD in a given educational population, may not be seen as a priority in many educational arenas.

A second factor interfering with the justification of need for a CAPD screening program is the existence of several test tools that purport to assess central auditory function and which are currently administered by psychologists, educational diagnosticians, and speech-language pathologists. These tools, which will be reviewed later in this chapter, often include "auditory perceptual" subtests that presumably provide descriptive information regarding a wide range of auditory abilities, from auditory memory and sequencing to auditory discrimination and attention. Given the fact that many of these test tools have been in use for several years within the educational setting, the question arises as to the need for additional testing that, on the surface, adds little or nothing to the overall picture.

Finally, it is our observation that the term *CAPD* has become a catch-all phrase used, often inappropriately, to explain a wide variety of learning and attention problems. We have found that, in many instances, if a child exhibits difficulty with verbal information processing or storage, the child automatically earns the label CAPD, regardless of whether valid central auditory tests have been performed. In recent months, we have had the experience of hearing the term CAPD linked automatically or used interchangeably with learning disabilities, dyslexia, attention deficit disorder (ADD), attention deficit hyperactivity disorder (ADHD), and receptive language disorders by professionals within the fields of psychology, neurology, speech-language pathology, and even audiology.

All of this creates a formidable task for the clinician devoted to developing a state-of-the-art assessment and management program for CAPD in the educational setting. **In order to obtain administrative support and funding for the project, the clinician must be able to show that (a) CAPD disorders do, in fact, exist as a separate entity and significantly impact a child's ability to learn; (b) current test tools in use may suffice for screening purposes—however, comprehensive central auditory testing remains a need for the purpose of defining the disorder and providing direction for management; and (c) remediation techniques are available that can assist in managing**

the disorder. Finally, it must be shown that the first, vital step in this process is a multidisciplinary screening program that will serve to identify those students at risk for CAPD while, at the same time, reducing the number of inappropriate referrals for costly comprehensive central auditory evaluation.

The succeeding chapters in this book will address the topics of defining CAPD, administering a comprehensive CAPD assessment, and developing a management program. The current chapter is concerned primarily with the need for a screening program that will provide preliminary information necessary in order to determine the need for further evaluation. Therefore, **the first question that must be addressed is the basic one of "Why screen?"**

Musiek, Gollegly, Lamb, and Lamb (1990) listed several reasons why a screening program for CAPD is necessary. Included in their rationale were that accurate screening and identification of CAPD would:

1. help to identify conditions that may require medical attention
2. foster increased educators' and parents' awareness of CAPD
3. reduce the shopping around associated with attempts to determine the cause of a particular child's listening and learning difficulties
4. minimize psychological factors on the part of the child arising from anxiety, stress, and fear of the unknown
5. allow for insightful educational planning based upon the individual child's auditory strengths and weaknesses.

Finally, the authors stated that it cannot be overlooked that audiologists have a basic responsibility to evaluate the entire auditory system. **Although traditional audiological evaluation procedures have focused primarily on the peripheral auditory system, the central auditory system cannot be ignored.**

We would add to this list that screening for CAPD would serve to reduce time and cost investments on the part of the special education team by reducing the number of overreferrals for comprehensive CAPD evaluation and other diagnostic assessments, and by helping to provide direction to special educators, speech-language pathologists, rehabilitative audiologists, and others entrusted with the task of developing a remediation program that will help to manage the child's disorder in the most efficient way possible.

Finally, a factor that must be taken into account in the justification of any screening program is the number of children potentially affected by the disorder. If, for example, only a very small number of children are likely to exhibit the disorder in question, it may not be cost-effective to develop a program designed to identify the disorder. If, however, the given disorder is likely to affect a large portion of the population, then the cost, in terms of time and money, of developing and implementing an identification program becomes much easier to justify.

Lewis (1986) estimated that **3 to 7% of all school-age children exhibit some form of learning disability. Although it is true that, due to the lack of adequate identification procedures to date, the number of children with CAPD within this population cannot be stated with any certainty, it is likely to be quite high** (Hurley & Singer, 1989). Therefore, if a program designed to identify the presence of CAPD is not in place, a good number of children exhibiting the disorder will be missed altogether or remain unidentified until long after effective management strategies might have been undertaken.

In conclusion, **the need for a CAPD screening program is justified when one considers the large number of school-age children who are likely to be affected with the disorder, combined with the need for a reduction in the number of inappropriate referrals for central auditory evaluation and/or additional diagnostic tests**. Appropriate identification of children with CAPD can assist not only in the development of effective management and educational strategies, but may also serve to reduce or eliminate the amount of shopping around and anxiety on the part of the child and the parents that occurs when the underlying reason for learning difficulties is not clearly understood. Finally, a CAPD screening program may help to identify those children in need of medical follow-up who might otherwise have gone undetected. The information discussed in this section is summarized in Table 4–1.

The Central Auditory Processing Team

The main purpose of assembling a mutidisciplinary CAP team is to allow its members to gather sufficient information about the child in question so that a preliminary understanding of his or her auditory abilities may be obtained. **A team approach to CAPD screening allows for the gathering of information regarding educational, social, speech-language, cognitive, and medical characteristics, and helps to reduce the time demand placed upon any one individual**. Finally, a team approach in which a multitude of data is collected

Table 4-1

Rationale for CAP Screening

Why Screen for CAPD?

- Many children likely are affected by the disorder.
- Screening will reduce the number of inappropriate referrals for comprehensive central auditory testing, thereby reducing long-term time and cost investment.
- Screening will help to identify children in need of medical intervention.
- Psychological effects of CAPD can be minimized.
- Appropriate identification of children with CAPD will allow for insightful educational planning.
- A screening program will help to foster awareness on the part of educational professionals and parents regarding CAPD.

allows for a more insightful answer to the question of whether additional testing is indicated to define the child's learning difficulties more fully. Bellis and Ferre (in press) emphasized that, regardless of whether audition, language, and learning are approached from a "bottom-up" or "top-down" perspective, it is important to realize that some degree of interdependency exists. Therefore, when attempting to determine the contribution of CAPD to learning and language difficulties in the educational setting, the whole child must be taken into account, and the identification process must reflect this interdependency.

To this end, a multidisciplinary team approach to CAPD identification should be implemented. A brief discussion of the relative contribution of various team members follows (Table 4–2).

The Audiologist

Typically, **the audiologist will be responsible for managing and coordinating the CAPD screening effort,** as it will fall to this professional to perform comprehensive central auditory assessment if the need for such is determined. Therefore, the audiologist should gather information from the other team members, evaluate and discuss the results of findings with the team, and aid in determining the need for comprehensive central auditory evaluation. In addition, the audiologist should perform standard audiological evaluations on children suspected of CAPD in order to rule out peripheral hearing loss as a possible contributing factor to listening or learning difficulties.

Table 4–2
The CAP Team

Member	Responsibilities
Audiologist	Manages and coordinates CAP effort; performs audiological evaluation to rule out peripheral hearing loss
Speech-Language Pathologist	Defines child's receptive and expressive language skills, as well as written language and associated abilities
Educator	Provides information regarding child's listening and learning behavior in the classroom
Psychologist	Determines child's cognitive skills and capacity for learning
Parents	Provides information regarding developmental milestones, auditory behavior in the home, and medical and academic history
Physician	Rules out presence of pathology that may affect learning abilities

The Speech-Language Pathologist

The speech-language pathologist is instrumental in defining the child's receptive and expressive language abilities. Using test protocols that are within their domain, these professionals can provide valuable information regarding relative strengths and weaknesses in the child's oral and written language abilities. Also, as will be discussed later, many of the speech-language test tools that are currently in use contain auditory perceptual subtests that help identify specific areas of auditory difficulty.

The Educator

The special education and classroom teachers are the primary source of descriptive information regarding the child's listening and learning behavior within the learning environment. Information that may be obtained from these professionals includes, but is not limited to, identification of specific subjects in which the child exhibits the greatest amount of difficulty, daily listening behaviors in group and individual learning situations, reading and writing competencies, comprehension of instructions, general problem-solving skills, and overall attitudinal and behavioral characteristics. In addition, the educator may administer basic skills testing that will serve to illuminate relative areas of academic strengths and weaknesses as well as cognitive functioning.

The Psychologist

The psychologist is the professional qualified to administer psychoeducational assessments, including IQ testing, which provide information concerning a child's cognitive skills and capacity for learning. Information regarding the possibility of attention-related disorders or emotional disturbances that may interfere with the learning process may be provided by the psychologist. In addition, portions of various psychological tests, like those of the speech-language pathologist, tap general auditory behaviors. Finally, as discussed in Chapter 3, a mental age of 7 or 8 years is required for the administration of many tests of central auditory function. Results of psychological testing may help to establish cognitive or mental age.

The Parents

Valuable information regarding developmental milestones, auditory behaviors and difficulties encountered in the home environment, medical history, and academic sequelae can be obtained only via inclusion of the parents in the screening process. The parent can provide valuable insight regarding the impact of the learning difficulties experienced on the overall well-being of the child as well as an analysis of family history of hearing or learning disorders, early history of otitis media or head injury, and other valuable information.

The Physician

The child's medical doctor, along with the school nurse, is a key player in ruling out the presence of pathological conditions that may cause learning difficulties in children. In many cases, referral to a physician may be indicated for diagnosis and/or treatment of otologic and neurologic disorders that threaten the health and well-being of the child.

The individuals discussed above may be considered the core members of the CAP team; however, it should not be overlooked that, in certain cases, additional persons significant in the child's life may be indicated. The inclusion of these individuals in the screening process allows for the efficient gathering of a wide variety of data so that a picture of the whole child begins to emerge. What would, in fact, be an overwhelming task for just the audiologist can be managed much more easily and effectively via a CAP team approach. In all but a few situations, the requirements for screening on the part of the team members would coincide with the duties they already perform in order to gather information for special education consideration.

Screening Test Tool Considerations

A key factor in considering tools for screening is the time involved in administration. As a general rule of thumb, **the time involved in gathering preliminary information, with respect to any team member, should not exceed the time needed for comprehensive central auditory assessment**. Fortunately, many of the tests recommended as screening tools either will have been administered already, or will be in the process of being administered, as part of a multidisciplinary evaluation resulting from a special education referral. Therefore, much of the information necessary for the determination of need for comprehensive central auditory evaluation already may be available for review. If current test results are unavailable, the audiologist may suggest that certain tests be updated in order to get a more timely picture of the child.

Additionally, it should be noted that many of the test tools discussed herein are not specifically designed to gather information regarding auditory processing abilities, but rather are used diagnostically within each discipline in order to rule out speech, language, cognitive, or other disorders. For example, the information obtained from IQ testing is designed to provide information regarding the child's cognitive capacity, not auditory processing skills. However, the data gleaned from such tests may provide useful information in determining whether a central auditory processing disorder is present, as well as in deciding whether the child possesses the cognitive ability to participate in central auditory assessment procedures.

Finally, although speech-language, psychoeducational, and cognitive tests exist that purport to assess auditory processing abilities, it should be recognized that most of these tests are confounded by language and other higher level neurocognitive variables, do not provide for sufficient acoustic control, or have no documented validity in the identification of disorders of the central auditory nervous system. Therefore, **these tests should be considered as screening tools from an auditory processing perspective and should never be utilized for CAP diagnostic purposes**. Chapter 5 will discuss validity and reliability of central auditory assessment materials, and the information provided there will help to guide the clinician in determining the relative worth of any test that claims to assess central auditory processing abilities.

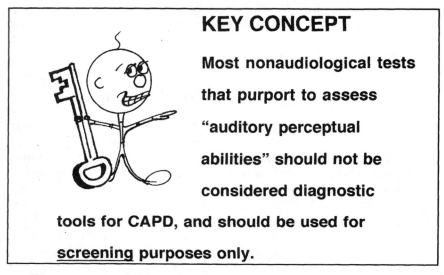

KEY CONCEPT

Most nonaudiological tests that purport to assess "auditory perceptual abilities" should not be considered diagnostic tools for CAPD, and should be used for <u>screening</u> purposes only.

We recommend that, whenever possible, the decision regarding which test or tests to utilize in the screening process be left up to the individual professional's discretion within his or her specific discipline. In other words, while measures of receptive and expressive language skills are important in the overall screening process, the audiologist should not presume to tell the speech-language pathologist which test(s) should be utilized in language assessment.

With that said, what follows is a general overview of some of the more commonly used tests within each discipline that may provide information regarding auditory perceptual abilities.

Audiological Tests

The only audiological test to date that has been designed specifically for the purpose of screening for central auditory processing disorders is the SCAN: A Screening Test for Auditory Processing Disorders (Keith, 1986). The test consists of three subtests: Filtered Words, Auditory Figure-Ground, and Competing Words. The SCAN is designed to be administered easily and quickly using a portable cassette tape deck with headphones and may be administered by virtually any individual on the screening team. In addition, results of the SCAN have been shown to correlate with findings on selected tests of auditory processing, and the test appears to demonstrate validity with regards to identification of learning disabilities. The SCAN is designed for use with children from 3 to 11 years of age.

The SCAN has been criticized for the absence of a measure of temporal processing and for the fact that there is no documented validity of the test with listeners with known lesions or disorders of the central auditory nervous system (Musiek, Gollegly, Lamb, & Lamb, 1990). In addition, the subtests within the SCAN have a limited number of items and may not allow for adequate investigation into the auditory functions that are assessed. Therefore, **results of the SCAN should be viewed in light of other data for determining if diagnostic evaluation is needed and cannot stand alone as a diagnostic test of central auditory function**.

An upward extension of the SCAN designed to screen auditory processing abilities in the adolescent and adult population, the SCAN-A, has recently become available (Keith, 1994b). In addition, Keith (1994a) has also designed a useful screening tool for looking at attention-related auditory abilities, the Auditory Continuous Performance Test (ACPT). Both of these tools may be administered by professionals other than the audiologist and may provide important preliminary information regarding a given child's auditory skills.

In addition to the possible administration of these screening tools, combined with serving as the CAP team leader, the greatest contribution to the screening process that the audiologist can make is the assessment of peripheral hearing sensitivity to rule out peripheral hearing loss as a contributing factor to academic or listening difficulties. To this end, **every child suspected of CAPD should undergo a complete audiological assessment prior to referral for comprehensive central auditory evaluation**.

Speech-Language and Psychoeducational Tests

The speech-language pathologist, psychologist, or special educator has a lengthy list of tests to draw from in the assessment of children's language abilities. It is not within the scope of this text to provide an overview of all of the speech-language, educational, and cognitive tools on the market, nor is such an overview necessary. Instead, we have attempted to identify some of the more commonly used test tools that include subtests that help to describe auditory perceptual abilities. However, it should be cautioned that these tests rarely provide useful information regarding the specific nature of an auditory deficit and, therefore, cannot be used diagnostically for central auditory assessment (Musiek, Gollegly, Lamb, & Lamb, 1990).

In addition to standard measures of speech, language, cognitive, and academic ability, the following tests may provide additional information regarding auditory-based capabilities in children. It is not our intention to imply that all of the following tests be included in the screening process, but rather to increase the reader's awareness regarding test tools on the market and to suggest that the addition of one or two of the following materials may help provide auditory-related data to the overall information-gathering process. For ease of reference, the tests discussed in this section are listed in Table 4–3.

Test of Auditory Perceptual Skills (TAPS)

The TAPS (Gardner, 1985) measures auditory perceptual skills in areas such as digit span (forward and reversed), sentence memory, word memory, dictation, and word discrimination. It is designed for use with children from 4 years to 11 years, 11 months of age.

Goldman-Fristoe-Woodcock
Auditory Skills Battery (GFWB)

The GFWB (Woodcock, 1976) is designed to measure several auditory perceptual skills including selective attention, discrimination, recognition memory, memory for content, memory for sequence, sound mimicry, recognition, analysis, blending, sound-symbol association, reading of symbols, and spelling of sounds. Therefore, the test relates auditory

Table 4–3
List of Selected Speech-Language and Psychoeducational Tests

- Test of Auditory Perceptual Skills
- Goldman-Fristoe-Woodcock Auditory Skills Battery
- Lindamood Auditory Conceptualization Test
- Auditory Discrimination Test
- Carrow Auditory Visual Abilities Test
- Token Test for Children
- Flowers-Costello Test of Central Auditory Abilities
- Auditory Sequential Memory Test
- Woodcock-Johnson Psychoeducational Battery—Revised
- Clinical Evaluation of Language Fundamentals—Revised

skills to reading and spelling ability. It is intended for use with children age 3 years to 8 years, 11 months, and uses tape-recorded materials in an attempt to provide for some acoustic control. As such, it is one of the more comprehensive psychoeducational tests on the market.

Lindamood Auditory Conceptualization Test (LAC)

The LAC (Lindamood & Lindamood, 1971) measures auditory skills in two primary areas: sound discrimination and sequencing of speech sounds in an attempt to relate auditory deficits in these areas to problems with spelling and reading as well as expressive speech. It may be used with ages 3 years to adult.

Auditory Discrimination Test (ADT)

The ADT (Reynolds, 1987) specifically measures auditory discrimination skills for fine differences between phonemes used in English speech. Intended for use with children 5 to 8 years of age, the ADT provides information regarding phonemic decoding abilities.

Carrow Auditory Visual Abilities Test

The Carrow (Carrow-Woolfolk, 1981) contains several subtests that may be used to help describe a variety of auditory perceptual abilities, including general auditory memory for related and unrelated stimuli, auditory sequencing, short-term auditory memory, digit span repetition (forward and reversed), auditory discrimination, sentence and word repetition, and auditory blending. In addition, this test may help to describe auditory-visual integration abilities in the child. The Carrow is designed for use with children ages 4 years to 10 years, 11 months.

Token Test for Children

The Token Test (DiSimoni, 1978) is primarily a measure of receptive language and assesses children's ability to understand verbal instructions of progressively increasing length and complexity. It is designed for use with children ages 3 years to 12 years, 6 months.

Flowers-Costello Test of Central Auditory Abilities

The Flowers-Costello (Flowers, Costello, & Small, 1973) consists of two subtests: Low-Pass Filtered Speech and Competing Messages. It utilizes tape-recorded stimuli and is designed to assess auditory skills in these two areas.

Auditory Sequential Memory Test (ASMT)

Based on the assumption that inability to remember and/or sequence auditory information will negatively impact a variety of academic skills, the ASMT (Wepman & Morency, 1973) is designed to assess auditory recall via a digit span approach. Normative values are presented in the test manual for children ages 5 to 8 years.

Woodcock-Johnson Psychoeducational Battery—Revised

The Woodcock-Johnson (Woodcock, 1977) test battery includes many subtests that relate to auditory perceptual abilities, as well as subtests regarding academic achievement in specific areas. It may be administered from kindergarten through adulthood.

Tests of Written Language Ability

Tests of reading and written language can provide valuable information regarding phonemic representation, word attack skills, reading comprehension, and other abilities. Some speech-language assessment tools include written language supplements, such as the Clinical Evaluation of Language Fundamentals-Revised (CELF-R; Semel, Wiig, & Secord, 1987). In addition, a multitude of oral reading ability tests is available. We suggest that information regarding reading and written language abilities be obtained for any child suspected of CAPD.

Determining the Need for Further Central Auditory Testing

The decision regarding whether to refer a given child for comprehensive central auditory assessment should be a team one and should be based on information gathered during the screening process. In general, three questions must be answered in order for this decision to be made: **(1) Is there a reasonable likelihood that the child exhibits CAPD? (2) Are the results of comprehensive CAP evaluation likely to lead to recommendations for management that are not already in place with the child? (3) Does the child have the capacity to partici-**

pate in comprehensive central auditory assessment procedures? If the answer to all three questions is affirmative, then referral for comprehensive central auditory evaluation is warranted.

Is There Reasonable Likelihood That the Child Exhibits CAPD?

Children with CAPD tend to exhibit certain common indicators of an auditory deficit. Often, the child will behave as if he or she has a peripheral hearing loss, particularly in noisy or other low-redundancy listening situations, even though hearing sensitivity is within normal limits. This is frequently the initial symptom that causes referral for CAPD screening. Once screening data have been collected, it is useful to look for general trends and patterns across the information obtained that are characteristic, in general, of the CAPD population.

Audiologically, the child with CAPD typically, but not always, exhibits normal hearing sensitivity. If a screening test such as the SCAN is used, the child may fail one or more subtests; however, it has been our experience that many children with CAPD pass the SCAN. The reverse is also true. Therefore, **a passing score on the SCAN should not be taken as evidence that further evaluation is unnecessary. Rather, it should be viewed in light of all other data obtained during the screening process.**

Often, the child with CAPD will demonstrate significant scatter across subtests within the domains assessed. For example, upon psychoeducational basic skills testing, the child may do quite well on the math subtests, but do poorly on reading and other language-based subtests. Likewise, in the classroom, the child is likely to perform more poorly in classes that are highly dependent on verbal language skills or are presented primarily via lecture format. On speech-language testing, the child with CAPD may or may not exhibit a language disorder; however, he or she is very likely to do poorly on subtests that tap auditory perceptual skills. In addition, depending on the underlying processing deficit, the child may show decreased performance in areas such as vocabulary, sequencing, and auditory discrimination/phonemic decoding.

Cognitively, the child with CAPD may exhibit normal or high IQ scores; however, verbal scores will nearly always be lower than performance scores. It should be noted, however, that not all children with CAPD exhibit normal IQ scores. Therefore, **we recommend that greater attention be given to any relative disparities between verbal**

and performance scores. Often, the child with CAPD will be classified as "learning disabled," because academic achievement does not meet the intellectual capacity of the child.

Information obtained from the classroom teacher typically will indicate that the child with CAPD is distractible in the classroom and requires a high degree of externally imposed organization in order to perform well. In addition, difficulty following multistep directions often will be noted. The child may be withdrawn or sullen and refuse to participate in classroom discussions, or may participate, but respond with comments that are inappropriate or demonstrate a lack of understanding of the discussion content. The child may say "Huh?" or "What?" a lot, and discrimination errors may be noted in which the child appears to understand what is said, but fails to respond in the correct manner. When taking spelling tests, the child may either exhibit difficulty in spelling in general, or may correctly spell words that sound like the target word, but are not.

Although many children with CAPD exhibit no significant neurologic or otologic sequelae, family history of learning disorders, or history of neurological trauma, it has been our observation that many children with CAPD do have a positive history of early chronic otitis media. In addition, if pressed, the parents often will acknowledge that either the father or the mother also had difficulties in school, were "slow readers," or struggled in some way academically. The child may have poor music and singing skills, although drawing and art skills often will be good.

Overall, the screening team should look for a general pattern in which skills and behaviors that rely upon listening and verbal language are relatively depressed when compared to those academic and personal pursuits that do not rely upon the auditory system. McFarland and Cacace (1995) discussed the need for modality specificity when defining and assessing central auditory processing abilities. Likewise, when reviewing information gathered during the screening process, the screening team should look for difficulties in those areas that particularly relate to audition.

Finally, it should be recognized that few children with CAPD will exhibit all of the above characteristics. It is not the task of the screening team to diagnose CAPD, but rather to calculate the likelihood, based on all of the data collected, that a CAPD is present. Methods of diagnosing and defining disorders of central auditory processing will be discussed in Chapters 5 and 6.

The key red flags to be on the alert for during the screening process, as discussed in this section, are summarized in Table 4–4.

Table 4-4
Common Indicators of CAPD

- Behaves as if peripheral hearing loss is present, despite normal hearing
- Demonstrates significant scatter across subtests within domains assessed by speech-language and psychoeducational tests, with weaknesses in auditory-dependent areas
- Verbal IQ scores often lower than performance scores
- Requires high degree of external organization in the classroom
- Exhibits difficulty following multistep directions
- Exhibits poor reading and spelling skills
- May refuse to participate in class discussions or respond inappropriately
- May be withdrawn or sullen
- Exhibits a positive history of chronic otitis or other otologic and/or neurologic sequelae
- May exhibit poor singing and music skills
- Fine and/or gross motor skills may be deficient

Are the Results of Comprehensive CAP Evaluation Likely to Lead to Recommendations for Management That Are Not Already in Place?

On occasion, a child will be referred for CAPD screening who, after having been determined to be eligible for special education services in the area of learning disabilities or language delay, is already receiving comprehensive special education services that target his or her disability area. For example, the child with reading difficulties, as well as difficulty hearing in noisy environments, may undergo daily therapy with a reading specialist who focuses on phonemic discrimination and speech-to-print skills. In addition, environmental modifications may already be in place for the purpose of improving the child's access to auditory information in the classroom. **It is possible that comprehensive central auditory evaluation, even if results of such an evaluation confirm the presence of a CAPD, may result in little or no contribution to the overall management of the child. In this situation, the screening team may prudently decide not to refer for comprehensive central auditory assessment at the present time, since the cost of such testing, in terms of time and money, may outweigh the potential benefit.**

This having been said, the reader should be cautioned that not all central auditory processing disorders are alike and, depending on the underlying dysfunctional process, recommendations for management will differ greatly. Therefore, the clinician should avoid at all costs blanket statements regarding what is an appropriate management strategy for all children with CAPD. Chapter 7 will discuss interpretation of central auditory assessment results, and management will be covered in Chapter 8. The clinician should be familiar with the range of possible profiles within the larger category of CAPD, as well as differential, deficit-specific management recommendations, before determining that intervention strategies currently in place for a given child are adequate.

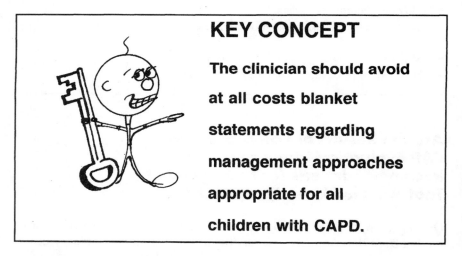

KEY CONCEPT

The clinician should avoid at all costs blanket statements regarding management approaches appropriate for all children with CAPD.

Does the Child Have the Capacity to Participate in Comprehensive Central Auditory Assessment Procedures?

Even if the likelihood of the presence of CAPD has been determined and it is felt that further evaluation is necessary, it may be determined that, for one reason or another, the child in question cannot be tested using present assessment tools.

As discussed in Chapter 3, a mental age of 7 or 8 is required for most tests of central auditory processing. Therefore, comprehensive evaluation of the very young child is not possible at the present time. Likewise, while children with hearing loss also may exhibit concomitant central auditory processing disorders, many of the assessment tools in current use require normal or near-normal peripheral hearing sensitivity (see Chapter 6).

Finally, the presence of significant cognitive or behavioral disorders may interfere with a child's ability to participate in comprehensive central auditory testing. Normal cognitive capacity is not necessary for participation in central auditory evaluation; however, the child must be able to follow the instructions and deliver the appropriate response required of each test used. In cases of children with very low cognitive ability, extreme hyperactivity that is uncontrolled by medication, or emotional and/or behavioral disorders that may result in refusal to cooperate, it may be impossible to administer a battery of central auditory processing tests.

It should be noted that, by deciding not to refer for comprehensive assessment based on these reasons, the screening team is not implying that a CAPD is not present. Rather, it should be acknowledged that, while the child may exhibit CAPD, the presence of such a disorder cannot be confirmed at the present time. More importantly, intervention should not be withheld simply on the basis of an inability to test reliably. Although a deficit-specific management program cannot be developed without the identification of the underlying dysfunctional process, many management strategies may be employed that address the child's most significant presenting complaints. Chapter 8 delineates various management strategies that may be implemented in these situations.

In conclusion, data collected from the screening process should be reviewed for trends across findings that suggest the presence of CAPD. Prior to referral for a comprehensive central auditory assessment, it should be ascertained that the child has the capacity to participate in the assessment procedure, and that the comprehensive evaluation will add sufficient additional information to the child's educational picture to justify the time and effort spent in such a pursuit. Finally, in those cases in which complete assessment procedures cannot be performed but a CAPD is likely to be present, the screening team should look for methods in which intervention strategies may be implemented in the absence of a confirmation of CAPD. Key factors in determining the need for further central auditory assessment are outlined in Table 4–5.

Final Considerations in Central Auditory Processing Disorders Screening

The importance of screening for CAPD has been discussed in this chapter, as have the methods through which screening for CAPD may

Table 4–5

Key Factors in Determining the Need for Comprehensive Central Auditory Assessment

---

- Likelihood of the Presence of CAPD
    Does the child exhibit several of the common indicators of CAPD?
- Need for Additional Management Recommendations
    Will the results of a comprehensive central auditory assessment contribute significantly to the child's overall educational plan?
- Ability to Evaluate the Child
    Does the child have the necessary cognitive ability to participate in a comprehensive central auditory evaluation?

---

be accomplished. However, it must be recognized that a screening program, no matter how efficient and well organized, is of no use unless a clear, workable plan for follow-through is implemented, as well. In particular, a comprehensive diagnostic assessment program must be in place and the outcomes of the screening process must be monitored.

In many geographical areas, resources for diagnosis and treatment may not be available, due either to lack of funding or lack of trained professionals to carry out the necessary steps involved in performing comprehensive central auditory evaluation and making recommendations for management. If the implementation of a CAPD screening program is under consideration, the availability of follow-up services for children identified by screening should be carefully investigated. As stated by Musiek, Gollegly, Lamb, and Lamb (1990), **even though procedures exist to diagnose most central auditory processing disorders, it should not be assumed that they will be available in a given locale**. Comprehensive central auditory evaluation is necessary in order to confirm and define the disorder, as well as for developing a deficit-specific management program. Therefore, **implementation of a screening program without the means of diagnostic and therapeutic follow-through is nothing short of a futile expenditure of time and effort**.

Unfortunately, considerable education on the part of special education professionals and audiologists is needed regarding the nature of CAPD and central auditory assessment in order to assure that an appropriate service delivery program is implemented. In our travels, we have encountered many regions throughout the country in which a screening program, such as the one described in this chapter, has been put into place without appropriate means of follow-through, and is used for diagnostic purposes. **It cannot be overemphasized that the procedures discussed in this chapter are for screening purposes only, and complete diagnostic procedures are a vital, integral portion of the overall CAPD service delivery system.**

A second consideration is that of monitoring the outcome of any screening program. Data should be collected regarding the number of children referred for screening, the number referred for comprehensive evaluation, and the number ultimately identified as exhibiting CAPD. In this manner, overall effectiveness of the screening program may be established, and directions for further modifications in the process may be suggested. Methods of data collection and outcome monitoring are discussed in Chapter 10.

Finally, the success of any screening program depends on cooperation from all persons involved. Therefore, efforts should be made to ensure coordination among all facets of the screening program, from administrative support, funding, data collection, decision-making, and follow-through. Only in this way can a CAPD screening program achieve its ultimate goal: the identification of children with CAPD.

Summary

This chapter has reviewed several basic considerations in screening for CAPD. The need for a CAPD screening program is evidenced by the prevalence of auditory processing disorders in the educational setting and the potential impact of such a disorder on a child's learning. The primary purpose of CAPD screening is to determine the need for referral for additional diagnostic testing.

Screening for CAPD should be approached from a multidisciplinary team perspective so that information can be collected that will reflect the whole child. In determining the need for further evaluation, the team should be on the alert for general trends across data that suggest relative difficulty in academic, cognitive, and behavioral areas that are most dependent on audition. In addition, the team should ascertain that further evaluation will add sufficient additional information to justify the time and effort involved in such a pursuit, and that the child in question is capable of participating in comprehensive central auditory evaluation procedures.

Finally, the implementation of a screening program will be of no use unless adequate resources are available for appropriate follow-through. Therefore, CAPD screening is just one component, albeit a vital one, of the entire CAPD service delivery system.

Review Questions

1. What is the primary purpose(s) of screening for CAPD?
2. Discuss the justification factors that help to document the need for a CAPD screening program.
3. Why should a multidisciplinary team approach be utilized in CAPD screening?
4. List the core members of the CAP screening team and discuss the relative contribution of each.
5. Discuss the reason(s) why the screening tools discussed in this chapter should never be used for diagnostic purposes.
6. Identify several speech-language, psychoeducational, or cognitive test tools that may provide valuable information to the CAP screening team.
7. What three factors must be taken into account when determining the need for comprehensive central auditory assessment?
8. Discuss the behavioral, academic, language, and cognitive characteristics typically associated with CAPD.
9. What should be done if a child is suspected of CAPD, but a comprehensive central auditory assessment cannot be performed due to age, cognitive ability, or other reasons?
10. Discuss the factors necessary to assure the success of a CAP screening program.

CHAPTER

FIVE

Overview of Central Tests

Once the likelihood of the presence of a central auditory processing disorder has been determined, it falls to the audiologist to perform assessments that will determine whether a CAPD is present and, if so, attempt to quantify and qualify the disorder. This chapter will provide a basic overview of central tests. The rationale for use of a test battery approach to assess auditory processing skills in children and the issues of validity and reliability of central tests will also be considered. Administration protocols for specific test tools as well as suggestions for choosing the components of the test battery based on individual need will be provided in Chapter 6.

Learning Objectives

After studying this chapter, the reader should be able to

1. Discuss the rationale for a test battery approach to CAP assessment
2. Distinguish between validity and reliability of central tests and discuss the importance of test validity in central assessment
3. Describe the major categories of central tests and discuss the purpose of each.

Rationale for Test Battery Approach

A question we often hear is, "What is the best test of central auditory processing?" This is a difficult, if not impossible, question to answer as there is no one test that is sufficient in scope to address the complexities of the CANS. As seen in Part One, the CANS is a highly redundant, complex system. Therefore, it is logical that the assessment of the CANS would, likewise, be redundant and complex.

The question to be answered by the central assessment is of paramount importance. If the question is simply, "Is a central auditory processing deficit present?" then the use of one or two valid test tools may be all that is needed to obtain an adequate answer. However, **if central assessment is undertaken with an eye toward identification of the underlying deficient processes and development of a deficit-specific management plan, then the assessment procedure must tap a variety of mechanisms.**

It is our opinion that the simple identification of the presence or absence of CAPD is insufficient. As will be seen in the next chapter, the outcome of a central assessment should be the development of an auditory profile that delineates the child's auditory strengths and weaknesses. Using this profile, a management program that will build upon the individual child's strengths and assist in overcoming the weaknesses may be designed. Therefore, the use of different tests that assess different processes is necessary. Again, it should be emphasized that knowledge of the underlying neuroanatomy and neurophysiology is essential in order to choose those test tools that will best provide the clinician with the information necessary to interpret the assessment results and make recommendations for management.

An additional purpose of CAP testing is the differentiation of site of lesion or dysfunction. It is our contention that this issue cannot be separated from that of describing auditory processing abilities in the clinical population. The identification of site of lesion, or level of dysfunction within the brain, will have a significant impact on recommendations for management, including the need for medical referral. The clinician should be aware that, although rare, neurological disorders requiring medical intervention can and do occur in the school age population. Therefore, the clinician engaging in central assessment must continually be on the lookout for symptoms that may indicate the need for neurological or other medical referral. Again, in order to investigate fully the system in question, it will be necessary to utilize tests that assess different processes and different levels and to examine the test results for trends and comparisons across assessment tools.

Finally, as stated by Musiek and Lamb (1994), the audiologist's job is the evaluation of hearing. Hearing does not end with the peripheral auditory system. Rather, peripheral acuity is merely the first step in the overall process of hearing. Therefore, from a philosophical perspective, **it is the audiologist's responsibility to assess all factors that affect hearing in the child or adult, and this includes evaluation of the central auditory system. The utilization of several test tools which assess a variety of processes represents the state of the art in current CAP assessment and should become the standard of care**.

It should be noted that we have been discussing specifically those tests designed for the evaluation of the CANS. However, when one considers comprehensive CAP assessment, the results of cognitive, speech/language, educational, and other measures should not be forgotten. Indeed, these findings will play a large role in the interpretation of CAP assessment findings as well as recommendations for management. Therefore, in a very practical sense, the assessment of central auditory processing abilities in the school-age child should be a multidisciplinary one, and the screening tools discussed in the previous chapter will become an essential part of the overall CAP test battery.

In conclusion, the utilization of one single test is rarely sufficient to explore dysfunction fully in any sensory system. Even when evaluating the peripheral auditory system, a test battery approach is utilized, including pure-tone air- and bone-conduction testing, word recognition measures, immitance testing, and other measures deemed necessary. The comprehensive assessment of central auditory processing abilities is certainly no exception. **Only through the use of a well-chosen test battery, in conjunction with information supplied by associated professionals and other individuals in a multidisciplinary manner, will the audiologist engaged in central auditory assessment be able to delineate those processes that are dysfunctional; evaluate the impact of the dysfunction on the child's educational, medical, and social status; and make appropriate recommendations for deficit-specific management that will address the individual child's needs**.

Test Validity and Reliability

The clinical validity and reliability of tests of central auditory function are often called into question, and rightly so. However, it is our experience that these issues are often poorly understood and frequently confused. An understanding of the meanings of these terms as well as the methods through which validity and reliability of a given test tool are determined will assist the clinician in critically evaluating literature pertaining to specific test tools on the market, wisely choosing tools for clinical use, and increasing confidence in the interpretation of results of a comprehensive assessment.

The terms validity and reliability are not interchangeable, although both are important when evaluating the clinical utility of a given test tool. Very simply, validity refers to the test's ability to assess that condition(s) which it purports to assess. **In other words, in order to determine the clinical validity of a test procedure, it must be demonstrated that the test typically will be abnormal in those subjects who present with the specific disorder in question and that the test typically will be normal in those subjects who do not present with the disorder. Reliability is the degree to which the test will yield the same results within the test session or upon repeat testing.**

Figure 5–1 provides an example of a decision matrix for use in determining the validity of diagnostic test tools. A *true positive* is a positive finding in subjects who do, in fact, have the disorder or disease, or an indication of the test's ability to identify correctly the presence of the disorder (hit). Conversely, a *false positive* is a positive find-

TEST RESULT

	ABNORMAL	NORMAL
DISORDER PRESENT	True Positive (hit)	False Negative (miss)
DISORDER ABSENT	False Positive (false alarm)	True Negative (correct rejection)

Figure 5–1. Sample decision matrix for determining the validity of diagnostic test tools.

ing on the test in subjects who do not have the disorder (false alarm). Likewise, a true negative is a negative finding in subjects who do not have the disorder, or an indication of the test's ability to identify correctly the absence of the disorder (correct rejection). Finally, a false negative is a negative finding in subjects who do, in fact, have the disorder (miss) (Turner & Nielsen, 1984).

The sensitivity of a diagnostic test is the number of true positives (hits) over the total number of true positives and false negatives (hits and misses). Therefore, *sensitivity* refers to the degree to which the test is able to identify correctly the presence of a disorder. The number of true negatives (correct rejections) over the total number of false positives and true negatives (false alarms and correct rejections) is referred to as *specificity*, or the test's ability to identify correctly those subjects who do not have the disorder. *Efficiency* refers to the test's overall degree of both sensitivity and specificity, or the test's ability to identify correctly both the presence and the absence of a disorder.

As sensitivity of a test increases, specificity decreases, and vice versa. The reason for this is quite simple. **The more sensitive a test is, the more likely it is to result in false alarms. The reverse is also true: The more specific a test is, the more likely it will be that some subjects who have the disorder will be missed**.

In making clinical decisions regarding the choice of test tools, the clinician will need to choose those tools that will best meet the needs of the individual situation. Therefore, depending on the question to be answered, the necessary degree of sensitivity and specificity of the test tool may change. For example, if the clinician is concerned that the presence of a life-threatening disorder is quite possible, it may be more prudent to err on the side of the conservative. In this situation, the clinician may decide that it would be better to have a false alarm than to miss the disease altogether. Therefore, the clinician is likely to choose a highly sensitive test tool even though the chance of a false positive finding may be greater.

On the other hand, if the disorder in question is unlikely to occur in the given population, specificity may be more important than sensitivity. Let us consider the current audiological issue of hearing screening of all newborns. As the likelihood of finding a significant hearing loss in a well newborn is quite low, choosing a test that yields a smaller degree of false positives may be more desirable as this would reduce the incidence of unnecessary referrals for further audiological evaluation.

The question to be answered by the diagnostic test is the critical factor. If the issue is to correctly identify the disorder *at all costs*, regardless of the number of false alarms, then the sensitivity of the test tool will be of paramount importance. If, however, one is charged with the task of identifying only those patients who do, in fact, have the disorder, even if it means missing some, then specificity will be the issue to consider. **In the majority of clinical situations concerning central auditory processing assessment, the clinician will want to choose those test tools that have the greatest sensitivity and specificity, or those that are most efficient, even though this will mean that some false alarms will occur and some subjects who do exhibit CAPD will be missed.**

A final, crucial issue in determining test validity is the standard against which test findings are compared. For example, if measures of validity are conducted for a test of central auditory processing using a population of children with *language impairment* and the test is shown to be highly efficient, the findings would suggest that the test is valid for language-impairment. The question of validity for disorders of central auditory processing cannot be adequately answered since the number of children in the validation sample who actually present with disorders of the CANS is unknown. The act of establishing validity for one type of disorder does not necessarily imply validity for other, related disorders. For this reason, the authors suggest that, **when considering validity of any tool that purports to assess central auditory processing, the clinician should examine critically the population upon which validation studies were conducted.** For a test to be considered a valid test of central auditory processing, data should be available that demonstrate validity utilizing a population with known CANS disorders or lesions. Only in that way can the clinician be sure that the test tool in question is a measure of central auditory processing and not some related disorder.

As mentioned previously, reliability refers to the repeatability of test results. Reliability of a given test tool is best estimated by using a sample population similar to the test population for which the test was designed (Franzen, 1989). A variety of factors may affect test reliability. For our purposes, we will separate these factors into two general categories: procedural variables, or those that relate to the test itself, and patient variables, or those that relate to the patient and/or disorder (Table 5–1).

Procedural variables, otherwise known as errors of measurement (Heise, 1969), may include issues such as calibration of equipment, practice effects, ceiling effects found when a test is too easy, and other variables directly related to the measurement being studied. One example of a procedural variable that should be familiar to most audiologists is that of the use of too few items, such as during standard word recognition testing. It is generally known within our field that, for years,

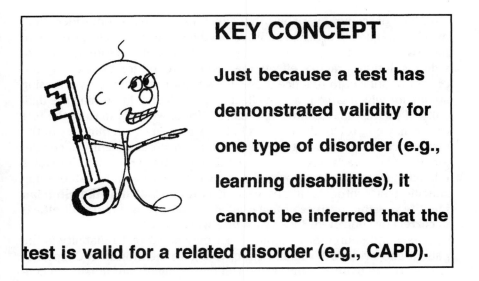

KEY CONCEPT

Just because a test has demonstrated validity for one type of disorder (e.g., learning disabilities), it cannot be inferred that the test is valid for a related disorder (e.g., CAPD).

debate raged regarding the use of full vs. half lists of phonetically balanced, monosyllabic word lists for clinical word recognition testing. While few of us would argue that the use of a 10-word list would provide sufficient test-retest reliability, it is our observation that the decision to use 25 or 50 words differs from clinic to clinic. Although the use of half lists for word recognition testing may be adequate for testing many populations, it may not be adequate for other, more involved, populations. Therefore, the use of fewer items on the test may affect test-retest reliability of word recognition measures in certain populations.

Table 5-1
Some Factors That May Affect Test Reliability

Procedural Variables	Patient Variables
Equipment calibration	Age
Practice effects	Degree and stability of hearing loss
Ceiling effects	Overall health
Floor effects	Attention
Use of too few items	Intelligence and linguistic ability
Other test-related factors	Presence of related disorder(s)

Many procedural variables that affect test reliability, once identified, may be modified in order to improve reliability. For example, if the use of too few items is a critical factor, then the addition of more items will provide a solution. Practice effects may be controlled for by allowing the patient or subject to practice those items prior to testing or by choosing stimuli for which large practice effects are not found. Increasing the difficulty of the test may control for ceiling effects, whereas making the test easier may control for floor effects in those tests in which difficulty of the test is a critical factor. Regular calibration of test equipment will control for procedural variables related to equipment standardization. Variables related to test administration and scoring can be avoided by establishing specific test protocols. In any case, **it is important that the clinician identify possible sources of test-related variability and make all efforts to correct or control for these variables when possible.**

A second source of variability that may affect test reliability is the patient and/or disorder itself (Heise, 1969). As mentioned in Chapter 3, the age of the patient being tested will have a significant impact on central test-retest reliability. The younger the population, the more variability noted, so that reliability of many central tests is quite poor when administered to children younger than approximately 7 years of age and age-appropriate normative data are required through the ages of 11 or 12 years. Degree and stability of peripheral hearing loss, if present, may have a significant impact on the reliability of many central tests. Issues such as overall health, attention, linguistic abilities of the patient, intelligence, and the presence of additional, related disorders may all affect central test reliability (Jerger & Jerger, 1975; Musiek & Lamb, 1994).

It has been suggested that the reliability of central tests may be difficult to determine using a population of subjects with CAPD due to the dynamic nature of central disorders as well as to the high degree of variability among these subjects (Musiek & Chermak, 1994). The argument was that, due to neuroplasticity and the fact that CNS pathology results in constant change within the brain, reliability continues to be an important issue in CAPD assessment. While this may well be the case, a review of the literature shows that very little research has been reported in which the reliability of specific CAP assessment tools in populations with known CAPD was studied. Therefore, **the issue of reliability of central auditory tests is an area of further, much-needed research. Furthermore, the clinician involved in central assessment must be familiar with possible sources of variability within the clinical population. Finally, central auditory assessment, interpretation of test results, and measures of treatment efficacy must take these factors into account.**

To summarize, validity is the test's ability to measure what it purports to measure, whereas reliability refers to the repeatability of test results. An understanding of issues surrounding validity and reliability of central tests is critical in order to determine the clinical utility of specific test tools as well as for the administration and interpretation of tests of central auditory function.

Overview of Central Tests

Historically, tests of central auditory function have been categorized in a variety of ways. For example, the ASHA Committee on Disorders of Central Auditory Processing (ASHA, 1990) divided central tests into monotic, dichotic, and binaural tests. Katz (1994) discussed nonspeech-based, monosyllabic, spondaic, and sentence procedures, and Bellis and Ferre (in press) separated tests of central auditory function into two broad categories: those that add information to the signal and those that take away information from the signal. For purposes of this text, we will follow the lead of Baran and Musiek (1991) and categorize central tests in the following manner: dichotic speech tests, temporal ordering tasks, monaural low-redundancy speech tests, and binaural interaction tests. In addition, a brief overview of electrophysiological procedures applicable to central auditory evaluation will be provided.

Dichotic Speech Tests

As discussed in Chapter 2, dichotic listening involves the presentation of stimuli to both ears simultaneously, with the information presented to one ear being different from that presented to the other. Kimura (1961a) is considered to be responsible for the initial introduction of dichotic speech tests into the field of central auditory assessment. Dichotic speech tasks differ from each other in terms of the stimuli utilized as well as the task required of the listener. Stimuli utilized in dichotic tests range from digits and nonsense syllables to complete sentences. **Depending on the test itself, the listener may be required to repeat everything that is heard (binaural integration) or to direct his or her attention to one ear and repeat what is heard in that ear only (binaural separation).** In addition, some tests of dichotic listening require the listener to perform a directed attention task in which he or she repeats what is heard in one ear first, followed by the stimuli presented to the other ear.

Stimuli utilized in dichotic speech tasks may be viewed on a continuum from least to most difficult. In general, the more similar and closely aligned the stimuli presented to the ears are, the more difficult the dichotic task will be. In addition, the issue of degree of linguistic loading of dichotic stimuli must be taken into account. As seen in Chapter 3, a greater right ear advantage (REA) will be observed in children when more complex, linguistically loaded dichotic stimuli are used than with the use of less complex stimuli. As the child matures, the REA will decrease, reaching adult values by approximately 11 to 12 years of age.

One of the most common dichotic tests in use today is the Dichotic Digits Test (DDT). Kimura (1961a) first utilized triads of digits presented dichotically for the assessment of central auditory function. More recently, a revised version of Kimura's procedure was introduced in which two digits from 1 through 10 (excluding 7) are presented to each ear simultaneously (Musiek, 1983a). The listener is required to repeat all four digits heard. On the continuum of least to most difficult, the DDT may be considered to be somewhat in the middle, as the stimuli are very closely aligned but lightly linguistically loaded. **The DDT has been shown to be sensitive to brainstem and cortical lesions (Musiek, 1983a), as well as to lesions of the corpus callosum** (Musiek, Kibbe, & Baran, 1984). In addition, the test is quick and easy to administer and score and appears to be relatively resistant to peripheral hearing loss (Musiek, 1983a; Musiek, Gollegly, Kibbe, & Verkest-Lenz, 1991).

A more difficult task than the DDT is the Dichotic Consonant-Vowel (CV) test developed by Berlin and colleagues (Berlin et al., 1972). In this test, stimuli consist of six CV segments (pa, ta, ka, ba, da, ga). Single CV segments are presented to each ear using a dichotic paradigm and the listener is asked to choose both segments heard from a printed list. Although the test is very lightly linguistically loaded, its difficulty lies in the high degree of similarity among the CV segments as well as the close acoustical alignment of the stimuli (Niccum, Rubens, & Speaks, 1981). In addition, the test may be administered so that the presentation of a CV segment to one ear may lag behind the presentation of a different CV segment to the other ear by 15, 30, 60, or 90 msec in order to investigate the effect of lag time on listener performance (Berlin et al., 1975). **The Dichotic CV test has been shown to be sensitive to cortical lesions; however, as in many central tests, laterality of dysfunction cannot be determined by the test results** (Berlin et al., 1975; Olsen, 1983). It should be noted that the difficulty of this test may preclude its use in some populations (Mueller & Bright, 1994). Our own experience indicates that this test is often too difficult for young children, and variability is high in the school age population.

Perhaps the most widely used dichotic speech test is the Staggered Spondaic Word Test (SSW), first described by Katz in 1962. This test involves the dichotic presentation of spondees in such a manner that the second syllable of the spondee presented to one ear overlaps the first syllable of the spondee presented to the other ear. The ear-specific spondees and the overlapping spondee form words. For example, when the word *upstairs* is presented to the right ear and *downtown* is presented to the left ear, the overlapping syllables will result in the dichotic presentation of the word *downstairs*. Specific details regarding administration and scoring of the SSW will be provided in Chapter 6. **The SSW has been shown to be sensitive to brainstem and cortical lesions** (Katz, 1962). In addition, the test is relatively resistant to peripheral hearing loss (Arnst, 1982; Katz, 1968), and is simple enough for use with a variety of ages (Katz, 1977).

Two commonly used dichotic procedures use sentences as stimuli. The first is the Competing Sentences Test (CST), developed by Willeford in 1968 (Willeford & Burleigh, 1994). The test consists of simple sentences presented dichotically. The target sentence is presented to one ear at a quieter level than the competing sentence, which is presented to the other ear. The listener is instructed to repeat the sentence heard in the target ear only and ignore the competing sentence, which assesses the process of binaural separation of auditory information. **The sensitivity of the CST as compared to other dichotic measures in the identification of cortical lesions has been questioned by a number of researchers (Lynn & Gilroy, 1972, 1975; Musiek, 1983b). However, it has been suggested that dichotic sentence tasks such as the CST may be valuable in investigating neuromaturation and language processing abilities** (Porter & Berlin, 1975; Willeford & Burleigh, 1994).

The second dichotic sentence procedure is the Synthetic Sentence Identification test with Contralateral Competing Message (SSI-CCM), described by Jerger and Jerger (1974, 1975). Stimuli for the SSI-CCM are 10 third-order approximations of English sentences. The stimuli resemble nonsense sentences, thus lightening the linguistic load of the test. The sentences are presented to the target ear while a competing message consisting of continuous discourse is presented to the contralateral ear. The listener is required to choose from a printed list which of the 10 sentences was heard. Like the CST, the SSI-CCM assesses the process of binaural separation of auditory information. **The SSI-CCM has been found to be useful in differentiating brainstem from cortical pathology** (Jerger & Jerger, 1975; Keith, 1977). The SSI with Ipsilateral Competing Message (SSI-ICM), in which both the sentence and the competing message are presented to the same ear, will be discussed in the section dealing with monaural low-redundancy speech tests.

A modification of the SSI-CCM entitled the Dichotic Sentence Identification test (DSI) was introduced in 1983 by Fifer and colleagues (Fifer, Jerger, Berlin, Tobey, & Campbell, 1983). The test uses the SSI sentences presented dichotically and requires the listener to identify both sentences heard from a printed list of all 10 sentences, thus tapping the process of binaural integration. The DSI was initially devised in hopes of providing a dichotic speech test that would be resistant to the effects of peripheral hearing loss. Although more research is needed into the clinical utility, **the DSI appears to show sensitivity to disorders of the CANS** (Mueller, Beck, & Sedge, 1987), **while being minimally affected by peripheral hearing loss** (Fifer et al., 1983). Therefore, the DSI may be a promising tool for the evaluation of central auditory function in the hearing-impaired population.

Monosyllabic words may also be used as stimuli in dichotic listening tasks. In the SCAN: A Screening Test for Auditory Processing Disorders (Keith, 1986), the Competing Words subtest is a directed attention dichotic task using monosyllabic words. During presentation of the first list, the listener is instructed to repeat the stimulus heard in the right ear first, followed by the left ear. During presentation of the second list, the instruction to the listener is reversed. **The SCAN test paradigm is reported to assist in determining ear differences related to neuromaturation** (Keith, 1986). The SCAN is a popular screening tool for CAPD due to its ease of administration; however, to date, no validation data have been presented in the literature regarding the SCAN using a population of subjects with known lesions of the CANS.

A second dichotic procedure using monosyllabic words has been presented in recent years. The Dichotic Rhyme Test (DRT), was introduced by Wexler and Hawles (1983) and modified by Musiek, Kurdziel-Schwan, Kibbe, Gollegly, Baran, and Rintelmann (1989). The DRT is composed of rhyming, consonant-vowel-consonant words, each beginning with one of the stop consonants (p, t, k, b, d, g). Each pair of words differs only in the initial consonant, (e.g., ten, pen). As such, the stimuli are almost perfectly aligned so that fusion takes place and the listener most often hears and repeats just one of the two words presented. **The DRT has been shown to be particularly sensitive to detection of dysfunction in the interhemispheric transfer of information via the corpus callosum** (Musiek, Kurdziel-Schwan, Kibbe, Gollegly, Baran, and Rintelmann 1989).

In conclusion, dichotic listening tasks involve the presentation of a different stimulus to each ear simultaneously. They may be viewed in a variety of different ways including type of stimuli used, level of difficulty, degree of linguistic loading, and the task required of the listener. Types of dichotic speech stimuli include CV segments, digits, monosyllabic words, spondaic words, and sentences, with the use of CV segments being the most difficult task due to the limited amount of linguistic information combined with the close temporal alignment of stimuli presentation. Sentence stimuli are considered to be heavily linguistically loaded whereas digits or CV segments carry a much lighter linguistic load. Finally, depending on the instructions given to the listener, dichotic tasks may assess the processes of binaural integration, binaural separation, or a combination of both (directed attention). Dichotic speech tasks have been shown to be sensitive to cortical and corpus callosal dysfunction, as well as, to a lesser degree, brainstem lesions, and are in wide clinical use today. A summary of the dichotic speech tasks discussed in this section is presented in Table 5–2.

Table 5-2
Summary of Selected Dichotic Speech Tests

Test	Process(es) Assessed	Sensitive to
Dichotic Digits	Binaural integration	Brainstem, cortical, and corpus callosal lesions
Dichotic Consonant-Vowels	Binaural integration	Cortical lesions
Staggered Spondaic Word Test	Binaural integration	Brainstem and cortical lesions
Competing Sentences Test	Binaural separation	Neuromaturation and language processing
Synthetic Sentence Identification Test With Contralateral Competing Message	Binaural separation	Cortical vs. brainstem lesions
Dichotic Sentence Identification Test	Binaural integration	Brainstem and cortical lesions
Dichotic Rhyme	Binaural integration	Interhemispheric transfer

Temporal Ordering Tasks

In Chapter 3, we discussed the effects of various pathologies, particularly lesions of the cerebral hemispheres and/or the corpus callosum, on temporal ordering abilities. These tasks require the listener to make discriminations based on the temporal order or sequence of auditory stimuli. For the most part, nonspeech stimuli such as tones or clicks are utilized in the evaluation of temporal ordering abilities. As mentioned in Chapter 3, temporal processing is critical to perception of speech and music. Temporal processing tasks, particularly temporal integration, two-tone ordering, gap-detection, and brief tone tasks, have been used for many years in order to investigate lesion effects on temporal aspects of audition (Carmon & Nachshon, 1971; Cranford et al. 1982; Efron, 1985; Efron & Crandall, 1983; Jerger et al., 1972; Lackner & Teuber, 1973; Swisher & Hirsh, 1972; Thompson & Abel, 1992a, b). However, perhaps due to the equipment-related difficulty involved in administering these tasks combined with the lack of standardized test protocols, temporal processing tasks such as these are not utilized in common clinical practice at the present time. Therefore, this section will focus on three tests of temporal ordering currently available for clinical use: Frequency Patterns, Duration Patterns, and the Psychoacoustic Pattern Discrimination Test.

Frequency Patterns, or the Pitch Pattern Sequence Test (PPST), was initially designed to investigate both pattern perception and temporal sequencing abilities in the listener (Pinheiro & Ptacek, 1971; Ptacek & Pinheiro, 1971). The test consists of 120 pattern sequences. Each sequence is made up of three tone bursts: two of one frequency and one of another. The frequencies utilized are 1,122 Hz and 880 Hz. Thirty items are presented to each ear, and the listener is instructed to report verbally each pattern heard. Six patterns are possible: high-high-low, high-low-high, high-low-low, low-high-low, low-low-high, and low-high-high. The test taps the processes of frequency discrimination, temporal ordering, and linguistic labeling. **The PPST is useful in the detection of disorders of the cerebral hemispheres, although laterality information cannot be obtained from this test** (Musiek & Pinheiro, 1987; Pinheiro, 1976; Pinheiro & Musiek, 1985). **In addition, the test has been shown to be sensitive to corpus callosal dysfunction** in that patients with disruptions in the interhemispheric transfer of auditory information exhibit improvement in performance when the linguistic labeling component of the test is removed by requesting the listener to hum the pattern rather than verbally describe it (Musiek et al., 1980). **Finally, results of the PPST may provide information**

regarding neuromaturation in the child with learning disability by indicating the degree of myelination of the corpus callosum (Musiek, Gollegly, & Baran, 1984).

A related test of temporal ordering is the Duration Pattern Test (DPT). Described by Pinheiro and Musiek (1985), the DPT is similar to the PPST except that the frequency of the tones is held constant at 1000 Hz and duration is the factor to be discriminated. Short (250 msec) and long (500 msec) tone bursts are presented in sequences of three-tone patterns and, like the PPST, the listener is asked to describe verbally the pattern heard (e.g., short-short-long, long-short-long, etc.) **The DPT appears to be sensitive to cerebral lesions while remaining unaffected by peripheral hearing loss** as long as the stimuli are presented at a frequency and intensity that can be perceived by the listener (Musiek, Baran, & Pinheiro, 1990). The DPT assesses the processes of duration discrimination, temporal ordering, and linguistic labeling.

Finally, an additional test of auditory pattern perception that is also a dichotic nonspeech task has been developed by Blaettner et al. (1989). The Psychoacoustic Pattern Discrimination Test (PPDT) assesses discrimination of temporal changes through the use of dichotically presented sequences of noise bursts or click trains. The listener is required to indicate discrimination of a monaural change in the pattern by pressing a button. Preliminary information indicates that, like other temporal patterning tasks, **the PPDT is sensitive to lesions of the cerebral hemispheres including the auditory association areas**. In addition, abnormal findings on the PPDT have been found to correlate with abnormal findings on middle and/or late evoked potential measures. While the PPDT holds great promise as a test for temporal processing, a drawback to the procedure is that it is not readily available in standardized format for clinical use at the present time.

To summarize, despite the use of temporal processing tasks in research and the importance of temporal processing in speech and music perception, very few tests of temporal processing are currently available for widespread clinical use. Those that are available include the Pitch Pattern Sequence Test and the Duration Pattern Test, both of which assess the processes of discrimination (frequency or duration, respectively), temporal ordering, and linguistic labeling. Both of these tests are currently available on compact disc (Musiek, 1994). A third test of temporal processing is the Psychoacoustic Pattern Discrimination Test, which assesses temporal patterning abilities without the need for linguistic labeling or verbal report. All three of these tests appear to be relatively resistant to the effects of peripheral hearing loss as well as being sensitive to cerebral pathology. The PPST, DPT, and PPDT are summarized in Table 5–3.

Monaural Low-Redundancy Speech Tests

Due to redundancy both within the auditory system (*intrinsic redundancy*) as well as in spoken language (*extrinsic redundancy*), the normal listener typically is able to achieve closure and make auditory discriminations even when a portion of the auditory signal is missing or distorted. This ability is often compromised in a listener with central auditory dysfunction. Electroacoustically modifying the temporal, frequency, or intensity characteristics of the acoustic signal reduces the amount of extrinsic redundancy and, because central pathology results in a reduction of intrinsic redundancy, auditory closure cannot be achieved. Therefore, **although a listener with CAPD will typically perform quite well when auditory stimuli are presented in an ideal listening environment, such as during standard phonetically balanced word recognition testing, he or she will often demonstrate significant problems when the task is made more difficult by distorting the signal in some way.** This section will discuss three methods of reducing the redundancy of the speech signal in order to assess central auditory function: low-pass filtering, time compression, and addition of reverberation. In addition, because the primary effect of the addition of noise is a reduction in the redundancy of the speech signal, speech-in-noise tasks also will be discussed in this section.

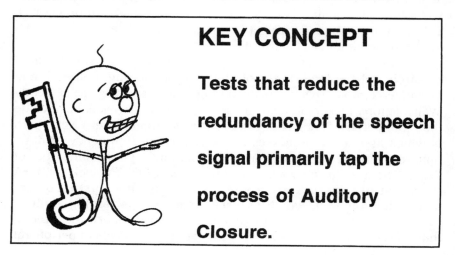

KEY CONCEPT

Tests that reduce the redundancy of the speech signal primarily tap the process of Auditory Closure.

Table 5-3
Summary of Selected Temporal Tests

Test	Process(es) Assessed	Sensitive to
Frequency Patterns	Frequency discrimination, temporal ordering, linguistic labeling	Cerebral hemisphere lesions, interhemispheric transfer
Duration Patterns	Duration discrimination, temporal ordering, linguistic labeling	Cerebral hemisphere lesions, interhemispheric transfer
Psychoacoustic Pattern Discrimination Test	Temporal discrimination	Cerebral hemisphere lesions including auditory association areas

Low-pass filtering of the speech signal in order to assess the integrity of the CANS has been employed since 1954 (Bocca, Calearo, & Cassinari, 1954). A number of studies have investigated the utility of low-pass filtered speech in the detection of CANS dysfunction, and the reader is referred to Rintelmann (1985) for a review. This section will describe two readily available, standardized filtered speech tests in clinical use today: the Ivey filtered speech test included in the Willeford central test battery (Willeford, 1977) and filtered NU-6 lists.

The Ivey filtered speech test of the Willeford central test battery is probably the most widely used low-pass filtered speech test in clinics today. The test consists of two 50-item lists of the Michigan consonant-nucleus-consonant (CNC) words with a 500 Hz cut-off and 18 dB/octave filter. The filtered words tend to be intelligible to normal listeners; however, listeners with central pathology perform poorly on this test.

In addition to the Ivey test, low-pass filtered versions of the Northwestern University No. 6 (NU-6) word lists are available (Tonal and Speech Materials for Auditory Perceptual Assessment, 1992; Wilson & Mueller, 1984). Low-pass versions of the test utilizing cut-off frequencies of 500, 700, 1000, and 1500 Hz may be used. Normative values for the 500, 700, and 1000 Hz cut-offs may be found in Wilson and Mueller (1984). The use of the 1500 Hz cut-off frequency is described in Bornstein, Wilson, and Cambron (1994). It should be noted that, when the 500 Hz cut-off is used, normal listeners have a great deal of difficulty with this test, indicating that this cut-off frequency probably would not be clinically feasible for use in a CAP test battery (Wilson & Mueller, 1984). Bornstein et al. (1994) also described the use of a high-pass filtered (2100 Hz cut-off) version of the NU-6. Further research into the use of the 1500 Hz low-pass and 2100 Hz high-pass NU-6 lists with listeners with neurological involvement remains to be completed.

Findings for low-pass filtered speech in general indicate that this procedure is sensitive to a variety of central disorders, including brainstem and cortical dysfunction. However, site of lesion cannot be determined from the use of filtered speech tests. These tests, like the other monaural low-redundancy speech tasks to be discussed in this section, primarily tap the process of auditory closure (ability to fill in the missing components) of degraded auditory information.

A second method of reducing the redundancy of the speech signal is time compression. In this technique, the temporal characteristics of the signal are altered by electronically reducing the duration of the speech signal without affecting the frequency characteristics (Fairbanks, Everitt, & Jaeger, 1954). Normative studies using time-compressed versions of the NU-6 word lists (30–70% compression) indicate that normal listeners demonstrate a reduction in word recognition scores as the degree of compression increases, culminating in a marked deterioration in performance with 70% compression (Beasley, Forman, & Rintelmann, 1972; Beasley, Schwimmer, & Rintelmann, 1972). Findings in subjects with neurological dysfunction indicate that **time-compressed speech tasks are most sensitive to diffuse patholo-gy involving the primary auditory cortex**, particularly at the higher degrees of compression (Baran et al. 1985; Kurdziel, Noffsinger, & Olson, 1976; Mueller et al., 1987).

Reverberation is the persistance of an acoustic signal, or echo, that occurs in an enclosed space. This term may be familiar to many clinicians, as it is reverberation that is most bothersome in rooms with poorly controlled acoustic characteristics and a preponderance of hard surfaces that enable sound to "bounce" for a period of time following the cessation of the signal. The degree of reverberation is defined by the time required for a signal to decay 60 dB following off-set of the signal (Wilson, Preece, Salamon, Sperry, & Bornstein, 1994). As reverberation time increases, recognition of subsequent words decreases (Helfer & Wilber, 1990). Thus, reverberation provides an additional method of reducing the redundancy of a speech signal for the purposes of central assessment.

Studies of the effects of signal distortion on word recognition abilities indicate that **a combination of disortion techniques results in greater effects than does the use of one disortion technique alone** (Harris, 1960).This is known as the *multiplicative* effect. For this reason, Wilson, Preece, Salamon, Sperry, and Bornstein (1994) have reported on the use of time compression combined with electronically induced, 0.3-second reverberation for use in central auditory assessment. The addition of reverberation to time-compressed speech resulted in the expected decrease in word recognition performance in a group of normal listeners; however, further research is needed using neurologically disabled populations. Time-compressed (45% and 65%) NU-6 word lists alone and combined with reverberation are available on the Tonal and Speech Materials for Auditory Perceptual Assessment compact disc (1992). It should be noted that the data provided by Wilson, Preece, Salamon, Sperry, and Bornstein (1994), as well as our own clinical experience, suggest that the **65% time-compression condition included on the compact disc appears to be difficult even for normal listeners. This suggests that the 45% time-compression rate may be more appropriate for clinical use**.

A final method of reducing the redundancy of the speech signal is to imbed the signal in a background of noise. Although speech-in-noise tests have been shown to be at least marginally sensitive to a wide variety of disorders of the CANS and related disorders (Chermak, Vonhof, & Bendel, 1989; Dayal, Tarantino, & Swisher, 1966; Heilman, Hammer, & Wilder, 1973; Morales-Garcia & Poole, 1972; Olsen, Noffsinger, & Kurdziel, 1975; Sinha, 1959), lack of standardized test tools and material-specific normative data have resulted in conflicting findings and questionable test reliability. Therefore, Mueller and Bright (1994) have suggested that **speech-in-noise tests may well be the most misused test of central auditory function**.

Of primary importance is the collection of normative data regarding whatever materials and signal-to-noise ratios are used in testing. Typically, monosyllabic words combined with the ipsilateral presentation of white or speech spectrum noise at signal-to-noise ratios of 0 to +10 dB are utilized. Some clinics also use "cafeteria" noise or multi-talker babble as the competing signal. The Synthetic Sentence Identification test with Ipsilateral Competing Message (SSI-ICM) (Jerger & Jerger, 1974), which presents the third-order SSI sentences described previously along with ipsilateral continuous discourse, is an example of a commercially available speech-in-noise test. **The SSI-ICM has been shown to be useful in the identification of lesions of the low brainstem** (Jerger & Jerger, 1974, 1975). We recommend that only tape-recorded speech materials be used due to the lack of acoustical control over monitored live-voice speech.

The clinician engaged in speech-in-noise testing should be warned that, **due to the great variability in scores seen in normal and lesioned listeners, speech-in-noise test results should be interpreted with caution**. In a study using NU-6 words presented in white noise at 0 dB signal-to-noise ratio, Olsen et al. (1975) found that a reduction in word recognition performance of at least 40% was required before the findings were considered to be significant. Even using this criterion, site of lesion could not be determined from the test results, and a number of listeners with temporal lobe lesions continued to perform within normal limits on the task. Therefore, we would recommend that speech-in noise tests only be used in conjunction with other, standardized tests of central auditory function.

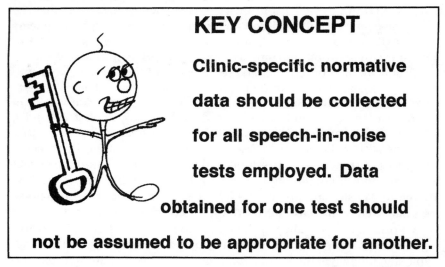

KEY CONCEPT

Clinic-specific normative data should be collected for all speech-in-noise tests employed. Data obtained for one test should not be assumed to be appropriate for another.

In summary, the inclusion of a monaural low-redundancy speech test in the central auditory test battery may be useful for the identification of central dysfunction. Methods of reducing redundancy of a speech signal include band-pass filtering, time compression, addition of reverberation, and addition of competing noise. All of these tasks assess the listener's ability to achieve auditory closure of degraded auditory information; however, information regarding site of lesion can rarely be obtained through the use of these tests alone. Finally, the clinician should use caution when engaging in speech-in-noise testing due to the lack of standardization and high degree of variability inherent in this type of task. Types of monaural low-redundancy speech tests are summarized in Table 5–4.

Table 5-4

Summary of Selected Monaural Low-Redundancy Speech Tests

Test	Process(es) Assessed	Sensitive to
Low-Pass Filtered Speech	Auditory closure	Brainstem and cortical lesions
Time Compressed Speech	Auditory closure	Diffuse pathology involving primary auditory cortex
Time Compression plus Reverberation	Auditory closure	More info needed re: neurological populations
Synthetic Sentence Identification Test With Ipsilateral Competing Message	Auditory closure	Low brainstem lesions
Speech-in-Noise	Auditory closure	Questionable sensitivity to low brainstem and cortical lesions

Binaural Interaction Tests

Tests of binaural interaction generally assess the ability of the CANS to process disparate, but complementary, information presented to the two ears. **Unlike dichotic listening tasks, the stimuli utilized in binaural interaction tasks typically are presented either in a nonsimultaneous, sequential condition, or the information presented to each ear is composed of a portion of the entire message, necessitating integration of the information in order for the listener to perceive the whole message.** This is considered to be a function primarily of the low brainstem, as discussed in Chapter 2. A variety of binaural interaction tasks has been used clinically, including rapidly alternating speech perception, band-pass and CVC binaural fusion tasks, interaural difference limen tasks, and the Masking Level Difference.

Rapidly alternating speech perception (RASP) is a procedure in which sentence material is switched rapidly between ears at periodic intervals, resulting in the alternating presentation of unintelligible, sequential bursts of information. In the normal listener, this rapidly alternating presentation of a speech message is easily understood. However, some listeners with lesions of the low brainstem demonstrate difficulty with the task (Lynn & Gilroy, 1977). The most commonly used version of the RASP was developed by Willeford (Willeford & Bilger, 1978). In their study, the authors found the test to be simple even for very young children. **Subsequent studies suggest that the RASP may not be sensitive to anything other than grossly abnormal brainstem pathology** (Lynn & Gilroy, 1977; Musiek, 1983c; Willeford & Burleigh, 1994). **Because of the availability of other tests that demonstrate greater efficiency with regard to brainstem pathology, such as the ABR and MLD, there is some question as to the clinical utility of the RASP in central assessment.**

Binaural fusion tasks involve the presentation of different portions of a speech stimulus to each ear, necessitating fusion of the information in order for the listener to perceive the entire word. Information may be band-passed so that only the high-frequency portion of the stimulus is presented to one ear and the low-frequency components are presented to the other, or CVC words may be utilized in which the consonants are presented to one ear and the vowel to the other in a sequential fashion.

Matzker (1959) used bisyllabic, phonetically balanced word lists for assessing binaural resynthesis. In his test, the low-pass band (500–800 Hz) was presented to one ear while the high-pass band (1815–2500 Hz) was presented to the other. The 41-word list was presented three times: twice using the filtered bands and once, during the second presentation, diotically so that fusion was not required. His results indicated that **listeners with cortical lesions performed normally on the binaural fusion task whereas listeners with brainstem pathology had difficulty with the resynthesis of the auditory information.** A modified version of the Matzker binaural fusion test was developed by Ivey (1969) and is included in the Willeford central test battery.

Smith and Resnick (1972) maintained that the use of monosyllabic words would reduce the redundancy of the signal and thereby improve the sensitivity of binaural fusion tasks. In their study, monosyllabic, CVC words were band-passed and presented using a variation of Matzker's resynthesis paradigm. Test results were interpreted by comparing the results of the diotic presentation of the stimuli with the two presentations requiring fusion. Diotic scores were significantly higher than resynthesis scores in 4 out of 4 cases of brainstem pathology.

More recently, a band-pass filtered, binaural fusion test using the NU-6 word list has been made available through Auditec of St. Louis, and in the Tonal and Speech Materials for Auditory Perceptual Assessment compact disc (1992). Normative data have been collected (Wilson & Mueller, 1984); however, further research needs to be done with populations exhibiting neurological disorders. Overall, **studies examining band-pass filtered binaural fusion tasks suggest that they are somewhat sensitive to brainstem lesions** (Lynn & Gilroy, 1977; Musiek, 1983c; Noffsinger et al., 1972). **In addition, abnormal binaural fusion or resynthesis performance has been seen in children with dyslexia and/or learning disability** (Welsh, Welsh, & Healy, 1980; Welsh, Welsh, Healy, & Cooper, 1982; Willeford, 1977).

An additional binaural fusion task currently available on the Tonal and Speech Materials for Auditory Perceptual Assessment compact disc (1992) is the Segmented-Alternated CVC fusion task developed by Wilson, Arcos, and Jones (1984) as a tool to assess central auditory function while remaining relatively unaffected by peripheral hearing loss. In this test, CVC words are segmented so that the consonant segments are delivered to one ear and the vowel is delivered to the other ear in an alternating manner. Data have been collected from 120 normal listeners (Wilson, 1994); however, further research is needed using pathological populations.

The concept of evaluating interaural time or intensity just noticeable differences (jnds) has existed for several years; however, it has not gained wide popularity as a clinical tool. Pinheiro and Tobin (1969, 1971) utilized an interaural intensity difference (IID) paradigm in which the degree of intensity difference between ears needed for lateralization of a signal was evaluated. Their results indicated that **subjects with central involvement demonstrated greater IIDs in the ear ipsilateral to the lesion.**

More recently, Levine et al. (1993a, b) described an interaural jnd task in which tonal stimuli were either high- or low-pass filtered and presented in pairs to both ears simultaneously. Either the onset time (time jnd) or the intensity (level jnd) of one half of the stimulus pair was altered in one ear. The listener was required to indicate when the signal lateralized to one side or the other. **The results of high-pass time jnd evaluation were found to be closely correlated with ABR results and, thus, appeared to be a good behavioral measure of brainstem integrity.** However, their test paradigm and that of Pinheiro and Tobin (1969) require greater acoustic control of the stimulus than is possible utilizing standard audiometric equipment. Therefore, clinical utility of these test paradigms is questionable at this time.

A final test of binaural interaction is the Masking Level Difference (MLD), described in Chapter 2. **MLDs may be obtained to speech or tonal stimuli, and have been shown to be highly sensitive to brainstem dysfunction.** Many commercial audiometers have the built-in capability to conduct MLD testing. In addition, The Tonal and Speech

Materials for Auditory Perceptual Assessment compact disc (1992) includes a spondaic MLD procedure (Wilson, Zizz, & Sperry, 1994).

Overall, and with the exception of the MLD, the clinical utility of the majority of binaural interaction tests has been questioned on the bases of sensitivity and/or ease of administration. Noffsinger et al. (1984) have suggested that the three primary responsibilities of the auditory brainstem are sound transmission, binaural integration of sound, and the control of reflexive behavior. These three areas may be tested reliably using the ABR, MLD, and acoustic reflex paradigms, respectively. **Therefore, the need for additional behavioral tests of brainstem integrity is questionable at this time and, indeed, the tests discussed in this section are not considered to be in widespread clinical use.** A summary of binaural interaction tests discussed in this section is provided in Table 5–5.

Electrophysiological Procedures

No discussion of central auditory tests would be complete without mention of electrophysiological procedures. Four of these procedures —the ABR, MLR, LEP, and P300—were discussed in some detail

Table 5-5
Summary of Selected Binaural Interaction Tests

Test	Process(es) Assessed	Sensitive to
Rapidly Alternating Speech Perception	Binaural interaction	Questionable sensitivity to low brainstem lesions
Binaural Fusion (Band-pass filtered)	Binaural interaction	Somewhat sensitive to low brainstem lesions, dyslexia and learning disabilities
Binaural Fusion (Consonant-Vowel-Consonant)	Binaural interaction	More info needed re: neurological populations
Interaural Just Noticeable Differences	Binaural interaction	Brainstem lesions

in Chapter 3. A fifth measure which appears to be promising for the neurophysiological evaluation of speech perception is the Mismatched Negativity (MMN) response, first described by Naatanen, Gaillard, and Mantysalo (1978). As originally described, **the MMN is a small negative deflection observed as a superimposition on the P2 wave of the late response following the presentation of a block of standard stimuli in which occasional deviant (target) stimuli occur.** Unlike the P300, conscious attention to the task is not required in order to obtain the MMN.

The MMN can be elicited by very small deviances in acoustic stimuli (jnds) that are close to the individual's conscious perceptual discrimination threshold (Kraus et al. 1993; Naatanen & Gaillard, 1983). In addition, virtually any acoustic stimuli may be used, including simple as well as complex, phonemic sounds, suggesting that **the MMN may provide an objective measure of speech perception ability** (Kraus, McGee, Carrell, & Sharma, 1995). Potential uses for the MMN include the prediction of speech perception abilities in infants, children, and other hard-to-test populations, as well as possible future use with hearing-impaired populations; however, further research is still needed in these areas. Kraus and her colleagues at Northwestern University have been responsible for a wealth of current research concerning the MMN, particularly as it relates to speech perception in children; however, the studies by these researchers are simply too numerous to cite here. For a recent overview of issues surrounding the clinical utility of the MMN, the reader is referred to Naatanen and Kraus (1995).

A topic of some controversy is whether electrophysiological measures are a necessary part of central auditory assessment. **While we realize that it is not practical to suggest that practitioners in the educational setting obtain the equipment and specialized training necessary for the administration of electrophysiological tests, we must emphasize that these tests may be an important adjunct to behavioral assessment of the CANS.**

Depending on the situation, the addition of one or more objective, electrophysiological measures may be indicated. For example, if a lesion of the low brainstem is suspected, the ABR continues to be the most efficient method of assessing low brainstem integrity and, thus, would likely be the test of choice. In cases where objective evidence of auditory processing dysfunction is necessary for special education classification, legal documentation, or other reasons, electrophysiology may provide that objective data. Finally, to assess the ability of the CANS to make subtle discriminations necessary for speech perception, particularly in hard-to-test populations, the MMN may provide information that cannot be obtained through behavioral testing. Therefore, the clinician should be familiar with electrophysiological measures of auditory function and make every attempt either to provide such services or to locate a source to which patients can be referred for such testing.

In conclusion, while we do not advocate the addition of electrophysiological measures to all central auditory evaluations, it should be recognized that they may provide useful information in certain situations. Therefore, electrophysiology should be considered an integral part of the central auditory test battery.

Summary

This chapter has discussed the topics of test validity and reliability, as well as provided an overview of assessment tools in five general categories: dichotic speech tests, tests of temporal processing, monaural low redundancy speech tests, binaural interaction tests, and electrophysiological procedures. The clinical validity of a given test tool may be calculated by evaluating the sensitivity and specificity of the test related to a specific standard. When tests of central auditory function are considered, it is suggested that the tests' ability to identify documented CANS lesions be the standard for determination of test validity. Reliability is determined by assessing the repeatability of test results in specific populations.

A variety of assessment tools is available within each of the five categories listed above, and each category is designed to assess different processes. Therefore, a comprehensive central auditory processing evaluation should include tests from more than one category as well as associated measures of speech/language, cognitive, and educational abilities, in a test battery approach. Only in this manner can an auditory profile delineating auditory strengths and weaknesses be developed and appropriate, deficit-specific recommendations for management made.

Review Questions

1.   List and discuss three reasons why a test battery approach to central auditory assessment should be utilized.
2.   Define the following terms related to test validity:

   false positive   true positive
   false negative   true negative

sensitivity   specificity
efficiency

3. Define test reliability and provide examples of procedural and patient variables that may affect test reliability.
4. List and give a brief description of five dichotic speech tests.
5. What auditory processes do the dichotic speech tasks described above evaluate?
6. List and give a brief description of three tests of temporal ordering.
7. What auditory processes do the temporal ordering tests described above evaluate?
8. List and give a brief description of four methods of reducing the redundancy of a speech signal for purposes of central auditory assessment.
9. Discuss the limitations of speech-in-noise testing.
10. What auditory process does monaural low-redundancy speech testing evaluate?
11. List and give a brief description of four methods of assessing binaural interaction abilities.
12. Discuss the limitations of binaural interaction tests in general.
13. Briefly describe the Mismatched Negativity response.
14. Discuss the value of including electrophysiological procedures in central auditory assessment.

CHAPTER

Comprehensive Central Auditory Assessment

This chapter will provide the reader with information necessary to plan and carry out comprehensive evaluations of central auditory function. Because of the practical nature of the information contained herein, the reader may be tempted to skip the earlier chapters in this book and approach central auditory assessment from a "cookbook" perspective, using this chapter as a guide. However, we cannot overemphasize the importance of understanding the scientific bases of central auditory assessment. Therefore, **we strongly recommend that the information provided in the previous chapters be studied carefully and internalized prior to entering into the assessment arena**. With an understanding of the scientific underpinnings, as well as the nature of the various types of central auditory assessment tools, this chapter can serve as a resource for information regarding specific assessment protocols. Test interpretation will be covered in Chapter 7.

Learning Objectives

After studying this chapter, the reader should be able to

1. Identify equipment needed for comprehensive central auditory assessment
2. Identify components of the assessment procedure
3. Discuss methods of choosing components of the central auditory test battery
4. Delineate assessment protocols for several commonly utilized tests of central auditory function.

Required Equipment

Although screening procedures for CAPD can and often are administered utilizing little more than a portable cassette tape deck, a table, and two chairs, **diagnostic tests of central auditory function should always be conducted in a sound booth so that adequate acoustic control of stimuli can be maintained**. A two-channel audiometer is required for many of the test procedures that will be discussed in this chapter. In addition, the clinician will need to procure a good quality tape player and/or a compact disc player. We recommend that both types of equipment be available as several commonly used tests are available only on magnetic tape, while others can be found on the Tonal and Speech Materials for Auditory Perceptual Assessment compact disc (1992), which provides higher quality and fidelity of auditory stimuli than can be obtained through the use of magnetic tape (Noffsinger, Wilson, & Musiek, 1994). As in all audiological assessment, equipment should be calibrated regularly and maintained in good working order.

The Assessment Procedure

Comprehensive central auditory assessment should be undertaken in such a manner as to maximize the child's abilities while controlling for confounding factors such as environmental distractions, attention, and fatigue. If at all possible, children should not undergo central auditory assessment when overly tired or ill. We have found it useful to schedule younger children in the morning so that they enter the clinic fully rested and alert.

The first portion of any central auditory assessment should be an interview with the child and accompanying parent(s) or caregiver. Often, the child and parent arrive at the clinic with varying degrees of apprehension. Before beginning formalized evaluation, it is advisable to explain the evaluation process fully so that the child and parent know what to expect and their apprehension can be minimized.

A complete history should be taken at the time of the interview, to include information related to the child's medical and educational history, auditory symptoms, and general behavior. The parent and child should be asked about those skills that require multimodality coordination and/or interhemispheric integration, such as art, music, and motor coordination. In addition, the presence of a family history of learning or hearing problems should be identified. In many cases, the clinician will hear, "Well, Johnny's father doesn't really think that this testing is all that important. After all, *he* had the same kinds of problems in school when he was Johnny's age." This comment may be taken as evidence of a possible familial transmission of auditory processing and/or learning disorders.

Like the assessment itself, the interview should be individualized. At times, the clinician may need to ask several, detailed questions in order to draw information from a reluctant parent or child. Conversely, one or two questions may prompt a descriptive monologue including a wealth of applicable information. **Regardless of the amount of information obtained from screening procedures and questionnaires, the face-to-face interview is necessary, as previously unknown details often will emerge.** In addition, the clinician will be able to get a feel for the parent's (and child's) attitudes toward the possible disorder as well as the its impact on social, emotional, and other aspects of the child's life.

Before beginning the assessment, the clinician should make sure that factors that may affect the child's ability to attend, including hunger, thirst, or needing to go to the bathroom, have been eliminated. Any extraneous environmental distractions should be kept to a minimum. For this reason, we have found it necessary to suggest that the parent not accompany the child into the sound suite for testing, except in select circumstances. Instead, we advise the parents to wait and assure them that they will be called when testing is completed, and that the results of our evaluation will be explained to them at that time.

The time required to complete the assessment will depend on the individual situation. The child undergoing evaluation should be monitored carefully for signs of fading attention or fatigue, and frequent breaks should be offered. In some cases, a complete evaluation may be completed within 45 minutes. When additional test procedures are deemed necessary or frequent breaks are required, testing may require as long as 2 hours.

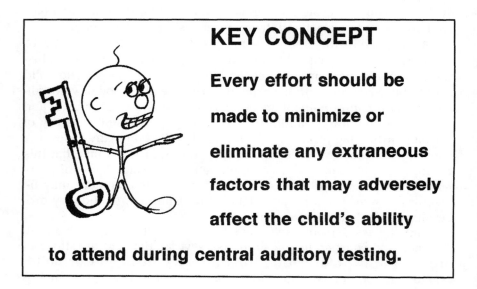

KEY CONCEPT

Every effort should be made to minimize or eliminate any extraneous factors that may adversely affect the child's ability to attend during central auditory testing.

When the test session has been completed, the clinician should sit down with the parents and child once again and explain the results of the evaluation as well as make preliminary recommendations for management. Questions and concerns should be addressed at this time. This practice helps to foster the parents' and child's understanding of the disorder and assists in ensuring that follow-through will occur, but does not take the place of a written report. Suggestions for report writing and imparting information to parents and educational professionals will be provided in Chapter 9.

In summary, the assessment procedure should include an interview with the parent and child, the assessment itself, and a discussion of evaluation results and preliminary recommendations for management. Therefore, the clinician will need to schedule comprehensive central auditory assessments in such a way as to ensure that sufficient time is available for all portions of the assessment procedure. Although this practice may prove to be time consuming, perhaps disheartening some clinicians for whom caseloads are already overwhelming, fostering an atmosphere of relaxation and thoroughness will help to increase the productivity of the test session itself, as well as assist in ensuring understanding of the disorder and follow-through on management recommendations.

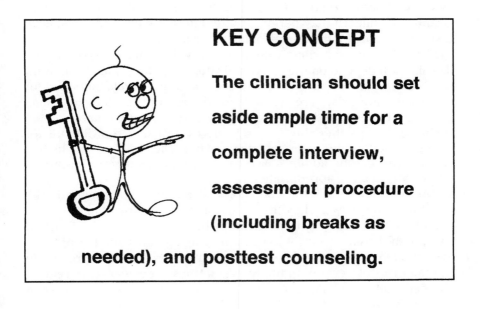

KEY CONCEPT

The clinician should set aside ample time for a complete interview, assessment procedure (including breaks as needed), and posttest counseling.

Choosing the Test Battery

In the previous chapter, the rationale for a test battery approach to central auditory assessment was presented. In addition, five general categories of central tests were discussed: dichotic speech tests, temporal ordering tests, monaural low redundancy speech tests, binaural interaction tasks, and electrophysiological procedures. However, the question of which tests would be appropriate for inclusion in a central auditory test battery remains.

Although the decision regarding how many and precisely which central tests to utilize should be based upon each individual case, we suggest the following rule of thumb: **Because it is desirable to ensure that the test battery assesses different processes as well as different**

levels of the CANS, it would be prudent to include one test from each category. An exception to this rule would be electrophysiological procedures, which should be recommended when the individual situation warrants their inclusion. **In addition, it is often helpful to include two tests of dichotic listening: one which is considered to be linguistically loaded (such as Competing Sentences or Staggered Spondaic Words), and one which carries a lighter linguistic load (such as Dichotic Digits).** The reason for this is that, as discussed in Chapter 3, children may perform quite differently on dichotic speech tasks depending on the degree of linguistic loading.

The decision regarding which test(s) within each category to utilize also will depend on the individual situation. The clinician will want to choose tests that have demonstrated validity and reliability and for which normative data are available for the age of the child. For example, older children and adolescents may perform quite reliably on the Dichotic CV test, but this test is likely to be much too difficult for younger children. In this case, a test such as Dichotic Digits, which is simpler and can be administered to children as young as 7 years of age, may be a more appropriate choice.

An additional factor in choosing test battery components is the question to be answered by the assessment. As discussed in the previous chapter, if the goal is to identify the presence of a CAPD *at all costs*, then the clinician will want to include a greater number of tests, even though the possibility of a false positive result will be greater. In the majority of central auditory evaluations, however, it is recommended that the clinician choose those tests that are the most efficient in terms of validity, time, and ease of administration.

Finally, it should be emphasized that **central auditory assessment is a dynamic process requiring ongoing interpretation *during* the evaluation process.** The assessment situation should be entered into with a basic "game plan" based on preassessment information in mind; however, that plan may, and often will, change depending upon the situation.

For example, a child may be referred for comprehensive central auditory assessment with the primary complaint of severe difficulty understanding speech in noise and preliminary screening information that indicates a strong likelihood of CAPD. Based upon this history, the clinician cannot predict which process or processes may be dysfunctional in this child. Therefore, the assessment plan will include a test from each category of central tests, as recommended above. However, it may be noticed during testing that, on a test of auditory closure such as Filtered Words, the child performs at a borderline-normal level. In this case, the clinician may decide to include a more difficult test of auditory closure, such as Time Compressed Speech plus Reverberation, in order to more fully tap the process of auditory closure. In addition, a speech-in-noise test may be given for the purpose of obtaining descriptive data although, as was seen in the previous chapter, speech-in-noise tests should be interpreted with caution and age-appropriate normative data must be available for the specific materials utilized.

In other words, individualization of the assessment procedure requires ongoing interpretation of the data, rather than simply collecting the data during assessment, and then scoring and interpreting the test results after the child has left the clinic. Decisions regarding additional assessment tools to include, as well as judgments of response reliability, must be made continually throughout the assessment procedure.

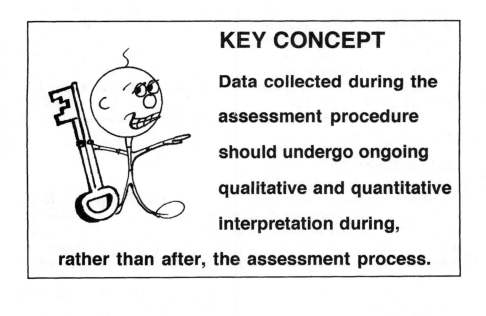

KEY CONCEPT

Data collected during the assessment procedure should undergo ongoing qualitative and quantitative interpretation during, rather than after, the assessment process.

Test Administration

This section will describe recommended assessment protocols for several commonly used behavioral tests of central auditory function. We do not intend to suggest that the following protocols are the only manner in which these tests may be administered. In addition, it should be reemphasized that age-appropriate clinic norms should be established for each assessment tool. A discussion of administration and interpretation of electrophysiological measures is not within the scope of this text, and the reader is referred to the References at the end of the book for further information regarding electrophysiological procedures. For information regarding statistical analysis and procedures related to the collection of normative data, the reader is referred to Chapter 10.

Dichotic Speech Tests

When administering any dichotic speech test, several procedural factors should be considered. By definition, a two-channel audiometer is required for dichotic listening. Because dichotic speech tests are interpreted in terms of ear effects, it is recommended that the clinician monitor only one channel at a time and keep careful track of which ear the monitored channel is being routed to so that scoring errors may be avoided. Finally, the administration of dichotic speech tests requires that the stimuli be delivered to both ears at equivalent intensities. Therefore, it is recommended that these tests only be administered in cases of bilaterally symmetrical hearing sensitivity. A summary of the dichotic speech tests described in this section is presented in Table 6–1.

Dichotic Digits (DD)

There are two commercial versions of the Dichotic Digits (DD) test: single digits and double digits. In the majority of situations, double digits will be the task of choice as it is more challenging while remaining simple enough even for young children. However, for cases in which double digits prove to be too difficult, single digits may be administered.

Both versions of the DD test are administered at 50 dB SL (re: spondee threshold), or, in cases of peripheral hearing loss, at the most comfortable loudness level (MCL). The listener is instructed that he or she will be hearing different numbers in each ear at the same time and is to repeat all of the numbers heard, regardless of order. The first three stimulus presentations are for practice. The test consists of 20 stimulus presentations or, for double digits, 80 digits in all (40 per ear). The test is scored in terms of percent correct per ear (for double digits, each digit is worth 2.5%).

Table 6-1

Summary of Selected Dichotic Speech Tests: Test Administration

Test	Stimuli	Presentation Level	Scoring
Dichotic Digits	20 presentations of 4 digits each (2 to each ear)	50 dB	% correct
Dichotic Consonant-Vowels	30 pairs of CV segments per ear	55 dB	% correct per ear
Staggered Spondaic Words	spondaic words presented in staggered format in 4 conditions: RNC, RC, LC, and LNC	50 dB	% of errors per ear; in each condition; and total
Competing Sentences	25 sentence pairs	target: 35 dB; competing: 50 dB	% correct per ear
Synthetic Sentence Identification Test With Contralateral Competing Message	10 third-order approximations of English sentences	primary: 30dB; competing: varies from 30–70 dB	% correct per ear
Dichotic Sentence Identification	same as SSI	50 dB (re: PTA)	% correct per ear, and interaural difference
Dichotic Rhyme Test	30 pairs of rhyming CVC words	50 dB	% correct per ear

The following normative values for children are provided in the accompanying test manual; however, as with all tests of central auditory function, clinicians are strongly urged to collect their own age-appropriate normative data.

7 years to 7 years, 11 months: 55% left, 70% right

8 years to 8 years, 11 months: 65% left, 75% right

9 years to 9 years, 11 months: 75% left, 80% right

10 years to 10 years, 11 months: 78% left, 85% right

11 years to 11 years, 11 months: 88% left, 90% right

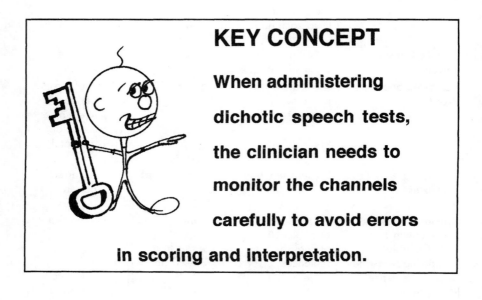

KEY CONCEPT

When administering dichotic speech tests, the clinician needs to monitor the channels carefully to avoid errors in scoring and interpretation.

Normative values for adults (two standard deviations below the mean) are 90% for both left and right ears. In addition, the DD test has been shown to be relatively resistant to cochlear hearing loss in adults when a criterion level of 80% for both ears is used (Musiek, 1983a).

Dichotic Consonant-Vowels (CV)

The recommended intensity for administration of the Dichotic CV test is 55 dB HL (75 dB peak equivalent SPL). All listeners should have hearing sensitivity within normal limits. The test consists of 30 pairs of CV segments. A response form is given to the listener, and he or she is instructed to indicate the segments heard.

Testing begins with monotic presentation of the stimuli so that the listener may practice. When the listener is able to identify 14 out of 16 CVs presented monaurally, test administration may begin. The test is given in three manners: (1) no lag (simultaneous) condition, (2) 90-

msec lag condition to one ear, and (3) 90-msec lag to the other ear. Like the DD test, Dichotic CVs are scored in terms of percent correct per ear, as well as double correct (occurrences in which stimuli presented to both ears are reported correctly).

Three measures may be obtained: (1) right ear advantage (REA), (2) lag effect, and (3) auditory capacity effect. The REA is computed by comparing right ear scores to left ear scores during the simultaneous presentation condition. Unlike more linguistically loaded tests of dichotic listening, the REA for Dichotic CVs does not show a significant maturational effect in normally hearing children ages 7 to 15 (Roeser, Millay, & Morrow, 1983).

The lag effect is computed by comparing performance during the 90-msec lag conditions to the performance during simultaneous presentation. Normal listeners tend to show a significant improvement in scores during the left ear 90-msec lag condition, whereas listeners with temporal lobe lesions do not.

Finally, auditory capacity may be determined by computing the double correct scores. The manual accompanying the magnetic tape version of the Dichotic CV test indicates that the double correct score improves from approximately 22% at age 7 to 43% at age 15. Normative values for the compact disc version of the Dichotic CV test indicate that the 90th percentile for single-ear performance (right or left) during the simultaneous presentation condition is at 56.7%. Therefore, **performance below 50% in an adult would be indicative of possible disorder** (Noffsinger, Martinez, & Wilson, 1994). Again, it should be stressed that each clinic needs to develop age-appropriate, normative data for the Dichotic CV test.

Staggered Spondaic Words (SSW)

The SSW is administered at 50 dB SL (re: pure tone average [PTA] or spondaic threshold); however, in cases of intolerance, the presentation level may be reduced to as low as 25 dB SL without significantly affecting test results. If a conductive hearing loss of 20 dB or greater is present, the presentation level to the affected ear should be lowered to 30 dB SL.

As described in Chapter 5, SSW stimuli are arranged in a manner such that spondaic words are presented in four conditions: (1) right noncompeting (RNC), (2) right competing (RC), (3) left competing (LC), and (4) left noncompeting (LNC). These four conditions are shown in Table 6–2 using the first item of the SSW test. Stimuli presentation is alternated between left leading and right leading; therefore, it is critical that the clinician carefully monitor which channel is routed

Table 6-2

Sample Item from the Staggered Spondaic Test

RNC	RC	
up	stairs	
	down	town
	LC	LNC

Note: RNC=Right Noncompeting; RC = Right Competing;
LC = Left Competing; LNC = Left Noncompeting.

to which ear and note this information on the score sheet. The listener is required simply to report the words heard.

The scoring procedure for the SSW is somewhat involved. Scores obtained include the Raw SSW Score (R-SSW), which indicates the percentage of errors obtained in each of the four conditions (RNC, RC, LC, and LNC); percentage of errors by ear; and total percentage of errors. These numbers are converted to the C-SSW score, using a correction chart provided with the test forms, for interpretation. In addition, scores may be interpreted quantitatively in terms of total-ear-condition (used only for site of lesion testing with adults), and qualitatively in terms of response bias (such as reversals, order effects, and ear effects), as well as listener behavior during testing (including response time). Because scoring and interpretation for the SSW are complex, the reader is referred to the manual that accompanies the test for detailed information (Katz, 1986).

Competing Sentence Test (CST)

The CST consists of 25 sentence pairs. The target signal is presented to one ear at 35 dB SL (re: PTA) and the competing signal is presented to the opposite ear at 50 dB SL. Ten target sentences are presented to one ear, followed by ten to the other. The remaining five stimulus items may be used for practice or in order to assess the patient's ability to repeat both sentences when they are presented dichotically at equal intensity levels (50 dB SL). During administration of the CST, the clinician needs to monitor carefully the channel through which the target sentence is being presented and to make sure that the intensity levels are correct for each ear. The listener is required to repeat the target sentence only and ignore the message in the other ear.

Willeford and Burleigh (1994) suggest that the CST be scored liberally when used with children. Paraphrasing of the target sentence is allowed. Responses are scored as incorrect when the child's response either includes significant intrusions of words from the competing message or the child fails to respond at all. Using this scoring method, normative values in children ages 5 to 10 years indicate scores of 100% in the "strong" (usually right) ear, whereas scores in the "weak" (usually left) ear may range from 0 to 100%, improving with increasing age of the child. **These findings suggest a significant effect of maturation on the CST, with the ear advantage decreasing as a function of an increase in the age of the child.** However, in our own experience, this liberal approach to scoring has resulted in confusion on the part of clinicians, as well as a significant lack of standardization among clinics using the CST.

For this reason, we use the following, more stringent, scoring method with the CST, adapted from F. E. Musiek (personal communication, June, 1994). Each of the 10 target sentences is assigned a value of 10 points and is divided into quadrants, each worth 2.5 points, or 25% of the total sentence score. The child's response is scored in terms of quadrants correct. Therefore, scores of 10, 7.5, 5, 2.5, or 0 are possible for each sentence, with a possible score of 100 for all ten sentences. Table 6-3 provides an example of how sample responses to the first item of the CST may be scored.

Table 6-3
Scoring of Sample Responses to the First Item of the Competing Sentences Test

Item 1

TARGET:	I think we'll have rain today.	
COMPETING:	There was frost on the ground.	
Responses:	I think we'll have rain today.	Score: 10
	We'll have rain today.	Score: 7.5
	I think we'll have frost today.	Score: 7.5
	There was rain today.	Score: 5
	I think we have frost on the ground.	Score: 5
	There was frost today.	Score: 2.5
	I think there was frost on the ground.	Score: 2.5
	There was frost on the ground.	Score: 0
	I don't know.	Score: 0

The total ear score is achieved simply by adding the 10 sentence scores, resulting in a percent correct score for that ear. For example, for a given child, the following sentence scores may be obtained: (1) 10, (2) 7.5, (3) 10, (4) 10, (5) 2.5, (6) 5, (7) 10, (8) 7.5, (9), 10, (10) 2.5. The total ear score is computed simply by adding the scores. Therefore, in this example, the ear score would be: 10 + 7.5 + 10 + 10 + 2.5 + 5 + 10 + 7.5 + 10 + 2.5 = 85, or 85%.

Using this scoring method with 150 listeners between the ages of 8 years to adult, we have developed the following normative values (two standard deviations below the mean):

8 years to 8 years, 11 months: 39% left, 82% right

9 years to 9 years, 11 months: 74% left, 90% right

10 years to 10 years, 11 months: 88% left, 90% right

11 years to 11 years, 11 months: 90% both ears

12 years to adult: 90% both ears

As can be seen from these figures, right ear scores on the CST reach adult values by age 9, whereas left ear scores demonstrate a maturation effect until age 11. Although further research is required using this scoring method with the CST, we have found that scoring the test in this manner reduces the variability of scores within the age groups being tested, as well as provides less ambiguous, more standardized recommendations for scoring the CST.

Synthetic Sentence Identification with Contralateral Message (SSI-CCM)

Both the ipsilateral and contralateral versions of the SSI test use the same sentence stimuli: 10 third-order approximations of English sentences. The competing message consists of continuous discourse (a male speaker reading a story about the life of Davy Crockett). During administration of the SSI-CCM, it is recommended that the primary message be presented at 30 dB HL to one ear, whereas the competing message presented to the other ear may be varied from 30 dB HL (0 dB signal-to-noise ratio [S/N]) to 70 dB HL (−40 dB S/N). The listener is given a list on which all 10 sentences are printed, and he or she is required to identify the sentence heard by number.

The score is reported in terms of percent correct per ear. The CCM score is considered to be either the score obtained in the most difficult condition (−40 dB S/N), or the average of the S/N conditions tested. If a score of 100% is achieved in the –40 dB S/N condition for a given ear, no further test conditions are necessary. The degree of asymmetry between ears on the SSI-CCM generally is a better indicator of central auditory dysfunction than is absolute test performance. Adults with normal hearing tend to perform at or near 100% in all conditions as do most listeners with brainstem lesions. Listeners with temporal lobe disorders tend to do poorly in the ear contralateral to the lesion (Jerger & Jerger, 1975).

It is recommended that the SSI only be administered in cases of normal hearing sensitivity at 500, 1000, and 2000 Hz.

Dichotic Sentence Identification (DSI)

The DSI test consists of the presentation of 30 pairs of the SSI sentences. It was designed for use with hearing-impaired listeners; however, **the listener's PTA should be no poorer than 50 dB for administration of the DSI**. The test stimuli are presented at a level of 50 dB SL (re: PTA of 500, 1000, and 2000 Hz). The listener is given a printed list of the sentences, and is instructed that he or she will hear two sentences presented simultaneously, and is to indicate (by number) which sentences were heard. Results are scored in terms of percent correct per ear, which may be computed by multiplying the number correct by 3.33.

The test may be interpreted in terms of individual ear performance as well as interaural difference. Normative values for the DSI are based on the degree of hearing loss, with individual ear scores of 75% or better considered to be within normal limits regardless of PTA. As the PTA increases, the normative values decrease, so that listeners with a PTA of 49 dB may achieve an individual ear score of only 23% and still be considered to have performed within normal limits.

Normative values for interaural difference scores are, likewise, based on the PTA of the poorer ear, and are as follows:

< 39 dB poorer ear PTA – < 16% difference between ears

< 40 dB to > 59 dB poorer ear PTA – < 39% difference between ears

Detailed information regarding normative values for the DSI may be found in the accompanying test manual, as well as in Fifer et al. (1983).

Dichotic Rhyme Test (DRT)

It is recommended that the DRT be administered at 50 dB SL (re: spondee threshold). The test consists of the presentation of 30 pairs of rhyming, CVC words. Because of the close temporal alignment of the stimuli, the listener typically will hear and report just one word for each stimulus presentation, resulting in an individual ear score near 50%. **As in all dichotic speech tests, it is critical that the clinician monitor one channel at a time and make careful note of which ear each channel is routed to.**

Scores are expressed in terms of percent correct per ear. Normative data collected in our clinic from 150 normal-hearing listeners ages 8 through adult indicated no significant effect of age or ear on the DRT. Normative values (two standard deviations above and below the mean) were 32–60% per ear. Scores below or above these values for a given ear are considered abnormal. It should be noted that our findings indicated a slightly smaller range of scores than those of Musiek, Kurdziel-Schwan, Kibbe, Gollegly, Baran, and Rintelmann (1989), who reported normative values of 30–73% for the right ear and 27–60% for the left ear in a group of 115 normal-hearing adults.

Temporal Ordering Tests

As we discussed in the previous chapter, temporal ordering skills may be assessed in a variety of ways; however, many of these methods require a degree of acoustic control that is not typically available from a standard audiometer. Therefore, this section will describe two tests of temporal ordering that are currently commercially available: Pitch Patterns and Duration Patterns. The reader is referred to the References at the end of this book for sources of additional methods of evaluating temporal processing abilities. Although methods such as gap detection, two-tone ordering, and brief tone detection may require additional equipment and planning for stimulus delivery, they are well worth investigating clinically as they assess processes within the temporal domain that may otherwise go untapped. Table 6–4 provides a summary of the two tests discussed in this section.

Frequency (Pitch) Patterns

The Frequency Patterns test should be administered at an intensity of 50 dB SL (re: 1000 Hz threshold). The test consists of 60 test patterns, and stimuli are presented monaurally. Generally, it is appropriate to use half lists (30 items) per ear; however, if scores are near the criterion for normal performance, making a clinical decision difficult, the full 60-item list should be administered (Musiek, 1994). It is critical that

Table 6-4

Summary of Selected Tests of Temporal Patterning: Test Administration

Test	Stimuli	Presentation Level	Scoring
Frequency Patterns	60 patterns of triads of tones differing in frequency	50 dB per ear	% correct
Duration Patterns	60 patterns of triads of tones differing in duration	50 dB per ear	% correct

detailed instructions to the listener be given and ample practice be provided to ensure comprehension of the task.

The listener should be instructed that he or she will hear sets of three tones each that will vary in terms of pitch. The listener is to report the tonal pattern heard (e.g., high-high-low, low-high-low). The clinician should then hum various patterns while visually cueing the listener. When the listener is able to perform the task with visual cues, the clinician should then hum various patterns without cueing the listener visually. If the listener is unable to perform the task without visual cues, he or she should be reinstructed and given hummed patterns, both with and without visual cues, once again in order to determine whether the inability to perform the task is due to a lack of understanding of the test protocol or to a possible processing deficit. Once the listener has been instructed and is able to perform the task without visual cues, six practice items chosen randomly from the test itself may be given.

One ear is tested first, then the other. Additional practice is rarely necessary for testing of the second ear. Test scores are expressed in terms of percent correct per ear. Only those patterns which are reported accurately are judged to be correct.

In situations where the listener is unable to perform the task without visual cues, or performs poorly on the task, he or she may be retested while humming or singing the pattern, thus removing the linguistic labeling component. In this manner, the clinician can compare the listener's performance on the two types of tasks, providing information regarding interhemispheric integration of auditory information. Some listeners will sing the responses from the outset. In this situation, the listener should be reinstructed simply to say, not sing, the required responses.

Normative values for the compact disc version of the Frequency Patterns test suggest a cut-off score of 78% for young, normal-hearing adults (Musiek, 1994). Our own clinic normative data, using 30-item half lists and collected from 150 listeners ages 7 through adult, are in general agreement with this suggestion, with no significant effect of ear tested. Our normative values (two standard deviations below the mean) are as follows:

8 years to 8 years, 11 months: 42%

9 years to 9 years, 11 months: 63%

10 years to 10 years, 11 months: 78%

11 years to 11 years, 11 months: 78%

12 years to adult: 80%

It should be noted that **the high degree of variability found in children ages 7 years or younger suggests that the Frequency Patterns test probably would not be an appropriate measure for children below the age of 8 years**.

Duration Patterns

The Duration Patterns test is administered and scored in the same manner as the Frequency Patterns test, except that the listener is to respond in terms of the length of the stimuli (e.g., short-short-long, long-short-long). Normative values using the compact disc version of this test suggest a cut-off of 73% for young, normal-hearing adults (Musiek, 1994).

It should be noted that, as long as the stimuli are detectable by the listener, both Frequency and Duration Patterns appear to be relatively resistant to mild to moderate degrees of cochlear hearing loss (Musiek, Baran, & Pinheiro, 1990).

Monaural Low-Redundancy Speech Tests

Monaural low-redundancy speech tests continue to be one of the most popular methods of assessing central auditory function, probably due to their ease of administration and scoring. All of the tests in this section are designed to be administered monaurally at a comfortable intensity level (usually about 50–70 dB HL), the listener is instructed to repeat the words (and to guess if he or she is not sure of the word), and the tests are scored simply by calculating the percent correct per ear. However, the clinician is reminded that normative values for these tests will differ depending on the specific stimuli used. Therefore, it is crucial that clinic norms be developed for each monaural low-redundancy speech test used.

With this caveat in mind, this section will provide information about the administration and scoring of the following general categories of monaural low-redundancy speech tests: low-pass filtered speech, compressed speech, compressed speech plus reverberation, and speech-in-noise tests. Because of the inherent distortion found in many peripheral hearing losses, **monaural low redundancy speech tests should only be used for central auditory assessment in cases of normal peripheral hearing**. For a summary of the monaural low redundancy speech tests discussed in this section, the reader is referred to Table 6–5.

Low-Pass Filtered Speech (LPFS)

Two of the most commonly used LPFS tests today are the Ivey filtered words test, recommended by Willeford (1976, 1977), and the filtered NU-6 lists, available on magnetic tape and on the Tonal and Speech Materials for Auditory Perceptual Assessment compact disc (1992). Although these are not the only filtered speech tests, our discussion will focus on these two tests.

As previously discussed, both low-pass filtered speech tests are to be administered monaurally at a comfortable intensity level. The listener is instructed to repeat the words heard, and the test is scored in terms of percent correct. For the Ivey test, normative data indicate a range of 74–98% for young, normal-hearing adults (Ivey, 1969). Normative values (two standard deviations below the mean) for the low-pass filtered, NU-6 lists, using a cut-off frequency of 1000 Hz, indicate that normal performance for young adults is 75%, 80%, 83%, and 78% for NU-6 lists 1–4, respectively (Wilson & Mueller, 1984). Our own clinic normative data, collected from 150 listeners ages 8 years through adult, and using the Auditec magnetic tape version of the 1000 Hz cut-off, low-pass filtered NU-6 words, at a presentation level of 50dB HL are as follows:

8 years to 8 years, 11 months: 70%

9 years to 9 years, 11 months: 68%

Table 6–5

Summary of Selected Monaural Low-Redundancy Speech Tasks: Test Administration

Test	Stimuli	Presentation Level	Scoring
Low-Pass Filtered Speech			
Ivey	Michigan CNC words— male speaker; 500 Hz cut-off	50 dB	% correct per ear
NU-6 (tape)	NU-6 words— male speaker; 500, 700, 1000, and 1500 Hz cut-off	50 dB	% correct per ear
NU-6 (disc)	NU-6 words— female speaker 1500 Hz cut-off	50 dB ;	% correct per ear
Time Compressed Speech	NU-6 words—female speaker; 45% and 65% compression	50 dB	% correct per ear
Time Compression plus Reverberation	same as above with reverberation added	50 dB	% correct per ear
SSI-CM	10 third-order approximations of English sentences	primary: 30 dB; competing: varied between 20 dB and 50 dB	average of % % correct at 0 dB S/N and –20 dB S/N

10 years to 10 years, 11 months: 72%

11 years to 11 years, 11 months: 75%

12 years to adult: 78%.

These scores are better than those reported by Bornstein et al. (1994), who used the compact disc version of the low-pass filtered NU-6 words. Their reported values for the 1500 Hz low-pass cut-off in a group of young, normal-hearing adults at a presentation level of 65 dB HL indicated a mean score of 66.5%, with a standard deviation of 8.5%.

A primary difference between the two versions of the filtered NU-6 lists is that the taped version uses a male speaker, whereas the compact disc version uses a female speaker. These findings underline the necessity of collecting test-specific normative data.

Time Compression and Time Compression plus Reverberation

Administration and scoring for Time Compressed Speech and Time Compressed Speech plus Reverberation are as previously discussed for low-pass filtered speech. The Tonal and Speech Materials for Auditory Perceptual Assessment compact disc (1992) includes the NU-6 word lists (female speaker) at 45% and 65% time compression, and combined with 0.3-sec reverberation. As reported by Wilson et al. (1994), normative values for these conditions (two standard deviations below the mean) for a group of young, normal-hearing adults are as follows:

45% compression (55 dB HL): 86.5%

45% compression plus reverberation (55 dB HL): 72.8%

65% compression (60 dB HL): 55.5%

65% compression plus reverberation (60 dB HL): 34.9%.

These findings indicate that **the 45% compression rate may be more useful as a clinical tool, because the 65% rate appears to be quite difficult even for normal listeners**.

Speech-in-Noise Tests

Of the many tests of speech-in-noise in use today, the most comprehensive normative and validity studies have been presented for the Synthetic Sentence Identification test with Ipsilateral Competing Message (SSI-ICM). Administration of the SSI-ICM is similar to that of the SSI-CCM, except that the primary signal and competing message are premixed at various S/N ratios for monaural presentation or, as an alternative, the clinician may choose to mix the SSI-CCM into one earphone. The accompanying test manual suggests that the primary sentences be presented at 30 dB HL, and the S/N ratio be varied in 10 dB steps from 20 dB HL (+10 dB S/N) to 50 dB HL (–20 dB S/N). As in the SSI-CCM, the listener is given a printed list of the stimulus sentences and is asked to indicate (by number) which sentence was heard. The individual ear score is calculated by taking the average of the percent correct at 0 dB S/N and –20 dB S/N.

The SSI-ICM score may be compared to the SSI-CCM score for interpretation purposes. Listeners with brainstem involvement tend to do poorly on the SSI-ICM as compared to the SSI-CCM. Again, it is important that listeners demonstrate normal hearing sensitivity in the frequency range of 250 through 2000 Hz for administration of the SSI-ICM.

Other speech-in-noise tests may be employed by the clinician involved in central auditory assessment. As discussed in the previous chapter, normative data should be collected for the specific stimuli, competing signal, and signal-to-noise ratios used, and interpretation of these tests should be undertaken with caution.

Binaural Interaction Tests

As previously discussed, many of the tests of binaural interaction have been criticized on the bases of ease of administration and sensitivity. For this reason, these tests do not enjoy widespread clinical use at the present time. This section will discuss two types of binaural interaction tests that currently are available commercially and for which normative data are available: binaural fusion tests and the Masking Level Difference (MLD) (Table 6–6).

Binaural Fusion (BF) Tests

By definition, all tests of binaural interaction require a two-channel audiometer. In order to administer BF tests, the stimuli delivered to the two ears must be at equal intensity levels. This section will discuss the administration of three BF tests: the Ivey adaptation of the Matzker BF test (Ivey, 1969), and the magnetic tape and compact disc versions of the NU-6 BF test. In addition, the CVC fusion task also found on the Tonal and Speech Materials for Auditory Perceptual Assessment compact disc (1992) will be described.

The Ivey BF test, recommended by Willeford (1977), consists of two lists of 20 spondees each. The stimuli are band-passed so that the low-pass segment of each word is presented to one ear and the high-pass segment is presented to the other. The listener is required to repeat the words heard, and the test is scored by calculating the percent correct.

Normative data were collected from adults using a presentation level of 25 dB SL (re: pure-tone thresholds at 500 and 2000 Hz), and

Table 6–6
Summary of Selected Binaural Interaction Tests: Test Administration

Test	Stimuli	Presentation Level	Scoring
Binaural Fusion			
Ivey	spondaic words; low-pass to one ear; high-pass to the other	25–30 dB SL	% correct per ear upon resynthesis
NU-6	NU-6 words; low-pass to one ear; high-pass to the other	30–35 dB SL	% correct per ear
CVC Fusion	segmented CVC words; consonants to one ear; vowels to the other	30 dB HL	% correct per ear
MLD	stimuli may be tonal or speech	levels and S/N ratios vary depending upon stimulus	SπNø threshold minus SøNø threshold

from children using a presentation level of 30 dB SL (Ivey, 1969; Willeford & Burleigh, 1985). These normative studies, as well as that done by White (1977), indicated that the words included in List 2 were less familiar and, thus, resulted in lower scores in children than did the use of List 1. Therefore, Willeford and Burleigh (1985) suggested that 10% be added to the score obtained from the use of List 2 for compensation purposes.

Normative data (with 10% added to the List 2 scores for children) indicate mean scores near or above 75% for children ages 6 through 8 years, near 80% for children age 9 years, and near 90% for 10-year-old children and adults (Willeford & Burleigh, 1985).

Administration of the monosyllabic BF task using the NU-6 word lists is similar to that of the Ivey BF test. As mentioned in the previous chapter, it has been suggested that the use of monosyllabic rather than spondaic words in BF testing may further reduce the redundancy of the signal and, thus, result in greater sensitivity (Smith & Resnick, 1972). Both the magnetic tape and the compact disc versions should be administered at a comfortable listening level. Normative data reported by Wilson and Mueller (1984) for the taped version suggest a cut-off (two standard deviations below the mean) of approximately 65% for young, normal-hearing adults.

Using the compact disc version, results of normative studies for the BF condition demonstrated a performance-intensity function essentially identical to that of standard NU-6 word recognition performance, with a cut-off (two standard deviations below the mean) of 86.6% at a presentation level of 36 dB HL for young, normal-hearing adults. When a presentation level of 30 dB HL was used, the normal cut-off was reduced to 66.4% (mean = 88.4%, standard deviation = 11.0%; Bornstein et al., 1994). Further research is needed in order to define normative values for children using the NU-6 word lists in a BF paradigm.

A final BF test that has recently been described by Wilson (1994) is the CVC fusion task included on the Tonal and Speech Materials for Auditory Perceptual Assessment compact disc (1992). In this task, the carrier phrase and vowel segment of the word is presented to one ear and the consonant segments are presented to the other ear, thus preserving the spectral characteristics of the stimulus. Therefore, unlike the other BF tests discussed in this section, the CVC fusion task was designed to be relatively resistant to peripheral hearing loss. Normative data suggest a cut-off of 87.4% (two standard deviations below the mean) at a presentation level of 30 dB HL for young, normal-hearing adults. Further research is needed using hearing-impaired and neurological populations. It should be noted that the utility of BF tests in central auditory assessment is questionable, as these tests characteristically are fraught with acoustic problems (F. E. Musiek, personal communication, November, 1995).

Masking Level Difference (MLD)

A listener's performance on MLD testing will depend on the type of stimuli and masker and the specific administration protocols used. All MLD testing, however, is designed to compare the listener's signal threshold for a variety of masking conditions. A description of the masking conditions used in MLD investigations has been provided in Chapter 2.

The MLD for pure tones may be as high as 10 to 15 dB, depending on the frequency of the signal and the characteristics of the masking stimulus. Many commercial audiometers are manufactured with the built-in capacity to perform pure-tone MLD testing, and the reader is referred to the equipment manual for specific administration protocols.

The MLD for speech typically is smaller than that for pure tones. This section will describe administration of the premixed, spondaic

MLD test included on the Tonal and Speech Materials for Auditory Perceptual Assessment compact disc (1992). For this test, the listener is given a printed list of the 10 spondees. First, testing in the SøNø condition is completed by routing one channel of the compact disc to one channel of the audiometer at a comfortable listening level (50 dB HL). The listener is asked to indicate which of the words was heard. Four words are presented for each of 16 signal-to-noise ratios, increasing in 2 dB increments from 0 dB S/N to –30 dB S/N. It should be noted that, due to the competing noise, clinician monitoring of the stimulus words is impossible; therefore, the words have been imbedded in noise bursts which allow the clinician to keep track of when the stimulus is being presented.

Testing in the SπNø condition is done by routing each channel of the compact disc to the corresponding channel of the audiometer (left channel to left earphone, right channel to right earphone) at the same presentation level as the SøNø condition and, again, beginning with the 0 dB S/N condition. Testing continues until the listener fails to respond correctly to all words at two consecutive signal-to-noise ratios. Thresholds in both conditions are computed using the following equation:

$$\text{Threshold} = (\text{dB HL}) + 1 - (\text{number of words reported correctly} / 2)$$

The MLD is calculated simply by subtracting the threshold value obtained in the SπNø condition from that obtained in theSøNø condition.

Wilson, Zizz, and Sperry (1994) reported mean MLD values of 7.8 dB and 8.8 dB for presentation levels of 65 dB SPL (45 dB HL) and 85 dB SPL (65 dB HL), respectively, in a group of young, normal-hearing listeners. Standard deviations were on the order of 2.1 dB and 2.7 dB for the two intensity levels. Because 90% of the normal listeners studied exhibited MLDs larger than 5.5 dB, the authors suggested that MLDs smaller than 5.5 dB should be considered abnormal for normal-hearing listeners.

Summary

This chapter has described recommended behavioral procedures for comprehensive central auditory processing assessment, including equipment needed, components of the assessment process, choosing test battery components, and specific administration protocols and normative values for several tests of central auditory function in common clinical use today. It was not our intent to imply that the tests listed in this section are the only ones that may be utilized, or that the assessment protocols described herein are the only manner in which central auditory evaluation may be conducted. Rather, the purpose of this chapter was to provide the clinician entering into central auditory assessment practical information for immediate use in the clinical arena. Again, it should be emphasized that the information contained in the previous chapters should be studied carefully prior to attempting any evaluation of central auditory function, and each clinician should collect normative data specific to the test tools used in his or her individual clinic for interpretation purposes.

Review Questions

1. List the equipment needed for comprehensive behavioral central auditory assessment.
2. List the steps that should be included in a comprehensive central auditory processing evaluation.
3. Discuss the factors that will affect the choice of which tests to include in a central auditory test battery.
4. Briefly outline the recommended stimulus presentation level, instructions to the listener, and method of scoring for the following behavioral tests of central auditory function:

Dichotic Digits	Dichotic CVs
Staggered Spondaic Words	Competing Sentence Test
SSI-CCM	Dichotic Sentence Identification
Dichotic Rhyme Test	Frequency Patterns
Duration Patterns	Low-Pass Filtered Speech
Time-Compressed Speech	SSI-ICM
Binaural Fusion	CVC Fusion
Masking Level Difference	

5. Which of the above listed tests may be suitable for use in cases of peripheral hearing loss?
6. In review, identify the process or processes assessed by each of the above-listed tests.

CHAPTER

SEVEN

Interpretation of Central Auditory Assessment Results

T he interpretation of central auditory assessment results may be undertaken with a variety of goals in mind and, depending on the desired outcome, the interpretation process may be involved and lengthy, or quick and simple. It is our contention that the simple identification of the presence of CAPD does not provide sufficient useful information upon which to base a rehabilitative program. Instead, interpretation should be entered into with the mind set of a detective attempting to solve a complex mystery, and all aspects of the assessment data should be analyzed so that the greatest amount of information may be obtained. To accomplish this task, the clinician must be able to relate the assessment findings to neuroscience, thus interpreting the given data in terms of how they deviate from the manner in which the typical CANS functions.

Because CAPD is a heterogeneous disorder, with a large degree of variability and individualization within it, it is not possible to address all possible combinations of findings for interpretation purposes. Therefore, this chapter will provide the reader with a variety of ways in which the assessment data may be looked at, from simple identification of a disorder to the development of an auditory learning profile. In addition, types of management recommendations appropriate for specific assessment findings will be included; however, actual examples of rehabilitative activities and management strategies will be provided in Chapter 8.

Learning Objectives

After studying this chapter, the reader should be able to

1. Identify several questions that may be answered by the assessment results
2. Discuss site-of-lesion interpretation of central auditory assessment results
3. Discuss process-based interpretation of central auditory assessment results
4. Identify and describe four basic subprofiles of central auditory processing disorders in children.

What Is the Question?

In Chapter 5, we discussed the rationale for a test battery approach to central auditory assessment. At that time, we emphasized that the question to be answered by the assessment process will have a major impact on the number and types of tests chosen. Logically, the question to be answered also will influence the manner in which the test results are interpreted.

In its simplest form, the central auditory assessment should provide information regarding the presence or absence of some type of central auditory processing disorder, thus answering the common question of whether the child in question "has CAPD." As we will see in the next section, however, identifying of the presence of a central auditory disorder is not as simple as it as it appears on the surface. Nor does simple identification aid the clinician in answering the question that will inevitably follow: Can we do anything about it?

To answer this question, several types of information must be obtained from the available assessment data. First, in order to develop a management plan that is as deficit-specific as possible, the clinician will need to determine what auditory process or processes are most likely dysfunctional in a given child. We call this procedure *process-based interpretation*. By identifying the dysfunctional process(es), we then are able to develop a management program that will build upon the child's auditory strengths while specifically targeting the weaknesses, thus resulting in greater efficiency and individualization.

Second, the clinician should be able to identify, as near as possible, the site-of-dysfunction within the CANS. This information is helpful in determining whether additional medical follow-up is indicated, as in the case of a possible neurological disorder or space-occupying lesion, as well as assisting in the development of management strategies.

Finally, assessment results should be related to information regarding educational, cognitive, speech/language, social, and other arenas. The use of subprofiles of auditory processing disorders is particularly helpful in determining the impact of a given CAPD on a child's quality of life, as well as providing direction for meaningful intervention.

In conclusion, **data from a central auditory assessment may be analyzed for the following four general purposes: identification of the presence or absence of a disorder, identification of underlying processes that may be disordered, site-of-lesion (or site-of-dysfunction) information, and, in conjunction with academic and other measures, the development of a CAPD subprofile.** By approaching the interpretation of central auditory assessment results from a variety of perspectives, the clinician helps to ensure that the information obtained from the assessment is as applicable and meaningful as possible, so that a deficit-specific management program that addresses the individual child's difficulties may be developed.

Identification of Central Auditory Processing Disorders

The decision as to whether results of a comprehensive central assessment indicate that a CAPD is, in fact, present will depend on a variety of factors. Perhaps the most important of these factors is the criterion for abnormal performance chosen by the clinician. Depending upon whether the criterion chosen is strict or lax, the interpretation of results of a test battery, on the whole, may differ significantly.

Choosing a criterion level for abnormal performance involves deciding how many, and to what extent, individual test measures should be positive for the disorder before a determination that the disorder is present may be made. To illustrate, let us consider a situation in which five central tests are utilized together in a test battery approach. If we decide that performance outside of the norm on any single test tool alone constitutes a positive finding on the entire battery, then this would be considered a *lax* criterion. If, on the other hand, results of all five tests must be abnormal for the battery to be positive, then the criterion is *strict*. Finally, if two, three, or four tests must be positive for CAPD before presence of disorder is determined, the criterion is said to be *intermediate*. Obviously, the choice of a strict, lax, or intermediate criterion will have a significant impact on the interpretation of the entire test battery.

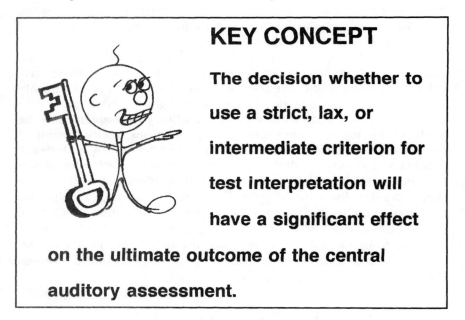

KEY CONCEPT

The decision whether to use a strict, lax, or intermediate criterion for test interpretation will have a significant effect on the ultimate outcome of the central auditory assessment.

Just as it is important for the clinician to choose individual tests that exhibit the greatest sensitivity, it is critical that the criterion for abnormal performance yield as many hits as possible, while avoiding false positives and misses. What, then, would be the ideal criterion for identifying CAPD in the educational setting? Again, the answer to this question would depend on the ultimate goal of the assessment process.

The obvious approach, and one that we hear advocated frequently by our fellow clinicians, is to establish an intermediate criterion in which results of at least two individual test tools, combined with educational findings, must be abnormal for a positive finding of CAPD to be made. However, there is an inherent drawback to this type of approach. One of the purposes of using a test battery approach to central assessment is so that different tests that assess different processes may be included. **If each test within the battery assesses a different process under the central auditory processing umbrella, is it not possible that, in a given child, one underlying process may be disordered while the others remain quite functional, resulting in abnormal performance on only one test measure?**

Indeed, we find this frequently to be the case when assessing children for possible CAPD. Two children with similar presenting behavioral characteristics of CAPD may exhibit dysfunction in different underlying processes, singularly or in any combination. Therefore, the establishment of an intermediate criterion for interpretation in which two or more tests must be abnormal for the finding to be positive would be inadequate for identifying the presence of a single disordered process that, nonetheless, significantly impacts the child's ability to function and learn.

For this reason, we advocate a lax criterion for interpretation in which an abnormal finding on any given test tool, *combined with significant educational and behavioral findings*, may be considered as evidence of CAPD. **Therefore, in order for the presence of CAPD to be identified, it must be established that (1) one or more underlying auditory processes are disordered or delayed, and (2) the disorder or delay, in all likelihood, has a significant impact on the child's ability to function and/or learn.**

There are some inherent difficulties in this approach, particularly in the determination of significant impact. It may not always be possible to establish a direct one-to-one relationship between a given presenting disorder and educational/behavioral findings. A child may exhibit concomitant physical or behavioral disorders, or disorders in other sensory processing systems, making it difficult or impossible to separate out the effects of the auditory complaint.

Nor is this separation of effects always necessary, or even desirable. When undertaking central auditory assessment from a whole child approach, it is important to realize that the auditory disorder may be merely one piece in the overall puzzle. The clinician's task, therefore, is not simply to identify the presence of an auditory disorder but to describe the disorder and help in determining which aspects of the child's overall presenting picture may be attributed, at least in part, to the given disorder. It is in these latter two tasks that process-based interpretation and the development of subprofiles of CAPD, to be discussed later in this chapter, come into play.

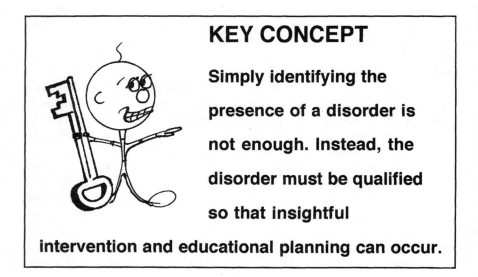

KEY CONCEPT

Simply identifying the presence of a disorder is not enough. Instead, the disorder must be qualified so that insightful intervention and educational planning can occur.

In conclusion, the identification of CAPD will depend on the criterion established for abnormal performance on a central auditory test battery. We recommend that the criterion for presence of CAPD be relatively lax, necessitating abnormal performance on one or more tests of central auditory function combined with significant educational and behavioral findings. The identification of CAPD, however, is just the first step in the overall interpretation process. To determine the relative impact of a given auditory processing disorder on a child's educational and behavioral functioning, as well as to develop a plan for management, the disorder must be described in functional, process-based terms, and the findings must be tied to the child's presenting educational and behavioral complaints.

Process-Based Interpretation

As mentioned in Chapter 2, The ASHA Task Force on Central Auditory Processing defined auditory processing as the auditory system mechanisms and processes responsible for behavioral phenomena such as sound localization and lateralization, auditory discrimination, auditory pattern recognition, temporal aspects of audition, and auditory performance decrements with competing and degraded acoustic signals (ASHA, 1995). **Process-based interpretation refers to the assessment** of these underlying processes with an eye toward the development of an individual auditory profile that will identify auditory strengths and weaknesses. Depending on the test tools chosen, process-based interpretation may provide information regarding the individual's processing ability in a variety of areas, including auditory closure and decoding, binaural separation and integration, temporal patterning or ordering, binaural interaction, and interhemispheric transfer of auditory information.

This section will discuss the main components of process-based interpretation. Again, the reader should be aware that interpretation of central auditory tests is not without limitations and should be undertaken with caution. In addition, we do not wish to suggest that the processes discussed herein are the only ones that may be assessed by tests of central auditory function, nor is the method discussed here the only manner in which tests of central auditory function may be interpreted. The information provided in this section will serve to provide the clinician with a starting point for approaching central auditory interpretation. Information regarding behavioral and academic characteristics will be provided in the section on subprofiles of auditory processing disorders, later in this chapter.

Auditory Closure (Decoding)

Auditory closure refers to the ability of the normal listener to utilize intrinsic and extrinsic redundancy to fill in missing or distorted portions of the auditory signal and recognize the whole message. The term *auditory decoding* refers to deciphering the components of an auditory message. Thus, both auditory closure and decoding play a part in the listener's ability to extrapolate the whole message from the individual components. For purposes of this section, we will refer to the act of deciphering and then filling in the missing components of an auditory message as auditory closure.

Auditory closure plays an important role in everyday listening activities. Rarely can our everyday listening environment be considered ideal. Instead, we must contend continually with background noise, regional dialects, conversation partners who speak with quiet voices or less than perfect diction, and other factors that make comprehension of auditory messages difficult. It is our ability to rely upon extrinsic and intrinsic redundancy of the signal that allows us to comprehend the overall message and engage in meaningful conversation.

Extrinsic factors that aid in our ability to achieve auditory closure include knowledge of the topic, familiarity with the vocabulary utilized, knowledge of phonemic aspects of speech, and familiarity with the rules of language, among others. Thus, if we are in a situation in which the topic of conversation is known, the speaker is using familiar vocabulary, syntax, and semantics, and the environment is acoustically adequate, then we need expend very little energy in order to follow the conversation. If, on the other hand, one or more of these factors is missing, then we must rely upon the other factors, as well as upon the repeated representation of characteristics of the auditory signal throughout the CANS (intrinsic redundancy), in order to achieve auditory closure.

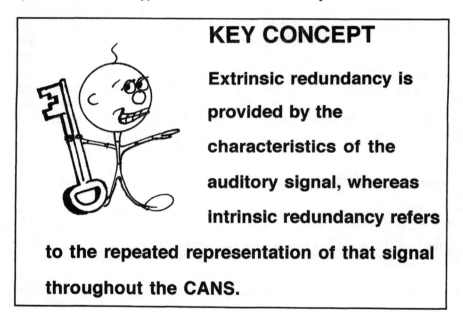

KEY CONCEPT

Extrinsic redundancy is provided by the characteristics of the auditory signal, whereas intrinsic redundancy refers to the repeated representation of that signal throughout the CANS.

For example, those of us in the field of speech and hearing often have been in the situation of conversing with a client who exhibits an articulatory speech impairment. Depending on the degree of distortion in the acoustic signal, the phonemic aspects of the signal will be available to us in varying degrees. Therefore, we must rely upon knowledge of the conversational topic, vocabulary, and rules of language in order to understand what the speaker is saying. If any of these factors are taken away as well, the listening task becomes much more difficult. Another familiar example would be the situation in which a parent is attempting to decipher the request of a small child in whom spoken language is just beginning to emerge. The child's articulation may be distorted, and he or she may utilize immature language forms and word approximations. If the topic also is unknown, the parent may be rendered completely unable to comprehend the child's request, resulting in frustration on both sides.

An individual with an auditory closure processing deficit exhibits a breakdown in the intrinsic redundancy of the CANS, thus reducing or eliminating the repeated representation of the incoming signal throughout the auditory pathways. Therefore, anything that reduces the extrinsic redundancy of the auditory signal may interfere with the individual's ability to achieve auditory closure. At its most basic level, an auditory closure deficit may interfere with the ability to decode the phonemic aspects of a speech signal. Conversely, the listener with an auditory closure deficit may have no difficulty understanding speech in an ideal listening environment; however, he or she may exhibit great difficulty in background noise or with unfamiliar speakers.

On tests of central auditory function, the individual with an auditory closure deficit will perform poorly on monaural low redundancy speech tests, such as Low-Pass Filtered Speech or Time Compressed Speech, as well as speech-in-noise tests. If the deficit is severe, word recognition skills in quiet may be affected.

Management of an auditory closure deficit would include methods of improving access to auditory information through environmental modifications, activities targeted at auditory closure from phonemic to sentence levels, preteaching of new concepts, and frequent repetition of key messages, among others. If phonemic decoding is affected, consonant and/or vowel discrimination training may be indicated. Specific management techniques will be provided in Chapter 8. Table 7–1 provides an overview of the characteristics of a deficit in auditory closure.

Table 7-1
Primary Characteristics of Deficits in Auditory Closure

Principle Feature:	A breakdown in the intrinsic redundancy of the CANS
Behavioral Characteristics:	Difficulty filling in the missing components when part of the auditory signal is inaccessible
Central Test Findings:	Poor performance on monaural low redundancy speech tasks
Suggestions for Management:	Improve acoustic access to auditory information. Phoneme training may be indicated

Binaural Separation and Integration

Binaural separation refers to the ability of a listener to process an auditory message coming into one ear while ignoring a disparate message being presented to the opposite ear at the same time. A different, but related, ability is that of *binaural integration*, or the ability of a listener to process information being presented to both ears simultaneously, with the information presented to each ear being different. The terms binaural separation and integration are not to be confused with the term *binaural interaction*, which is a brainstem function and will be discussed later in this section. Rather, the terms binaural separation and integration, as used here, specifically refer to processes that are typically assessed through the use of dichotic speech tests.

Binaural separation and integration are processes that are critical to everyday listening, particularly in a school environment. Situations arise continually in which a listener is required to ignore linguistic information from one source while focusing his or her attention on a primary message. Consider, for example, the situation in which a child is sitting quietly in a classroom, attempting to listen to the teacher provide instructions while, at the same time, a student next to the child is talking either to the child or to another student. In order for the child to hear the information being presented by the teacher, he or she must be able to ignore the adjacent student's verbalizations, an activity that relies, in part, upon the process of binaural separation.

Binaural integration, likewise, comes into play in everyday listening situations. An example of a listening situation in which the process of binaural integration would be relied upon might be that of a mother who is attempting to carry on a phone conversation while simultaneously listening to the demands of her child, a situation that occurs frequently during the normal course of parenting. In this situation, the mother must be able to process information from both sources, thus utilizing the process of binaural integration.

Therefore, **dysfunction in the processes of binaural separation and integration may be expressed in the behavioral symptom of difficulty hearing in background noise or when more than one person is talking at the same time**. It should be noted that the behavioral characteristic of difficulty hearing in noise has been mentioned previously as a symptom of auditory closure deficit and will be mentioned again as a symptom of a deficit in binaural interaction. In fact, difficulty hearing in noise is one of the most common complaints of individuals with CAPD. The clinician cannot automatically assume the cause of such a complaint, as **two children who present with the identical behavioral symptom may exhibit dysfunction in two entirely different underlying processes.** It is for this reason that careful, systematic assessment be undertaken in a test battery approach, so that identification of the underlying deficit may be attained in each case.

The child with binaural separation/integration dysfunction will perform poorly on dichotic speech tests. The determination of which underlying process is disordered (e.g., separation, integration, or a combination of both) may be made by the behavioral requirements of the tests themselves. For example, test tools such as Dichotic Digits and Dichotic Consonant-Vowels (CVs) require the listener to report all auditory information heard, thus tapping the process of binaural integration. Conversely, Competing Sentences requires the listener to ignore the information being presented to one ear while reporting the sentence heard in the target ear, thus assessing binaural separation abilities.

A further purpose of dichotic speech tests such as those mentioned above is in the evaluation of neuromaturation and interhemispheric transfer of information, which will be discussed later in this chapter.

Approaches appropriate for management of binaural separation and/or integration dysfunction would include environmental adaptations that improve the listener's access to target auditory information while decreasing competing signals, and the teaching of compensatory strategies to assist the listener in directing attention. Again, specific management strategies will be discussed in Chapter 8. Characteristics of a deficit in binaural separation and/or integration are presented in Table 7–2.

Table 7–2

Primary Characteristics of Deficits in Binaural Separation and/or Integration

Principle Features:	Difficulty in processing an auditory message in one ear while ignoring a competing message in the other (separation)
	Difficulty processing information presented to both ears simultaneously (integration)
Behavioral Characteristics:	Difficulty hearing in background noise or when more than one person is talking at the same time
Central Test Findings:	Poor performance on dichotic speech tests
Suggestions for Management:	Decrease signal-to-noise ratio within the environment; teach compensatory strategies re: directing attention

Temporal Patterning

The term *temporal patterning*, as used here, specifically refers to a listener's ability to recognize acoustic contours. Several auditory processes contribute to this ability, including discrimination of differences in auditory stimuli, sequencing of auditory stimuli, gestalt pattern perception, and trace memory (Musiek & Chermak, 1995; Musiek et al. 1980). Of the tests of central auditory function discussed in Chapter 6, only Frequency Patterns and Duration Patterns may be considered tests of temporal patterning.

The ability to recognize the acoustic contour of a signal greatly contributes to a listener's ability to extract and utilize prosodic aspects of speech, such as rhythm, stress, and intonation. Relative differences in stress within a sentence allow the listener to identify the key words. Alterations in stressed words within a sentence may change the meaning of the sentence as a whole (e.g., *You* can't go with us vs. You can't go with *us*), and changes in syllabic stress may alter the meaning of an individual word (e.g., *pro*ject vs. pro*ject*). Intonation provides clues regarding the intent of the message as well as the emotional status of the speaker (e.g., surprised, happy, angry, sad). Rhythm of speech may also affect the meaning of the utterance (e.g., He saw the *snowdrift* by the window vs. He saw the *snow drift* by the window). In short, prosody provides a wealth of information that cannot be obtained from the words of a message alone.

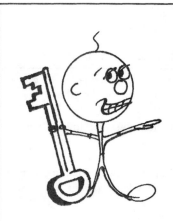

KEY CONCEPT

Cerebral lesions typically result in contralateral deficits on dichotic and monaural low redundancy speech tests, as well as bilateral deficits on tests of temporal patterning.

Children with deficits in acoustic contour recognition and temporal patterning may exhibit difficulty recognizing and using prosodic aspects of speech. They may have difficulty extracting key words from a spoken message and may be unable to discriminate subtle differences in meaning brought about by changes in relative stress and intonation. In addition, these children may, themselves, be "flat" readers or be somewhat monotonic in their own speech. Sequencing of critical elements within a message, as well as individual speech sounds within a word, may be an issue. These children tend to perform poorly on Frequency Patterns and Duration Patterns testing in both the linguistic labeling and humming response conditions.

Management approaches that may be useful for children with temporal patterning difficulty include prosody training and instruction in the extraction of key words from a message. In addition, reading aloud daily with specific emphasis on intonation, stress, and rhythm may help to enhance awareness of prosodic aspects of speech. The reader is referred to Chapter 8 for specific management suggestions. Table 7–3 summarizes the information presented in this section.

Binaural Interaction

As discussed in Chapter 2, auditory functions that rely upon binaural interaction include localization and lateralization of auditory stimuli, binaural release from masking, detection of signals in noise, and binaural fusion. Of these functions, **two are particularly important in everyday listening situations: localization of auditory stimuli and detection of signals in noise**.

Table 7-3

Primary Characteristics of Deficits in Temporal Patterning

Principle Feature:	Difficulty recognizing acoustic contours
Behavioral Characteristics:	Difficulty recognizing and using prosodic features of speech
Central Test Findings:	Poor performance on tests of temporal patterning in both the linguistic labeling and humming conditions
Suggestions for Management:	Prosody training

It has been shown earlier in this section that the ability to understand speech in noise is affected by the processes of auditory closure and binaural separation. However, to understand a signal in noise, the signal must first be detected. For this to occur, the listener must, at a preconscious level, be able to localize the sources of both the target and competing signal. As previously discussed, the further apart the target and competing signals are, the easier this task is. As the target and competing signals move closer together, it becomes more difficult to locate the sources of the stimuli. Therefore, detection of the target signal, likewise, becomes more difficult.

Localization and lateralization of an auditory stimulus is a function of binaural interaction, or the way in which the two ears work together. This ability may be significantly affected by peripheral hearing loss, particularly when the hearing loss is asymmetrical. In addition, an auditory processing disorder at the brainstem level may affect the listener's ability to localize auditory stimuli. **The primary behavioral characteristic of this type of processing disorder is the inability to detect speech in a noisy background**.

Tests of brainstem function, including the Masking Level Difference (MLD), may be used to identify brainstem dysfunction that may affect localization and lateralization ability and, thus, the ability to detect speech in noise. In addition, speech-in-noise tests, while not without significant limitations, may provide descriptive information regarding the listener's ability to recognize words in a background of noise.

Management of auditory processing disorders that affect the listener's ability to detect speech in noise should focus primarily on environmental adaptations that will improve access to the target signal while reducing the background competition. In addition, specific skills training in localization and lateralization of varied auditory stimuli, as well as selective attention training, may be useful. Characteristics of binaural interaction deficits are summarized in Table 7–4.

Neuromaturation and Interhemispheric Transfer of Information

As discussed in Chapter 3, the final portion of the CANS to attain maturation is the corpus callosum, which is responsible for interaction between cerebral hemispheres. Theoretically, a neuromaturational delay will result in findings on tests of central auditory function that

Table 7-4

Primary Characteristics of Deficits in Binaural Interaction

Principle Feature:	A breakdown in the brainstem's ability to process binaural cues
Behavioral Characteristics:	Difficulty localizing and lateralizing auditory information, leading to difficulty in detecting signals in noise
Central Test Findings:	Abnormally reduced Masking Level Differences, abnormal findings on Auditory Brainstem Response
Suggestions for Management:	Decrease signal-to-noise ratio within the environment; refer for medical follow-up to rule out neurological pathology

are similar to those of corpus callosal involvement. **Specifically, the pattern that is characteristic of delayed neuromaturation and/or corpus callosal involvement is left ear suppression on dichotic speech tasks combined with poor performance on tests of temporal patterning**, although performance on these tests may improve when the listener is asked to hum the responses, thus removing the linguistic labeling component (Musiek, Kibbe, & Baran, 1984).

A child with delayed neuromaturation may present with any combination of behavioral auditory complaints. Therefore, it is critical that management strategies be designed that target the individual child's auditory and educational difficulties specifically. In addition, rehabilitative exercises that require interaction between cerebral hemispheres may be useful in improving interhemispheric processing. Examples of interhemispheric exercises are provided in Chapter 8. Finally, enrolling in singing and musical instrument lessons, both of which require efficient interhemispheric interaction, would be an appropriate recommendation for a child with a neuromaturational delay. A summary of behavioral characteristics and suggested management approaches for neuromaturational delay can be found in Table 7–5.

Determination of Site of Lesion

The high degree of redundancy within the CANS makes absolute determination of site-of-lesion difficult when tests of central auditory func-

Table 7-5
Primary Characteristics of Delayed Neuromaturation

Principle Feature:	Delay in myelination, particularly of the corpus callosum
Behavioral Characteristics:	Behavioral symptoms are variable and can include any combination of auditory complaints
Central Test Findings:	Left ear deficit on dichotic speech tests combined with bilateral deficit on temporal patterning tests requiring linguistic labeling of stimuli
Suggestions for Management:	Management should target specific auditory and educational difficulties; interhemispheric exercises may be useful to speed maturation

tion are relied upon for this determination. However, it is possible to consider general trends in the central auditory test data and, in many circumstances, to determine the level of the CANS at which the dysfunction is occurring. This determination is important for a number of reasons, including identification of the need for a medical referral, as well as in monitoring effects of rehabilitative activities and tracking changes in the effects of lesions (Musiek & Lamb, 1994).

This section will provide an overview of general trends of central auditory tests that are characteristic of dysfunction at the brainstem, cerebral, and interhemispheric levels of the CANS. It should be noted that, if a neurological lesion or any condition requiring medical follow-up is suspected, the clinician should refer the individual for such follow-up.

Brainstem Lesions

As previously mentioned, many of the behavioral tests of brainstem function have been criticized on the bases of poor sensitivity and specificity. Three behavioral measures of central auditory function have demonstrated good sensitivity for brainstem lesions: the Synthetic Sentence Identification Test with Ipsilateral Competing Message (SSI-ICM; Jerger & Jerger, 1975), Masking Level Difference (MLD; Olsen & Noffsinger, 1976), and Staggered Spondaic Words (SSW; Katz, 1977). In addition, Musiek and Guerkink (1982) reported that, while the sensitivity of procedures such as rapid alternating speech perception (RASP) and binaural fusion appeared questionable for identifying brainstem dysfunction, other tests of central auditory function did appear to be sensitive to both brainstem and cortical lesions, including Dichotic Digits, Competing Sentences, and Low-Pass Filtered Speech. However, differentiation between brainstem and cortical dysfunction could not be determined on the basis of performance on these latter three tests.

When undertaking brainstem assessment, the clinician also should keep in mind other tests of brainstem function, including acoustic reflex measures and speech audiometry. In addition, **the value of electrophysiological measures, particularly Auditory Brainstem Response (ABR), in the assessment of brainstem function cannot be overemphasized**. Musiek, Gollegly, Kibbe, and Reeves (1989) reported that, when using a battery of seven central tests in listeners with multiple sclerosis, the combination of ABR along with either the MLD or Dichotic Digits test demonstrated the same sensitivity for brainstem dysfunction as did the use of the entire battery.

ABR results in cases of pontine brainstem lesions, in general, tend to be abnormal for the ear ipsilateral to the lesion (Chiappa, 1983). On the other hand, a large degree of variability in behavioral tests may be found depending on the location, size, and type of the lesion, and abnormal findings may be contralateral, ipsilateral, or bilateral.

When assessing central auditory function in children, it should be kept in mind that, although rare, space-occupying lesions and other neurological involvement of the brainstem can and do occur. Therefore, we rely on the following rule of thumb: **If results of our behavioral test battery, along with acoustic reflex measures, suggest the possibility of brainstem involvement in a school-age child, we routinely refer the child for ABR and additional medical follow-up**.

Cerebral Lesions

The term *cerebral* is used to denote lesions that affect the gray and/or white matter of the brain. Musiek and Lamb (1994) used the terms *cortical* and *hemispheric* to differentiate between the two types of cerebral lesions. Cortical refers to the gray matter of the brain alone, whereas hemispheric refers to lesions that affect both the white and gray matter.

Typically, cerebral lesions manifest themselves in deficits in the ear contralateral to the lesion. This is true for dichotic listening tasks as well as for monaural low-redundancy speech tasks. However, performance on temporal patterning tests, such as Frequency and Duration Patterns, typically is nonlateralizing. That is, cerebral lesions tend to result in bilateral deficits on these types of tests, regardless of the site of lesion. Therefore, laterality information cannot be obtained from tests of temporal patterning.

Qualitatively, performance of listeners with temporal lobe lesions may differ from that of normal listeners or listeners with brainstem lesions. Thompson and Abel (1992a, b) reported that listeners with temporal lobe lesions generally demonstrated greater difficulty on temporal patterning and consonant discrimination tasks than did listeners with acoustic tumors and normal controls. In addition, listeners with temporal lobe lesions required a greater response time than did the other two groups. In all cases, listeners with lesions of the left temporal lobe tended to demonstrate greater performance deficits.

Interhemispheric Lesions

As shown in Chapter 1, the fibers of the corpus callosum, responsible for interhemispheric transfer of information, extend well into the cerebral hemispheres. Therefore, it is quite possible that a cortical lesion may affect fibers of the corpus callosum, as well.

Typically, lesions of the corpus callosum result in a left ear deficit on dichotic speech tasks combined with a bilateral deficit on tests of temporal patterning when the listener is required to respond verbally. As discussed in the previous section regarding neuromaturation, performance on temporal patterning tests improves when the linguistic labeling component of the response is removed by requiring the listener to hum the response. Monaural low-redundancy speech tests remain generally unaffected by corpus callosal lesions (Musiek, Kibbe, & Baran, 1984).

Subprofiles of Central Auditory Processing Disorders

It has been emphasized again and again throughout this book that the whole child must be taken into account in order to assess the contribution of a given CAPD to academic, communicative, and associated difficulties. Myklebust (1954) stated that, when assessing children with auditory problems, a differential diagnosis is necessary because children having different types of auditory problems will vary greatly in their individual needs. To address these individual needs, we must first strive to define the underlying problem in as precise a manner as possible. Likewise, Luria (1973) wrote that all activity results from the combined interplay of interdependent brain units. Regardless of whether we approach audition, language, and learning from a bottom-up or top-down approach, it must be recognized that some degree of interdependence exists in both models. Therefore, our interpretation of central auditory findings and recommendations for management should reflect this interdependency. In other words, **a multidisciplinary approach which takes into account the individual child's auditory, language, learning, and associated characteristics is critical to appropriate interpretation and management** (Ferre, 1994).

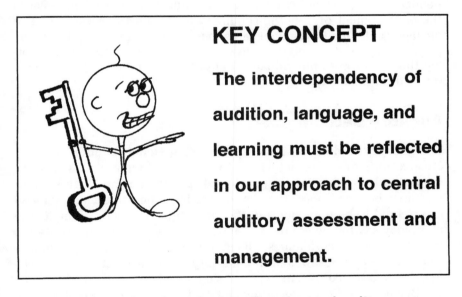

KEY CONCEPT

The interdependency of audition, language, and learning must be reflected in our approach to central auditory assessment and management.

In recent years, the use of subprofiles of central auditory processing deficits has begun to gain wider acceptance clinically (Ferre, 1992; Katz, 1992; Katz, Stecker, & Masters, 1994; Musiek, Gollegly, & Ross, 1985). Each of these authors has approached subprofiling of CAPD from a slightly different perspective. For example, Katz et al. (1994) suggested that categories of CAPD be made up of skills that cluster with specific language and communication deficits. In their "Buffalo Model," the authors separated CAPD and language/communication deficits into four categories: Phonemic Decoding, Tolerance-Fading Memory, Integration, and Organization.

A similar system of categorizing CAPD was introduced by Ferre (1987; 1992) and expanded upon by Bellis and Ferre (in press). In this model, electrophysiological and anatomical data are combined with educational, communicative, behavioral, and central auditory processing findings to separate children with CAPD into the following four categories or subprofiles: Auditory Decoding Deficit, Integration Deficit, Associative Deficit, and Organization-Output Deficit.

This section will provide a description of each of these subprofiles, as well as suggestions for management for each category. It should be noted that the use of the subprofiles discussed herein is not intended to suggest that this is the only manner in which CAPD may be categorized. Rather, this method is delineated only so that it may provide the clinician with a useful way in which to view the interdependency of CAPD and education/communication, as well as assist in the development of a multidisciplinary approach to assessment and management. Finally, the clinician should be reminded that these subprofiles may exist singularly or in any combination, further underscoring the need for an individualized approach to interpretation of central auditory findings.

Auditory Decoding Deficit

The primary finding in Auditory Decoding Deficit is poor auditory closure abilities, characterized by poor performance on tests of monaural low-redundancy speech and speech-in-noise. Right ear performance is often poorer than left ear performance on these tests, and errors tend to be phonemically similar to the target. For example, the child may say bite when the stimulus was bike, or may substitute hip for ship. This deficit manifests itself in the inability to achieve auditory closure when portions of the auditory signal are distorted or missing, due to a breakdown in the intrinsic redundancy of the CANS.

Because Auditory Decoding Deficit reduces a child's phonemic representation ability, sound blending, discrimination, and retention of phonemes are often poor. Therefore, the child with Auditory Decoding Deficit often exhibits difficulty in reading, particularly when an auditory phonics approach to reading is applied. Likewise, speech to print skills will also be affected, resulting in poor writing/spelling skills, and vocabulary, syntax, and semantic skills may also be weak. Behaviorally, the child will exhibit difficulty understanding speech in noisy listening environments and often may ask for repetition. These children tend to perform well in subjects where phonemic decoding is not required, such as math computation.

Management approaches for a child with Auditory Decoding Deficit are similar to traditional aural rehabilitation. Consonant and vowel training are often indicated, as is specific training of speech to print skills. Vocabulary building and other auditory closure activities designed to teach the child to use contextual cues often will be appropriate. The learning environment may need to be modified so that the child has the greatest access to auditory information without interference from background noise. Therefore, the use of preferential seating and auditory equipment to improve signal-to-noise ratio in the classroom will be useful with this profile. The child will need to learn to use visual cues to augment auditory information.

A recommendation that is frequently made for teachers who have a child with CAPD in their classrooms is to repeat or rephrase information. However, it should be emphasized that **the utility of repetition or rephrasing will depend upon the characteristics of the CAPD**. For children with Auditory Decoding Deficit, repetition may be helpful, but only if the repetition is acoustically clearer than the original presentation of the message. The child's ability to comprehend the message is good as long as the child is able to decode the message. Therefore, repetition of the message will allow the child another chance at filling in the parts of the message he or she did not get the first time. Rephrasing, on the other hand, is useful only if sufficient information is added to clarify the original message. In addition, preteaching of new information, particularly new vocabulary, will greatly aid the child in becoming familiar with new subjects and associated terminology so that closure may be achieved more easily.

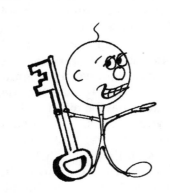

KEY CONCEPT

Whether the repeating or rephrasing of auditory information is effective will depend upon the individual characteristics of the CAPD and the way in which the repeating and/or rephrasing is carried out.

Although it is not possible to pinpoint the anatomical site-of-dysfunction with certainty in any of the CAPD subprofiles discussed in this chapter, electrophysiological and site-of-lesion research implicates the primary auditory cortex as the probable site of dysfunction in Auditory Decoding Deficit (Katz, 1994; Kraus et al., 1995).

Integration Deficit

Integration Deficit is characterized by difficulty in tasks that require interhemispheric communication. This difficulty may be within and/or across modality. For example, the child with Integration Deficit may have difficulty integrating auditory and visual functions, or in integrating linguistic-based auditory information with nonlinguistic auditory information, such as rhythm and pattern perception. Therefore, the child with Integration Deficit may present with a wide variety of behavioral auditory complaints, some which are difficult to pin down precisely.

On tests of central auditory function, children with Integration Deficit typically demonstrate abnormal left ear suppression on dichotic listening tasks combined with bilateral deficits on tests of temporal patterning when verbal report is required. The child's performance on temporal patterning tests often improves when he or she is asked to hum the response, thus removing the linguistic labeling component of the test.

Academically, these children often exhibit difficulty in reading recognition, spelling, and writing. **In contrast with Auditory Decoding Deficit, children with Integration Deficit exhibit these difficulties not because the ability to develop a phonemic representation of the letters is affected, but rather because the ability to recognize and utilize gestalt patterns, which is necessary in sight word recognition and spelling, is dysfunctional.** Likewise, tasks that require the use of symbolic language, such as math application, may be affected. Use of prosodic aspects of speech, including rhythm, stress, and intonation, will often be impaired. At its most severe, Integration Deficit may result in an inability to perceive prosody, with the result that spoken sentences sound like strings of unrelated words, with no relative stress to emphasize key words and other important cues. In this situation, comprehension of spoken messages is severely affected.

Behaviorally, the child with Integration Deficit also may exhibit difficulty with multimodality tasks that require interhemispheric cooperation. Therefore, skills such as taking dictation, which requires auditory and visual integration, may be poor, as will tasks that require multisensory pattern perception. For example, the child may be unable to draw a picture from verbal or written instructions, dance to the beat of the music, sing or play a musical instrument, or perform other tasks that require interhemispheric integration of multisensory functions.

The child with Integration Deficit may benefit from management approaches designed to improve interhemispheric transfer of information. These approaches need not always be auditory. Rather, any activity that requires interhemispheric integration may be utilized. Therefore, linguistic labeling of tactile stimuli, music, singing, and dance activities, and following verbal instructions to complete art projects all may be appropriate remediation activities. In addition, training in the use of prosodic aspects of speech, including key word extraction, often will be indicated. Reading aloud daily while emphasizing rhythm, stress, and intonational patterns is a good home-based activity for children with Integration Deficit.

In the classroom, children with Integration Deficit will exhibit difficulty with a teacher who is quiet, reserved, or monotonous. Therefore, placement with an animated teacher will be desirable, as prosodic cues will be more accessible to the child. **The use of multimodality cues, such as visual and tactile aids, may not always be appropriate for a child with Integration Deficit, as the addition of other sense modalities may result in confusion rather than clarification**. Therefore, the use of visual, tactile, or other multimodality augmentations will be effective only if concrete examples and repeated modeling of the desired outcome are provided.

Neurophysiologically, the child with Integration Deficit probably is exhibiting behavioral manifestations of delayed or impaired development of the corpus callosum or other structures necessary for adequate interhemispheric transfer of information. Therefore, children for whom a primary causative factor is delayed neuromaturation will probably fall, at least in part, into the category of Integration Deficit.

Associative Deficit

The primary feature of Associative Deficit is an underlying inability to apply the rules of language to incoming acoustic information. For example, the child with Associative Deficit often exhibits difficulty with sentences presented in the passive voice (e.g., The ball was thrown by the girl), compound sentences, and other linguistically complex messages. At its most severe, Associative Deficit can manifest itself in the inability to attach linguistic meaning to phonemic units of speech, as in receptive childhood aphasia.

On tests of central auditory function, children with Associative Deficit often will demonstrate bilateral deficits on dichotic listening tasks. Performance on tests of temporal patterning (i.e., Frequency and Duration Patterns) is often good. Speech sound discrimination typically is quite good; however, word recognition itself may be poor.

Behaviorally, the child with Associative Deficit may exhibit receptive language deficits in vocabulary, semantics, and syntax. In addition, pragmatic and social communication skills may be poor. For many of these children, early academic achievement appears to be age-appropriate. However, as the linguistic demands within the classroom begin to increase, often around the third grade, general academic difficulties may begin to become apparent.

Management approaches indicated in cases of Associative Deficit likely will contain elements of language intervention, and speech-language services are often a key component of remediation. Metacognitive techniques designed to strengthen the memory trace and aid in item recall are helpful. These would include training the child to utilize verbal rehearsal, chunking, tag words (e.g., first, second, before, after), and other organizational aids. Classroom management strategies useful in cases of Associative Deficit would include preteaching of new information and imposition of external organization within the classroom. These children often have difficulty with independent work, whole language approaches, and other classroom techniques that require self-monitoring of learning behavior.

The child with Associative Deficit often is able to repeat verbatim instructions he or she has been given. This behavior can be deceptive, as the ability to repeat an instruction does not necessarily imply comprehension of the instruction. Therefore, **repetition as a clarification strategy is rarely effective for the child with Associative Deficit.** Instead, instructions or other verbal messages should be rephrased using simpler language. Comprehension should be checked by asking the child to paraphrase or demonstrate what is expected of him or her, rather than requesting simple repetition of the instruction.

Based on neurophysiological information to date, inefficient communication between primary and associative cortical regions (i.e., inefficient intrahemispheric communication) may be an underlying basis for Associative Deficit.

Output-Organization Deficit

Output-Organization Deficit is as its name implies: a deficit in the ability to sequence, plan, and organize responses. In this profile, receptive auditory skills are good; however, the difficulty lies in the ability to act upon incoming information. Children with Output-Organization Deficit often will demonstrate poor performance on any task that requires report of more than two critical elements. Therefore, performance on monaural low-redundancy speech tasks will remain unaffected, as the child is required simply to repeat one word at a time. However, performance on tests such as Frequency and Duration Patterns, Dichotic Digits, Competing Sentences, and SSW likely will be poor, because all of these tests require the child to report multiple elements. The deficit found on these tests is not due to difficulty in receptive skills, but rather to the inability to formulate the appropriate response. In addition, abnormal contralateral acoustic reflexes and extremely poor speech-in-noise skills are often found in children with Output-Organization Deficit.

Behaviorally, the child with Output-Organization Deficit may demonstrate poor organizational skills, difficulty following directions, reversals, and poor recall and word retrieval abilities. Expressive speech errors often consist of perseverative responses in which the target is substituted by a previously heard word. Sequencing errors and sound blending difficulties are not uncommon. Academically, children with Output-Organization Deficit may demonstrate good reading comprehension; however, spelling and writing skills are often poor due to the multi-element nature of these tasks. Finally, motor planning abilities often are affected in these children, resulting in poor fine and gross motor skills.

As previously discussed in Associative Deficit, children with Output-Organization Deficit will benefit from management strategies designed to aid in organization, including imposition of external organization within the classroom and use of metacognitive techniques. Because of the expressive language component in this profile, speech-language services will likely be an important component in the overall management of the child. Finally, both repetition and rephrasing of critical messages and instructions may be useful for the child with Output-Organization Deficit, but only if the message and required response is broken down into smaller linguistic units of no more than two critical elements.

The precise site-of-dysfunction within the CANS of Output-Organization Deficit is not certain at this time. However, because motoric tasks are an efferent nervous system activity, and the efferent system plays a role in the detection of signals in noise, it is possible that Output-Organization Deficit is the behavioral manifestation of impaired efferent function. This hypothesis is supported by the finding of abnormal contralateral acoustic reflexes in many of these children. The four subprofiles of CAPD discussed in this section are summarized in Table 7–6.

Summary

This chapter has provided the reader with a variety of ways in which results of a comprehensive central auditory assessment may be interpreted. No one method of interpretation is considered to the only correct method. Rather, we encourage the clinician to look at the assessment data from as many different perspectives as possible so that the full value of the information may be realized.

Based on central auditory test findings, the clinician should be able to make a determination regarding presence or absence of disorder. We recommend that the identification of CAPD be based on abnormal findings on one or more test tools, combined with significant educational and behavioral findings.

In addition to identifying the presence of the disorder, all attempts should be made to identify the underlying process or processes that are dysfunctional in order to develop a deficit-specific management plan. Thus, it should be determined whether a deficit exists in auditory closure, binaural separation or integration, temporal patterning, binaural interaction, interhemispheric communication, or a combination thereof. If possible, information regarding site-of-dysfunction within the CANS should also be obtained, most importantly to determine whether further medical follow-up is warranted.

Finally, results of central auditory tests should be related to the academic, communicative, and behavioral characteristics of the individual child so that a multidisciplinary management program that will address the child's functional difficulties may be developed. To this end, the use of subprofiles or categories of CAPD may be useful. This chapter has presented descriptions of four subprofiles of CAPD: Auditory Decoding Deficit, Integration Deficit, Associative Deficit, and Output-Organization Deficit. Directions for management for each of the subprofiles and underlying dysfunctional processes have been provided, and the reader is referred to Chapter 8 for specific management activities.

Table 7-6

Characteristics of the Four Subprofiles of CAPD

Type	Primary Sequelae	Central Test Findings	Management
Auditory Decoding Deficit	Sound recognition, blending, reading, and writing skills adversely affected. Poor auditory closure abilities.	Poor performance on monaural low redundancy speech tests and speech-in-noise. Site of dysfunction: primary auditory cortex.	Phoneme training, preteach new information, improve acoustic clarity of signal.
Integration Deficit	Difficulty in multimodality tasks, reading, spelling, writing, and use of symbolic language and prosody. Poor music skills.	Left ear deficit on dichotic speech tasks combined with bilateral deficit on tests of temporal patterning requiring verbal report. Site of dysfunction: corpus callosum.	Interhemispheric exercises, reduce use of multimodality cues, prosody training, key word extraction, music training.
Associative Deficit	Receptive language deficits, pragmatic skills may be poor. Academic difficulties may not become apparent until the 3rd grade.	Bilateral deficit on dichotic speech tasks, poor word recognition skills Site of dysfunction: primary and associative cortical regions.	Language intervention combined with compensatory strategies.
Output-Organization Deficit	Deficit in sequencing, planning, and organizing responses. Poor organizational skills, reversals, poor recall and sequencing abilities. Motor skills often affected.	Difficulty on any task requiring report of more than 2 critical elements. Site of dysfunction: efferent system	Similar to associative deficit, including training of organizational skills and language intervention.

Review Questions

1. Identify four questions that may be answered by the results of central auditory testing.
2. Differentiate between strict and lax criteria for the interpretation of test results.
3. What two components are recommended to be present in order for identifying the presence of a CAPD?
4. Define process-based interpretation.
5. Identify the behavioral auditory characteristics of dysfunction in the following underlying auditory processes:

> Auditory Closure (Decoding)
> Temporal Patterning
> Interhemispheric Transfer
>
> Binaural Separation and Integration
> Binaural Interaction

6. What findings would be expected on tests of central auditory function for dysfunction in each of the processes listed above?
7. What management approaches may be appropriate for deficits in each of the processes listed above?
8. What is the clinical utility of determining the site of lesion?
9. What central auditory test findings are indicative of dysfunction in the following areas of the CANS?

> brainstem   cerebral
> interhemispheric

10. List the behavioral, academic, and central auditory test characteristics of each of the following subprofiles of CAPD:

> Auditory Decoding Deficit   Integration Deficit
> Associative Deficit   Output-Organization Deficit

11. What management approaches might be appropriate for each of the CAPD subprofiles listed above?

CHAPTER
EIGHT

Management of Auditory Processing Disorders

There is a paucity of empirical data regarding the efficacy of management approaches to CAPD. In fact, it would not be unreasonable to suggest that treatment efficacy may be the area of greatest need for further research within the field of auditory processing disorders. However, recent research in neuroplasticity, as discussed in Chapter 3, suggests that neuroplasticity and neuromaturation are dependent, at least in part, on stimulation. Therefore, a comprehensive approach to management of CAPD, including auditory stimulation designed to bring about functional change within the CANS, should be undertaken in all cases of CAPD (Chermak & Musiek, 1992).

While further data are sorely needed within this area, logic tells us that the decision regarding what should be included in a comprehensive management program is one that should be based on the child's individual presenting profile and should be as deficit-specific as possible. In other words, all attempts should be made to remediate auditory areas that have been shown to be dysfunctional, while building upon the child's auditory strengths. In addition, the management program also should address behavioral, educational, and communicative sequelae so that maximum functional benefit may be achieved. Therefore, **management of CAPD, like assessment, should be multidisciplinary in nature**. Speech-language pathologists, psychologists, audiologists, neuropsychologists, learning disabilities specialists, social workers, teachers, parents, and others may all be involved in the child's overall care. The extent of each team member's contribution will depend on the nature of the disorder, the functional manifestations of the disorder, and the degree to which the problem may be medically treatable.

This chapter will provide the reader with suggestions regarding the development of a deficit-specific management program that will address a given child's auditory, educational, and communicative needs. Suggestions regarding remediation activities, recommendations for classroom-based modifications, and strategies for compensation will be given. The reader is referred to the previous chapter for information regarding management approaches appropriate for specific processing deficits and CAPD subprofiles. In addition, Chapter 10 will discuss methods of determining treatment efficacy utilizing statistical analysis.

Learning Objectives

After studying this chapter, the reader should be able to

1. Discuss the general principles of CAPD management
2. List the three components of any CAPD management program
3. Delineate specific management approaches and activities appropriate for children with CAPD
4. Give examples of management approaches appropriate for very young children for whom definitive diagnostic central testing is not possible.

Overview of Central Auditory Processing Disorders Management

CAPD management in the educational setting may be divided into three main categories: (1) environmental modification and teaching suggestions designed to improve the child's access to auditory information, (2) remediation techniques designed to enhance discrimination, interhemispheric transfer of information, and associated neuroauditory functions, and (3) provision of compensatory strategies designed to teach the child how to overcome residual dysfunction and maximize use of auditory information. In other words, **management of CAPD should focus on changing the environment, remediating the disorder, and improving the child's learning and listening skills**. Every management program should include components from each of these three categories; however, the overall management plan should be individualized based on the individual child's specific presenting profile and sequelae.

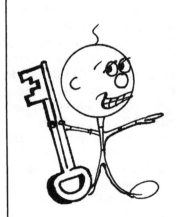

KEY CONCEPT

CAPD management may be viewed as a tripod: without all 3 "legs" (environmental modifications, remediation activities, and compensatory strategies), the tripod cannot stand.

As clinicians working with CAPD on a daily basis, frequently we are asked for general recommendations appropriate to all children with CAPD. It may surprise the reader to find that, in truth, very few management recommendations apply to CAPD in general. Let us take, for example, the situation in which the teacher is instructed to augment auditory information with visual and other cues. As seen in the previous chapter, this seemingly innocuous recommendation, while appropriate for some listeners, may actually confuse a child for whom the ability to integrate auditory and visual information is dysfunctional. Likewise, it is commonly suggested that teachers repeat or rephrase information. As also seen in the previous chapter, whether repetition and/or rephrasing of auditory information will be effective will depend upon the specific presenting deficit as well as the manner in which the repeating or rephrasing is accomplished.

On the other hand, frequently we see the use of an auditory trainer or other assistive listening device routinely recommended for children with CAPD. While this recommendation may be appropriate for some, it is likely to be a complete waste of time and money for others. Only those children for whom access to and decoding of auditory input is an issue will benefit significantly from auditory equipment designed to improve access to auditory information. Children with Integration Deficit or the latter two language-based deficits discussed in Chapter 7 will probably demonstrate the same difficulty with auditory information regardless of whether access to the initial message is improved.

Therefore, **we urge clinicians entering into the CAPD arena not to surrender to the urge to make general recommendations to classroom teachers and others regarding management of CAPD and to avoid at all costs preprinted lists of "general" suggestions without first analyzing the list to ensure that each suggestion contained therein is, in fact, appropriate for the specific child in question.**

That having been said, a few recommendations may be generalized as being useful, not only for all children with CAPD, but for listeners in general. These recommendations may be referred to as Smart Listening suggestions, and would include reduction in or elimination of obvious adverse noise sources within the listening environment, education of educators and other significant individuals regarding listening and the nature of auditory disorders, and optimization of the learning environment based on the individual child's needs.

For children with CAPD, **the primary goal is to increase the child's ability to use information presented in the auditory mode.** Therefore, management suggestions for classroom use would focus on environmental modifications and the child's use of *compensatory* *strategies* to increase the redundancy of the learning environment, thereby improving access to and use of new information.

In contrast, remediation techniques for CAPD are designed to provide direct intervention for specific deficit areas and to teach compensatory strategies that will be used in the classroom. In order to do this, the remediation environment should be challenging and varied, so that adequate auditory stimulation occurs and the child has ample opportunity to practice new skills that will ultimately be used in everyday listening situations. Therefore, the only effective management approach for a child with CAPD is to combine a highly redundant learning environment with a highly challenging, low-redundancy, therapy environment.

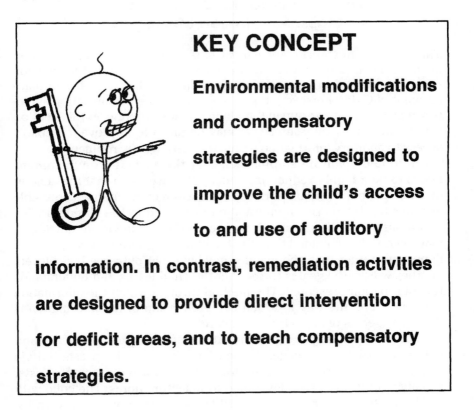

KEY CONCEPT

Environmental modifications and compensatory strategies are designed to improve the child's access to and use of auditory information. In contrast, remediation activities are designed to provide direct intervention for deficit areas, and to teach compensatory strategies.

Finally, the child's own internal motivation often will need to be addressed. Many children with CAPD are considered to be passive listeners, or listeners who do not take an active part in their own comprehension. By the time a child is identified as having CAPD, he or she may have experienced failure in listening situations for so long that a prevailing attitude exists in which the child feels that he or she is stupid and nothing can be done to remedy the situation. To the extent that the child is helped to understand the nature of the disorder, and helped to analyze difficult listening situations, a sense of control may be achieved. The child will need to be taught to be an active participant in his or her own listening and learning experience to maximize the efficacy of the overall management program and enhance the child's sense of motivation and control.

Environmental Modifications and Classroom-Based Strategies

This segment of CAPD management is the one that is probably most familiar to clinicians. In our experience, we have found that many clinicians are able to provide good suggestions for classroom-based management of CAPD; however, it is in the area of direct remediation activities that the need for outside guidance arises. Therefore, this section will briefly discuss measures that may be taken to improve the child's access to auditory information within the learning environment.

It should again be emphasized that **the learning environment needs to be a highly redundant one**. By this, we mean that the child in question should be required to expend as little extra energy as possible in order to obtain critical information presented in the classroom. To accomplish this, the classroom teacher and other involved individuals may need to be reminded that it is the ultimate desired outcome that is important, rather than the manner in which that outcome is achieved. In other words, the goal is to see that the child learns and understands the information presented. The method through which the information is learned, and the way in which comprehension of the information is demonstrated, is of much lesser concern.

For example, beginning in the later elementary school years and continuing through college, information begins to be presented via lecture format, and notetaking often becomes a requirement. Tests, usually written, are often developed from lecture notes. The child with CAPD is often a poor writer, as well as exhibiting difficulties with listening. The division of attention that ensues from attempting to listen to a message, write the message in a coherent manner, and return attention to the speaker may be detrimental for the child with CAPD. The writing often lags behind the spoken message, with the result that the next piece of information is simply missed. In addition, the inability to direct full attention toward the spoken message and invoke listening strategies virtually ensures that the child will not comprehend much of the spoken message. The final result, of course, will be that the child does not learn the critical information presented.

In this situation, the classroom teacher will need to realize that, while lecture format and notetaking may be a standard requirement for the class, accommodations will need to be made for the child with CAPD to be able to demonstrate the desired learning outcomes. Provision of lecture notes by the teacher prior to the class presentation may be helpful, as the child can become familiar with the lecture content prior to class time and can use the notes for studying at a later date. If teacher-made lecture notes are not available, a notetaker may be provided. This could be accomplished simply by providing carbon paper to another student within the class, but the teacher should take pains to check the chosen student's notes and ensure that the critical information is reflected accurately. Finally, it may be helpful for the child with CAPD to tape-record each lecture, using the tapes later for studying purposes. Whatever the method or combination of methods chosen, the goal is to allow the child with CAPD to focus all attention on the speaker during lecture time, thus avoiding the division of attention and loss of information that occurs during notetaking.

A second concern in the classroom is acoustic access to and clarity of the spoken message. Children with deficits in the areas of auditory closure, phonemic decoding, binaural separation or integration, and binaural interaction characteristically demonstrate difficulty hearing in noise. Although, as discussed in the previous chapter, the mechanism by which this difficulty occurs is different in each of these disorders, the final result is the same. Even if a notetaker or tape recorder is provided so that the child may focus all attention on the speaker, comprehension of the spoken message will be adversely affected if the acoustic signal is contaminated by competing noise or lack of clarity. Therefore, **measures should be taken that improve the child's access to target information, while simultaneously decreasing background noise. Preferential seating**, so that the child may make use of visual cues and facial expressions, should be encouraged. If there is a significant noise source within the classroom, such as an aquarium or a fan, the child should be seated away from the source of the noise.

Finally, the **use of an auditory trainer or other assistive listening device** may be helpful in improving signal clarity. In recent years, sound field amplification systems have also become available that are likely to benefit everyone in the classroom, not just the child with

CAPD. However, the fitting of an assistive listening device should never be undertaken lightly. We recommend that use of an assistive listening device begin with a trial period in order to evaluate effectiveness. The trial period should begin with baseline information regarding listening and comprehension behaviors, as well as a baseline audiogram obtained prior to fitting. The decision to use the device on a regular basis should be made only after posttrial data indicate benefit, and serial audiograms should be obtained on a regular basis during equipment use in order to monitor for possible adverse effects on peripheral hearing sensitivity. **It must be emphasized that under no circumstances should an auditory trainer or other assistive listening device be provided simply on the basis of a diagnosis of CAPD, without further corroborating evidence of need and careful, ongoing documentation of efficacy**.

The teacher should be encouraged to **make frequent checks for understanding** after giving the child instructions. These checks may be visual, watching to see if the child in question follows the instructions, or they may be verbal. However, simply asking the child to repeat the instruction is rarely effective, because many children with CAPD are able to repeat verbatim what was said without actually understanding the content of the message. Therefore, the child should be asked to paraphrase the instruction or to demonstrate the action requested. If it is clear that the instruction was not understood, repetition or rephrasing may be necessary. However, as discussed in the previous chapter, the decision regarding whether to repeat or rephrase should depend on the underlying deficit, and the manner in which the repetition or rephrasing is carried out will have a significant impact on the efficacy of the attempt at clarification.

Likewise, the use of **multimodality cues and hands-on demonstrations** may be an effective aid to understanding, but only if utilized correctly. The multimodality cues should match precisely, in content and timing, the spoken information. For example, if, during a discussion about transportation, the teacher is describing types of cars and a slide is presented showing a truck, confusion may result from the lack of agreement between the spoken and visual messages. Also, it should be remembered that not all children with CAPD will benefit from a multimodality approach. Children with Integration Deficit, for example, may find the addition of tactile and visual cues confusing unless they are guided, step by step, through the use and application of the additional cues.

A classroom-based management approach that is often effective for children with CAPD is **preteaching of new information and new**

vocabulary. The teacher should be encouraged to provide introductory information and new vocabulary to the child before presenting the subject in the classroom. By doing this, the teacher helps to ensure that the child will be familiar with the subject to be discussed, thus increasing the external redundancy of the information.

Perhaps the most critical factor in ensuring efficacy and follow-through of classroom-based management approaches to CAPD is obtaining teacher support and cooperation. The teacher who is unconvinced about the need for classroom modifications, or who feels that such modifications may be "unfair" to the other students, is unlikely to implement management suggestions on a daily basis. Therefore, the classroom teacher should be included in all aspects of assessment and management of CAPD, and every effort should be made to educate teachers and other professionals regarding the nature of the disorder and the underlying theoretical bases for suggested management approaches. The more these individuals understand, the more likely they will be to cooperate with any recommendations made. Suggestions regarding methods of imparting information to teachers and other significant individuals are provided in Chapter 9.

Finally, it should be recognized that not all sources of classroom-based difficulties will be readily apparent by the differential diagnosis. Therefore, it is helpful for the clinician to visit the child's classroom and analyze the listening environment in order to better make classroom-specific suggestions. Through classroom observation, issues that had previously gone unnoticed may surface. For example, it may be discovered that the teacher speaks very rapidly or in a very soft tone of voice. It may be found that, due to the unique characteristics of a specific classroom, preferential seating actually means seating toward the back, rather than the front, of the classroom. Unnoticed sources of external noise may be identified and eliminated. A myriad of issues may become apparent to the clinician simply through the act of observing the child in the classroom.

In conclusion, a variety of classroom-based management suggestions may be made for the child with CAPD. However, not all suggestions will be appropriate for every child. **Therefore, it is critical that the clinician approach the management of each child from an individualized perspective and that the teacher be involved in the decision-making process.** By working closely with the teacher, the clinician can help to ensure that the learning environment is a highly redundant one, thus improving the child's access to information and opportunity for success.

Obviously, this section did not discuss all possible recommendations for classroom management. The clinician is encouraged to gather as much information as possible and to use common sense combined with knowledge of the underlying auditory deficit when providing guidance to classroom teachers. The suggestions discussed in this section are briefly outlined in Table 8–1.

Remediation Activities

The purpose of remediation is to attempt to alleviate the disorder through specific therapeutic activities, either by training the recipient how to perform a specific auditory task, or by stimulating the auditory system in hopes of facilitating a structural, and concomitant functional, change. The degree to which the dysfunction will be ameliorated through these activities varies and, indeed, cannot be estimated for any given child. In fact, many of the activities that will be discussed here are based primarily on what is currently known about how the brain and auditory system function and have little documented efficacy at this time.

For example, if a child presents with an Auditory Decoding Deficit, demonstrating difficulty in phonemic decoding and speech-to-print skills, it is logical that remediation will center around phoneme training. Conversely, if a child exhibits an Integration Deficit, with auditory skills closely mimicking that of a younger child, then remediation activities logically will include interhemispheric activities to stimulate the corpus callosum in hopes of improving interhemispheric communication.

Table 8-1

Overview of Classroom-Based Management Suggestions for CAPD

Note: The utility of each of the following suggestions is dependent upon the characteristics of the individual child's CAPD:

- Provide a notetaker or allow the child to tape-record lectures
- Use preferential seating
- Consider use of an FM auditory trainer or other assistive listening device
- Check frequently for understanding
- Make appropriate use of multimodality cues and hands-on demonstrations for students who are likely to benefit from these adaptations
- Preteach new information and vocabulary
- Repeat and/or rephrase information when appropriate

As was seen in Chapter 3, recent research in neuroplasticity has shown us that, **just as lack of stimulation may result in structural and functional neurophysiological alterations within the CANS, increased stimulation may, likewise, result in structural changes and functional improvement.** Just as an unused muscle will atrophy and wither, a muscle that is exercised regularly in a challenging manner will grow in size and strength. So it may be with structures within the brain, if recent findings in neuroplasticity are any indication. It should be remembered, however, that the degree to which any remediation technique will serve to remedy the dysfunction will depend on the individual child, and efficacy of treatment activities awaits further research and validation.

As with all of the information contained in this book, the presentation of the following remediation activities is not intended to suggest that these are the only techniques that may be utilized, nor that the activities discussed are equal in effectiveness. In addition, it should be remembered that therapeutic techniques typically utilized by the speech-language pathologist and associated professionals may also be useful for a child with CAPD, particularly if the child exhibits a language-based disorder. These activities are presented in order to provide the clinician with a starting point for therapeutic intervention once a diagnosis of CAPD has been made.

Auditory Closure Activities

The purpose of Auditory Closure activities is to assist the child in learning to fill in the missing parts in order to perceive a meaningful whole. As such, context plays an important role in auditory closure, since prediction of the complete word or message often depends on the surrounding context. Therapeutic activities that focus on auditory closure are most appropriate for those children who have demonstrated reduced performance on tests of central auditory function that challenge the process of auditory closure, such as monaural low-redundancy speech tasks.

The activities discussed herein are presented in sequential fashion, from least to most difficult. The child in question should demonstrate mastery of one level before moving on to the next.

Missing Word Exercises

These exercises are designed to teach the child to use context to fill in the missing word in a message. It is best to begin with very familiar

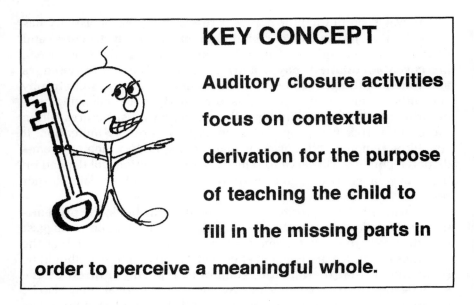

KEY CONCEPT

Auditory closure activities focus on contextual derivation for the purpose of teaching the child to fill in the missing parts in order to perceive a meaningful whole.

subject matter and then move to new information. For example, when working with a very young child, the clinician may wish to begin with familiar songs or nursery rhymes in order to familiarize the child with the task of listening to the whole in order to predict the missing part. For example, the following rhymes may be used:

> Twinkle, twinkle, little _____. (star)
>
> Little Jack Horner sat in the _____. (corner)
>
> Hey diddle diddle, the cat and the _____ . (fiddle)

In these examples, the child's task would be to fill in the missing word. It may surprise some clinicians to find that, even with a great amount of external redundancy due to familiarity of the message, some children will exhibit difficulty with even this simple task. In this case, and at all stages of auditory closure activities, the child should be talked through the process and prompted with questions such as, What is the sentence talking about? What word comes next when you sing the song? What word would rhyme with "Horner" and make sense in this sentence?

A slightly higher level activity might be prediction of rhyming words. For example, the clinician may ask the child, "Can you name an animal that rhymes with house?" If the child is unable to perform the task, prompts should be given that guide the child in solving the puzzle. For example, the child may be instructed to begin at the beginning of the alphabet and substitute the initial consonant of the word with different letters until the correct consonant is reached (aouse, bouse, couse, douse, etc). If the child is demonstrating difficulty with the concept of rhyming, the initial consonant of the target word, in this case *m*, may be provided for the child, requiring him or her to add it to the remainder of the word *ouse* to derive the whole *mouse*. A third method of *prompting*, useful when the child correctly chooses an initial consonant and combines it with the remainder of the word to derive a meaningful, but incorrect, word (e.g., *douse*), may be to draw the child's attention to the key word or words in the clue. In this situation, the clinician would remind the child that, while *douse* is, indeed, a word that rhymes with *house*, what is wanted here is an animal. Some examples of stimuli that may be used in this activity are as follows:

Color that rhymes with bed. (red)

Family member that rhymes with other. (brother or mother)

Fruit that rhymes with beach. (peach)

Once mastery of these steps has been demonstrated, the clinician may move to new, unfamiliar messages in which the child must utilize the context of the phrase, sentence, or paragraph in order to predict the missing component. When using this approach, the clinician should begin with simple sentences (e.g., When I'm hungry, I _____), then move to more complex material, such as paragraphs in textbooks or popular novels. In addition, the clinician should progress from omitting the subject or object of the sentence or phrase (e.g., Jill hit the _____ with a bat), to omissions of verbs, adjectives, and other portions of the message (e.g., Jill _____ the ball with a bat; The water was so _____, it took his breath away). The child should be prompted continually to use context in order to predict missing components, as well as to derive meaning from the whole message. In addition, materials appropriate for this exercise can be taken from classes in which the child is demonstrating difficulty, in order to assist the child further in understanding the class material.

Missing Syllable Exercises

Once the child has demonstrated that he or she can predict a missing word based on context, the clinician may move to omission of syllables. As with missing words, missing syllable exercises should be presented in a progression from least to most difficult. Initially, the context should be familiar so that the child is best able to fill in the missing components of the target word. The clinician may find that, even if the child is able to predict an entire missing word from a sentence easily, he or she may have great difficulty when only a portion of the target word is omitted. In addition, achieving closure for words in which the initial syllable is omitted is a more difficult task than for words in which the final syllable is omitted. Therefore, the clinician should begin by omitting the final syllable of the target word and, once mastery is achieved, move to omission of medial and initial syllables.

The clinician may begin with sentences in which the target word is imbedded (e.g., There are 26 letters in the al-pha-_____), and then gradually move to single words in which the only contextual cue may be a category designation (e.g., Sports: base_____, soc_____, ten_____). Through repeated drills such as these, the child learns to become less dependent on hearing and decoding every component of the target word and more aware of the need for contextual derivation when the complete acoustic signal is inaccessible.

Missing Phoneme Exercises

Exercises in which specific phonemes are omitted may be carried out in a similar fashion to the missing syllable exercises. Again, it is best to use a progression of least to most difficult, moving to the next stage only when the child has demonstrated mastery of the previous stage. Therefore, the child should be able to supply the missing phonemes in words with contextual cues (e.g., I like to (w)atch (t)ele(v)ision), before moving on to isolated words. With these exercises, tape-recording the target sentences or words may be useful, as it may be difficult to perform the necessary phonemic omissions using a live voice approach. Again, when focusing on isolated words, it is helpful to provide general categories as a contextual cue (e.g., Animals: ti(g)er, (m)on(k)ey), and to require mastery with final phonemes prior to moving on to medial and initial phonemes.

Other Auditory Closure Activities

Virtually any method whereby the external redundancy of the acoustic signal is reduced may be utilized to train auditory closure skills. Therefore, auditory closure activities such as those discussed in the previous sections may be undertaken in distracting or noisy situations to increase the difficulty of the task further. In addition, variations in speakers, such as the introduction of regional dialects, misarticulations, and other speaker-related characteristics may be utilized to help train the child to use context to achieve auditory closure.

It should be noted that, as discussed in the previous chapter, difficulty understanding speech in noise may be due to an Auditory Decoding or Closure Deficit, or it may be due to dysfunction at the brainstem level affecting the listener's ability to lateralize and localize auditory information, thus interfering with the detection of signals in noise. For this reason, it may be beneficial in some cases to include *localization training* in a comprehensive management program. Localization training may be conducted in a sound booth or in a quiet room, and stimuli should be varied and challenging. In addition, localization activities should also progress from least difficult (greatest separation of sources of auditory stimuli) to most difficult (minimal separation of stimuli sources).

Vocabulary Building

A final activity that falls within the category of auditory closure activities is Vocabulary Building. Just as a word may be indecipherable due to missing syllables or phonemes, requiring the listener to use context to predict the word, a word may be indecipherable due to the child's lack of familiarity with the word or subject itself. As in all of the other auditory closure activities discussed in this section, the ability to derive or predict word meaning for an unfamiliar term depends on the ability to utilize context effectively.

Miller and Gildea (1987) delineated several important points in describing how children learn new vocabulary. First, the child must be able to associate the sound of the word with its meaning. Later, many new vocabulary words are encountered and learned through reading. Most importantly, the child must be exposed to the new word in several different contexts in order to internalize the meaning of the word fully. The authors emphasized that **the most effective vehicle for learning the meaning of new vocabulary is through contextual derivation, or utilizing the surrounding context to predict meaning of the unfamiliar term**.

Therefore, when approaching Vocabulary Building from an auditory closure perspective, it is important that the child learn to use the context in which the word appears to deduce its meaning. First, the child should learn to say the word aloud a few times, a technique known as *reauditorization*, so that the sight and sound of the word becomes familiar. Then, the child should be encouraged to attempt a definition of the new word based on the context in which it appears.

Next, the actual definition of the word should be provided to the child. It should be noted that, while dictionary skills are encouraged in academic pursuits, the goal of Vocabulary Building is to help the child achieve closure. This can only occur if the context is kept in the forefront of the child's mind and the child's motivation to learn the meaning of the word remains high. **Therefore, immediate problem solving in the form of providing the definition, rather than telling the child to look it up in the dictionary, is necessary**.

Finally, the child should be encouraged to define the new word in his or her own way, thus assuring that comprehension of the provided definition has been achieved. By following this process, the child has learned to recognize the new word visually and auditorily, utilize contextual cues to achieve closure, and has added a new word to his or her internal vocabulary store.

Materials for Vocabulary Building should be interesting and encourage maintenance of a high level of motivation. Therefore, popular novels and stories are often good choices for this activity. In addition, since vocabulary is frequently a weak area for children with CAPD, it may be useful to utilize new vocabulary from the student's specific academic classes so that the child is able to become familiar with the new terminology prior to its introduction in the classroom setting.

Finally, while Vocabulary Building is a beneficial activity in and of itself, in the context described here it serves as a vehicle for emphasizing the skills learned in all auditory closure activities - namely, the use of context to predict missing or unfamiliar components of the whole. Therefore, the use of contextual cues to deduce word meaning is an appropriate addition to a comprehensive CAPD management plan (Chermak & Musiek, 1992), particularly when the child exhibits a deficit in the area of Auditory Closure.

The Auditory Closure activities discussed in this chapter are summarized in Table 8–2.

Phoneme Training

The child with Auditory Decoding Deficit likely will not only demonstrate difficulty with auditory closure, but, by definition, phonemic decoding skills will be deficient, as well. For these children, specific consonant and vowel training often will be indicated. **The purpose of phoneme training is to help the child learn to develop accurate phonemic representation and to improve speech-to-print skills**.

Sloan (1995) details a comprehensive program for consonant discrimination training. In her program, she emphasizes that the most

Table 8-2
Summary of Auditory Closure Activities

- Missing word exercises
  - familiar songs or rhymes
  - prediction of rhyming words
  - new, unfamilar messages in which context is used to fill in the missing word
- Missing syllable exercises
  - sentences in which the target word is embedded
  - single words
- Missing phoneme exercises
  - sentences in which the target word is embedded
  - single words
- Repeating above activities in noisy or distracting situations
- Vocabulary Building
  - reauditorization
  - contextual derivation of word meaning
  - immediate provision of definition
  - reinforcement of definition

important feature of this type of therapy is not only to teach the child to discriminate speech sounds correctly, but, even more crucial, to help the child know when he or she has perceived a sound incorrectly or is unsure. In these situations, the child can put into use additional strategies he or she has learned throughout the course of therapy in order to resolve the uncertainty, resulting in an improvement in confidence and self-esteem.

Sloan's program, which focuses primarily on consonant discrimination skills, involves the presentation of minimal contrast phoneme pairs, or phoneme pairs that are very similar (e.g., /t/ versus /d/). Phonemes are presented to the child in isolation, and the **child must demonstrate mastery of minimal contrast pair discrimination**, in terms of both accuracy and promptness of response, before adding new pairs.

Following discrimination of phonemes presented in isolation, activities move to discrimination of minimal contrast pairs of phonemes in consonant-vowel and vowel-consonant syllables, and then to words of increasing complexity. The final portion of Sloan's program focuses on *speech-to-print skills*, and involves demonstrating the connection between the phoneme

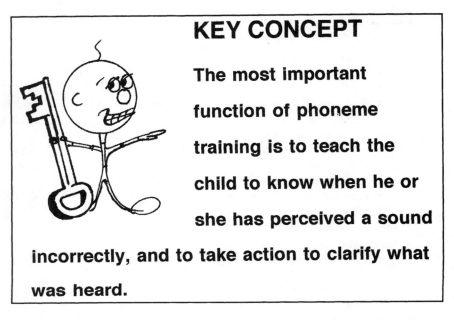

KEY CONCEPT

The most important function of phoneme training is to teach the child to know when he or she has perceived a sound incorrectly, and to take action to clarify what was heard.

segments previously trained auditorily with their corresponding printed letter symbols. Thus, the word attack difficulty often exhibited by children with Auditory Decoding Deficit is addressed, as well.

It should be noted that, although Sloan's program deals primarily with consonant discrimination, the need for vowel training should not be overlooked. As in consonant discrimination activities, vowel discrimination can be facilitated through the presentation of contrast pairs in isolation, followed by syllables and words. The speech-to-print activities previously discussed may also be used effectively with vowels. For further information, the reader is referred to Sloan (1995).

Prosody Training

Children with Temporal Patterning deficits who exhibit difficulty on the Frequency Patterns Test may also exhibit difficulty recognizing acoustic contours. Therefore, **specific training in recognition and use of prosodic aspects of speech, such as rhythm, stress, and intonation, may be indicated** (Musiek & Chermak, 1995).

Prosody Training may begin with words in which a change in the syllabic stress pattern changes the meaning of the word (e.g., con*vict* versus *con*vict, re*cord* versus *rec*ord, sub*ject* versus *sub*ject) (Musiek &

Chermak, 1995). Each version of the word should be introduced to the child and, if the word is unfamiliar, the steps delineated in Vocabulary Building should be utilized to familiarize the child with the sight, sound, and meaning of the new word. The change in meaning brought about by relative syllabic stress should be pointed out clearly. Once the child is able to define both versions of the word in isolation, the word may be imbedded in a sentence, so that the child must listen for relative stress within the word as well as use contextual cues to determine which meaning of the word is appropriate.

Following work with words, training may focus on sentences in which subtle differences in stress, temporal cueing, or other prosodic features alter the meaning of the entire sentence (e.g., Don't touch that *book* versus Don't touch *that* book. He saw the *snowdrift* by the window versus He saw the *snow drift* by the window). At first, the stress and rhythm characteristics of each sentence will need to be exaggerated; however, once the child becomes familiar with the task, the activities may be undertaken in a more normal tone of voice. The child should be led, step by step, through analyzing the sentences for meaning depending on relative stress and rhythm characteristics. For example, in the sentence "Don't touch that book," the implication is that the listener is not to touch books, although he or she may be permitted to touch other items. Conversely, in the sentence "Don't touch that book," it is clear that the listener is not to touch one book in particular, although other books may be allowed.

Another example of a sentence in which changes in prosodic cues may alter the general meaning is "You can't go to the movies with *us*," versus "*You* can't go to the movies with us." In this example, emphasis on the word *us* implies that, while the listener is welcome to go to the movies, he or she cannot join the speaker's group. Emphasis on the word *you* implies a rejection of the listener; although others may be invited to go to the movies with the group, the listener will not.

It is interesting that many children with deficits in Temporal Patterning often misunderstand or misconstrue what they hear, resulting in hurt feelings as they jump to an often erroneous conclusion about the intent of the message. This may be attributed to the difficulty these children experience in extracting and using prosodic features of speech correctly, which contribute not only to meaning, but to emotion and intent, as well. For these children, Prosody Training may help in determining intent of a message, as well as understanding the overall meaning of the message.

In addition, many of these children exhibit difficulty in sequencing and following directions, understanding complex messages, and so forth. If, in fact, the child's perception of prosodic features is dysfunctional, the child may well hear a message simply as a string of equally stressed words, so that remembering the message for dictation or follow-through purposes becomes a task of memory, rather than comprehension. Many of these children, when taking dictation, tend to write down sentences that make little or no sense, and articles and other filler words may be transcribed accurately, while key words in the message are left out.

For these children, training in the *detection of key words* within a message is very helpful. The child may need to be taught to listen specifically for subject, verb, and object, while placing less emphasis on articles, conjunctions, and other, less important words. After being given a complex direction, the clinician may prompt the child with questions such as, What was the action word? Who or what are you supposed to do it to? When? and so on. Training in key word extraction, a component of Prosody Training, may greatly help the child to remember and understand complex directions or messages.

Finally, many children with CAPD are described as flat or monotonic readers. This may be due to their lack of awareness of prosodic features of speech. **Reading aloud daily, with special emphasis on animation, is a good task for these children that may be done at home or school. Reading aloud serves not only to increase reading aptitude but also to reauditorize and reinforce the use of rhythm, stress, and intonation in expressive language**. The components of Prosody Training are summarized in Table 8–3.

Table 8-3
Components of Prosody Training

- Words in which change in syllabic stress changes the meaning (e.g., con*vict* vs *convict*)—isolation
- Words in which change in syllabic stress changes the meaning—sentences
- Sentences in which differences in prosodic features alter the meaning (e.g., He saw the *snowdrift* by the window vs He saw the *snow drift* by the window)—exaggerated prosodic features
- Sentences in which differences in prosodic features alter the meaning —normal tone of voice
- Key word extraction
- Reading aloud with exaggerated prosodic features

Temporal Patterning Training

Temporal Patterning Training is an activity that is closely related to Prosody Training, but is more basic in nature. If the child in question has significant difficulty with discriminating subtle changes in stress or rhythm or is unable to sequence information, these activities may be indicated.

As in all training activities, Temporal Patterning Training should be organized so that the least difficult activity, usually discrimination of same versus different, is mastered before going on to analysis and imitation of rhythm patterns. Virtually any auditory stimulus may be used for Temporal Patterning Training, but it is recommended that nonverbal stimuli be utilized first and linguistic stimuli be added only after the child has demonstrated success.

The goal of Temporal Patterning Training is for the child to first discriminate differences in, and then analyze and imitate, rhythmic patterns of auditory stimuli. The clinician may begin with short (three elements) patterns that may be clapped, tapped on the table, or done in any manner that will hold the child's attention. The patterns may be presented in pairs, requiring the child to report if the two patterns are the same or different, or the child may be required to imitate the pattern exactly. The patterns should be altered in terms of speed (by increasing or decreasing the inter-tap interval), relative loudness (by placing more emphasis on one or more taps than the others), and rhythm (by including silent intervals). In addition, the rhythms may be made gradually more complex by adding more elements, up to seven or eight.

Once the child has mastered discrimination and imitation of nonverbal rhythmic stimuli, the clinician may move on to word sequences. The child's task may be to determine which of three words was different (e.g., tick, tack, tick). The clinician should begin with words that are easiest to discriminate, then move to more difficult stimuli (e.g., pen, pin, pen).

Next, the clinician may introduce sentences of three or four elements in which one word is stressed more than the others. At this point, the child's task is not to derive relative meaning from the sentences, but merely to indicate which of the four words was emphasized. The same sentence may be used over and over again, each time stressing a different word (e.g., *You* are going home. You are going *home*. You *are* going home. You are *going* home). Once the child has demonstrated that he or she can detect relative stress within a sentence, the clinician may move on to Prosody Training, discussed previously, in order to attach meaning to relative differences in stress.

It should be noted that not all children with deficits in Temporal Patterning will need to undergo training in this area before moving on to Prosody Training. These activities may be quite simple for many children, whereas recognition of very subtle prosodic features of speech is a much more difficult task. However, if the child in question is unable to discriminate relative stress in a sentence, even when the stress features are exaggerated, the clinician may wish to backtrack and work on temporal patterning skills before returning to the more challenging task.

Interhemispheric Exercises

The child who exhibits a neuromaturational delay or Integration Deficit may benefit from exercises designed to stimulate the corpus callosum and improve interhemispheric transfer of information (Musiek & Chermak, 1995). **These exercises need not always be linguistic in nature. Rather, the key factors in these activities are that a single or double transfer across the corpus callosum must occur, and the exercises must provide enough opportunity for repetition so as to stimulate the corpus callosum efficiently**. Even the simple act of throwing a ball from hand to hand meets these criteria.

Interhemispheric Exercises are particularly appropriate for home-based therapy activities and lend themselves easily to parent or sibling involvement. Verbal-to-motor transfers may be utilized, in which the child is instructed to find a particular object or shape with his or her left hand from a grab bag or behind a screen, where he or she cannot see the objects. A motor-to-verbal transfer occurs when this process is reversed: The child finds an object with his or her left hand and is instructed to label it verbally in terms of shape, texture, identification, and so on.

Singing to music is an activity that requires rapid transfer of information across the corpus callosum. We suggest that any child with a neuromaturational delay or Integration Deficit be encouraged to pursue singing and/or musical instrument lessons, and to practice daily. Many of these children report, upon clinician interview, that musical skills are particularly weak. Music therapy is a fun, repetitive way in which to facilitate interhemispheric communication.

In conclusion, remediation activities should be chosen that are specific to the individual child's deficit area(s) and level of mastery. They may include techniques to facilitate auditory closure, phoneme discrimination, awareness and use of prosody, temporal patterning skills, and interhemispheric interaction, singularly or in any combination. In addition, for children in which the deficit is language-based, traditional speech-language intervention may be indicated. The remedial activities discussed in this chapter, and the purpose of each, are reviewed in Table 8–4.

Compensatory Strategies

Perhaps one of the most important components of any CAPD management program is that of teaching the child to become an active rather than a passive listener. The child must learn to accept responsibility for his or her listening comprehension and to invoke strategies for determining and retaining the content and meaning of each message.

Chermak (1992), and Musiek and Chermak (1995) outlined several strategies for effective listening that children with CAPD may be trained to utilize. These strategies include *linguistic, metalinguistic,* and *metacognitive abilities,* and are intended to aid the child in actively monitoring and self-regulating his or her own message comprehension abilities, as well as in developing general problem-solving skills.

Table 8–4
Overview of Remediation Activities for CAPD

Activity	Purpose
Auditory Closure Activities	To assist the child in learning to fill in missing components of a message in order to arrive at a meaningful whole
Phoneme Training	To help the child develop accurate phonemic representation and speech-to-print skills
Prosody Training	To help the child learn to recognize and use prosodic aspects of speech (e.g., rhythm, stress, and intonation)
Temporal Patterning Training	To train the child to discriminate differences in, analyze, and imitate rhythmic patterns of auditory stimuli
Interhemispheric Exercises	To stimulate the corpus callosum in order to improve interhemispheric transfer of information

For some children, **training in the rules of language may be necessary**. Children who exhibit difficulty applying linguistic rules to incoming auditory stimuli, as in Associative Deficit, may benefit from specific training in the use and meaning of tag words (e.g., first, last, next, before, after), causal words (because, since), adversative terms (but, however, although), and other terms that imply relationships between parts of the message. Once the child has become adept at identifying and interpreting these terms, he or she will be better able to separate the message into smaller linguistic units dependent on the relative relationship between and among portions of the message. This ability aids in comprehending and retaining information as well as in sequencing critical elements.

Other strategies that may aid in the retention of complex messages include *chunking* (breaking long messages into smaller component parts and grouping like concepts together), *verbal rehearsal* (repetition and reauditorization of a message, in much the same way as one repeats a phone number over and over in order to retain the number until it can be dialed), and *paraphrasing* (having the child reiterate the message in his or her own words). These strategies are likely to be most effective with children who exhibit an Associative or Output-Organization Deficit; however, all children with CAPD may benefit from training in these approaches.

The use of external aids to organization, as well, should not be overlooked. Teaching the child to use notebooks, calendars, computerized diaries, and other aids may be effective in training overall organizational learning skills. The child who demonstrates an inability in initiation and follow-through of complex projects due to inefficient planning and sequencing skills, as is often seen in Organization-Output Deficit, will benefit from training in the use of files and other organizational devices that will allow him or her to separate steps of a project into distinct units to be dealt with one at a time.

Regardless of the underlying deficit, the child with CAPD most often will benefit from activities designed to increase motivation and self-confidence. **The first step in increasing motivation and returning control of the situation to the child is to educate the child regarding the nature of his or her disorder**. Simply putting into words the cause of the difficulties that are experienced in listening situations can begin the process of convincing the child that he or she is not stupid or worthless, but that specific deficits exist that, with awareness and effort, can be overcome.

The situations in which understanding spoken language are most difficult should be precisely identified and discussed openly. If, for example, the child exhibits an Auditory Decoding Deficit and has difficulty decoding the spoken message, particularly in noisy situations, the reasons underlying his or her difficulty may be discussed. Through Phoneme Training, specific phonemes with which the child has the most difficulty can be identified. The child, along with the clinician, may develop a list of suggestions that he or she can use when in a difficult listening situation, as well as tips for predicting when a listening situation is likely to be problematic. In addition, the child can identify when skills learned in therapy, such as key word extraction, vocabulary building, and phonemic discrimination, may need to be invoked in daily listening situations.

For example, the child (with the clinician's assistance) may be able to recognize that certain classes are most difficult due to specific acoustic characteristics (e.g., the softness of the teacher's voice, the presence of poor acoustics, or significant sources of noise). As a result, the child can predict in advance that he or she will experience difficulty in understanding lectures or instructions in these specific classes. Therefore, the child may plan to be prepared to sit in a seat from which he or she can best hear the teacher and utilize visual cues, ask questions to clarify messages about which uncertainty exists, and request a list of new terms and information prior to class lecture. The child may wish to read assignments in advance in order to be better prepared for in-class discussions and activities. Finally, the child may request the use of an assistive listening device in order to improve access to auditory information.

In this manner, the clinician is involving the child in general problem-solving decisions designed to help alleviate the problem. Although many of these recommendations are those that may have been made without input from the child in question, by involving the child in the problem-solving process, the child is empowered and made to realize that many of the factors governing his or her ability to hear and comprehend spoken messages are under the child's control. Therefore, the child becomes less likely to enter a listening situation with a passive, ready-to-fail attitude, and becomes an active participant in his or her own listening and learning experience.

In conclusion, management of the child with CAPD should include modifications of the learning environment, remediation activities directed toward specific deficit areas, and compensatory strategies to include teaching the child how to analyze and approach problematic listening situations. **Although each of the three components of CAPD management are dealt with separately in this chapter, the clinician should realize that they are interwoven and interdependent.** Skills taught in therapy must be voluntarily evoked by the child in the everyday listening environment, which requires awareness and education on the part of the child. Likewise, recommendations for environmental modifications may be developed along with the child, thus involving him or her in the overall management process and helping to ensure the most important component of all: motivation to succeed.

Central Auditory Processing Disorders Management in the Very Young Child

Much has been made in previous chapters of the need for an age of 7 or 8 years before diagnostic central auditory testing can be conducted. What, then, of the very young child? Are we to wait until the disorder can be confirmed before beginning intervention for young children that are clearly exhibiting many of the behavioral signs and symptoms of CAPD?

Although it is true that comprehensive central auditory assessment cannot be undertaken in preschool-age children, the fact remains that early and aggressive intervention is imperative as soon as the presence of CAPD is suspected. Musiek and Chermak (1995) suggested that children suspected of CAPD be involved in a program that focuses on auditory skills development. A variety of activities may be used with children that maintain a high interest level while improving auditory perceptual skills.

The Phoneme Training activities discussed earlier in this chapter can be adapted for use with the very young child in much the same manner in which auditory training activities are carried out with the preschooler with hearing-impairment. Instead of associating the sound with the printed letter symbol, pictures may be used to illustrate the minimal contrast pairs (e.g., a picture of a tiger for /t/ and a dog for /d/). The remainder of the activity may be carried out as with older children, although the speech-to-print activities probably would not be necessary with preschoolers.

Musiek and Chermak (1995) suggested that reading aloud, a popular activity for young children, be conducted with specific goals in mind; namely, selective listening for designated target words identified prior to the story being read. In this manner, the child must listen carefully to all aspects of the story in order to hear and identify the target words. To ensure comprehension of the story, the reader should ask comprehension questions throughout and at the end of the story presentation. Games such as "Duck, Duck, Goose," and variations of "Musical Chairs" can also foster selective listening skills in the very young child.

Likewise, additional remediation activities provided in this chapter may be adapted for the very young child so that they may be conducted in the preschool classroom as a fun, group activity. Interhemispheric exercises such as grab bag activities offer an interesting diversion for any preschool child. Activities that require the child to guess the emotion based on intonational characteristics may foster awareness of prosodic features of speech, and elementary verbal scavenger hunts and variations of "Simon Says" assist in the development of skills necessary for following verbal directions. Even Temporal Patterning activities can be developed that build on the young child's inherent love of imitation and body movement.

The child who is suspected of CAPD should be watched carefully in the classroom in order to identify areas of functional difficulty. As many preschool classrooms are experiential in nature, involving multimodality stimulation every step of the way, the child should be monitored carefully for signs of confusion when more than one modality is introduced, a possible sign of Integration Deficit. The teacher or clinician may discover that the child in question does much better when information is presented via one mode at a time, thus providing useful insight into the possible underlying deficit as well as into the child's primary learning mode.

In conclusion, although valid and reliable test procedures to diagnose CAPD in the preschool-age child are not available at the current time, early intervention can and should be undertaken with children suspected of CAPD. As with other auditory disorders, early intervention may help to dilute or avoid entirely later difficulties that will inevitably appear when a child exhibits CAPD.

Summary

This chapter has discussed management strategies appropriate for children with CAPD. The clinician should remember that the management program should be individualized and should be as deficit-specific as possible.

Any CAPD management program should consist of three parts: environmental and classroom-based modifications to improve the child's access to auditory information, deficit-specific remediation activities designed to overcome or remedy the disorder, and compensatory strategies to aid the child in becoming an active listener. If any of these three components is missing, the management program cannot be considered comprehensive.

Finally, although absolute diagnosis of CAPD is not possible with children younger than 7 or 8 years, intervention should not be delayed until diagnosis can be accomplished. Instead, management principles appropriate for the older child may be adapted for the preschool child and may be implemented in the preschool classroom in a manner that is fun and educational for all children involved.

Finally, it should be remembered that, although the management approaches discussed in this chapter are based on current knowledge regarding the way the auditory system develops and functions, further research is needed in order to demonstrate treatment efficacy of the techniques discussed herein.

Review Questions

1. What are the three main categories of CAPD management in the educational setting, and what is the goal of each?
2. What general recommendations for management may be made for all children with CAPD?
3. List three classroom-based management recommendations that may be appropriate for the child with each of the following four CAPD profiles:

   Auditory Decoding Deficit   Associative Deficit
   Integration Deficit   Output-Organization Deficit

4. Briefly discuss the following remediation techniques, including what type of CAPD the activity would be appropriate for use with:

   Auditory Closure Activities   Vocabulary Building
   Phoneme Training   Prosody Training
   Temporal Patterning   Interhemispheric Exercises
       Training

5. List at least five compensatory strategies that may be of use for children with CAPD.
6. Discuss the role of the child's internal motivation in the success or failure of a CAPD management program.
7. Outline activities that may be undertaken with very young children suspected of CAPD.
8. Johnny is a 10-year-old male who is exhibiting significant difficulties in the classroom. His teachers report that he

has difficulty following directions, appears confused much of the time, and exhibits difficulty in noisy situations. Upon central auditory assessment, Johnny exhibits a left ear deficit on Dichotic Digits and a more pronounced left ear suppression on Competing Sentences. In addition, his performance on the Frequency Patterns test indicates a bilateral depression when verbal report is required; however, the scores revert to within normal limits when Johnny is asked to hum his responses. His performance on Low-Pass Filtered Speech is within normal limits for his age.

    a. Is it likely that Johnny exhibits a CAPD and, if so, what underlying processes appear to be dysfunctional?

    b. What CAPD subprofile(s) does Johnny exhibit characteristics of?

    c. Design a management program based on Johnny's specific deficit(s), if any.

9. Mary is a 12-year-old female with difficulty understanding speech in noise. Although she is in the sixth grade, she reads at a second- to third-grade level, and her word attack skills are significantly depressed. Upon central testing, Mary scored within the normal range for her age on Dichotic Digits, Dichotic CVs, the SSW, and Frequency Patterns; however, her performance on Low-Pass Filtered Speech was abnormally low bilaterally. When a Com-pressed Speech test was administered, Mary scored just above the chance level for both ears.

    a. Is it likely that Mary exhibits a CAPD and, if so, what underlying processes are likely to be dysfunctional?

    b. What CAPD subprofile does Mary exhibit characteristics of?

    c. Design a management program for Mary.

10. Fred is a 9-year-old male who is enrolled in speech-language services for receptive language delay. He exhibits receptive language deficits in the areas of vocabulary, semantics, and syntax. His early academic history is unremarkable, but he began having difficulty in school upon beginning the fourth grade. Fred is looked upon as a social misfit by many of his peers and teachers. Central testing indicates bilateral deficits on Dichotic Digits and Competing Sentences; however, performance on all other tests is within normal limits.

    a. Is it likely that Fred exhibits a CAPD and, if so, what underlying processes are likely to be dysfunctional?

    b. What CAPD subprofile does Fred exhibit characteristics of?

    c. Design a management program for Fred.

11. Alex is a 14-year-old male who seems to understand what is being said to him, but exhibits difficulty in carrying out instructions. His teachers and parents have postulated that he has a memory problem, as his ability to recall directions and words is poor. He reads well, but has difficulty with writing and spelling. In addition, Alex is doing poorly in Shop class, in which he is completing assembly of a bookshelf. Upon central auditory evaluation, Alex exhibits bilateral deficits on all tests administered except for Low-Pass Filtered Speech, upon which he performs within normal limits.

    a. Is it likely that Alex exhibits a CAPD and, if so, what underlying processes are likely to be dysfunctional?

    b. What CAPD subprofile does Alex exhibit characteristics of?

    c. Design a management program for Alex.

PART

THREE

Developing a Service Delivery Program

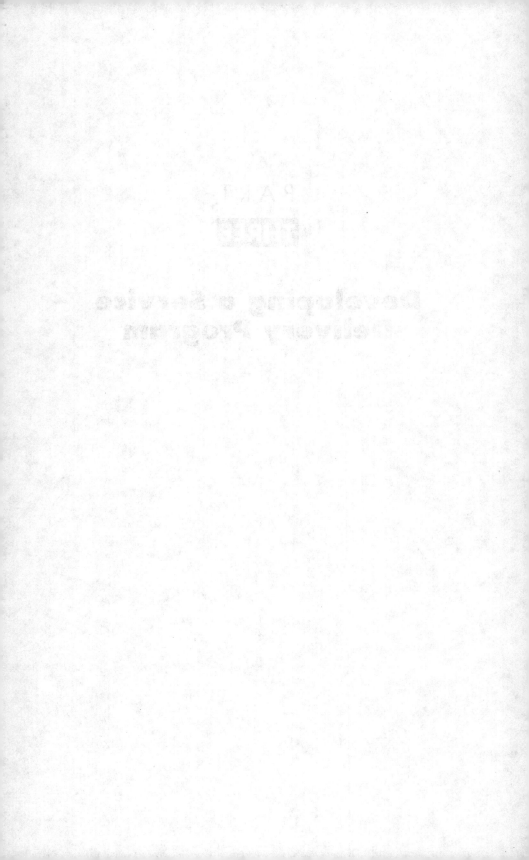

CHAPTER

NINE

Considerations in Central Auditory Processing Service Delivery

entral auditory processing disorders do not exist in a vacuum, and neither does the clinician invoved in the assessment and management of such disorders. Instead, the clinician involved in the field of CAPD must interact with other professionals in the special education arena, medical personnel, administrators, parents, and additional key individuals in order to ensure the success of any CAP program.

This chapter will provide recommendations for the development and implementation of a service delivery program. Included will be methods of educating appropriate individuals as to the nature of CAPD and the justification for a comprehensive program to address CAPD, suggestions for report writing and other means of imparting assessment and management information to referral sources, the use of the Child Study process to detail management recommendations and foster appropriate follow-through on management suggestions, and the presentation of a model service delivery program that includes all levels of CAPD assessment and management, from screening to follow-through.

Learning Objectives

After studying this chapter, the reader should be able to

1. Provide justification for the need for a comprehensive CAP service delivery program
2. Identify methods of addressing questions and concerns most likely to be raised by colleagues, associated professionals, and parents
3. Discuss methods of conveying salient information to referral sources and other appropriate parties
4. Identify components necessary in any CAP service delivery program.

Education of Key Individuals

The first step in the success of any CAP service delivery program is the education of all individuals involved regarding the nature of CAPD, state-of-the-art methods of assessing and managing such disorders, and the justification underlying the necessary expenditures of time and money to ensure the quality of a comprehensive program.

It cannot be denied that there exists a general consensus regarding the need for means of addressing CAPD in the educational setting. Audiologists throughout the country are deluged by phone calls requesting information about CAPD. Special education professionals are hungry for recommendations regarding management of such disorders. Journal articles concerning CAPD proliferate in every professional arena, and CAP workshops and conferences are springing up in every region.

Therefore, it may surprise the enthusiastic clinician who charges to the forefront of his or her educational setting like a knight in shining armor that many of the recommendations made regarding assessment and management of CAPD are met with resistance, reluctance, and perhaps even complete dismissal.

It appears that what is wanted is not just a method for addressing CAPD in the educational setting, but a method that is simple to implement, costs no additional money, and involves little additional time or training on the part of the individuals involved, yet will still yield the desired results. When confronted with the complexity of CAPD itself, combined with the need for training, equipment, and clinical time to implement a comprehensive, state-of-the-art CAP program, audiologists and other educational professionals may question whether the return is worth the cost. These individuals, already struggling with inflated caseloads and insufficient funding, may unconsciously search for ways to look the other way, while still expressing a desire for answers to the continuing problem of CAPD.

Citing the lack of consensus among special education professionals regarding best methods of assessment and management, these individuals may decide to wait until all the answers are in before taking action. Referring to screening tools already available and in use in many regions, they may determine that little additional information would be gained by the employment of assessment techniques such as those described in this book and, therefore, decide that the screening tools already in use are sufficient for diagnostic purposes. Emphasizing their own full schedules, combined with poor prospects for funding for additional personnel, they may decide that they simply don't have the necessary time or interest to engage in comprehensive CAP service delivery.

Flying in the face of the growing body of literature in the areas of neurophysiology, neuroplasticity, reliability and validity of assessment measures, management techniques, and the like, the search continues for the easy answer to the CAPD question.

It must be emphasized that **there is no easy answer nor, in our opinion, is there likely to be one, for the sheer complexity of the central auditory system precludes a simplistic approach to the identification and treatment of disorders of that system.** In addition, the heterogeneity of the CAPD population disallows the existence of one, easy, right way of addressing the needs of the population. And, as more and more is learned about auditory processing and its disorders, the entire topic of CAPD undoubtedly will become even more complex than it is currently.

However, it should be recognized that great strides have been made in the field of CAPD in recent years and, while recommendations for assessment and management will no doubt continue to change and evolve as more data are collected, sufficient information exists today to help us refine our identification and treatment approaches. Assessment procedures, such as those described in Chapters 6 and 7, are available that have demonstrated validity in detecting disorders of the CANS. Likewise, there is increasing evidence that language, auditory, and educational management approaches, undertaken as early as possible, are likely to be of benefit to the child with CAPD.

Therefore, despite the complexity of the subject, **the only effective means of providing services to children with CAPD in the edu-**

cational setting is through the development and implementation of a CAP service delivery program that incorporates current state-of-the-art diagnostic and therapeutic techniques while, at the same time, providing for continuing education so that modifications to the program may be made based on emerging data and recommendations for best practice.

This is not an easy task. The clinician entering into the field of central auditory processing must be prepared to invest time and energy in the education of fellow audiologists, speech-language pathologists, psychologists, educators, administrators, and other associated individuals. In addition, each of these individuals is likely to bring to the table different questions and concerns related directly to his or her area of expertise and involvement. Therefore, what follows is a discussion of common concerns likely to be raised by each of the disciplines involved in the implementation of a comprehensive CAP program and also suggestions for addressing those questions and concerns with an eye toward ensuring transdisciplinary cooperation and support.

The Audiologist

Not surprisingly, the audiologist is the professional most likely to raise concerns regarding the components necessary in the implementation of a comprehensive CAP program, primarily because it is the audiologist to whom the task of leading the project will fall. Several concerns may be raised by the audiologist; however, they will tend to fall into two general categories: lack of time and lack of training.

The audiologist in the educational setting has a formidable task. Often, he or she is responsible for a given district's hearing screening program, including the provision of diagnostic audiological services to those children who fail the screening, as well as monitoring the audiological status of at-risk and hearing-impaired students. Staffings must be planned for and attended, and inservices must be given. Amplification and assistive listening devices used by the hearing-impaired, school-age population must be monitored and repaired. And, to perform all of these duties, many school districts employ only one full-time, or even one part-time, audiologist.

There is no evading the fact that serving as the team leader for a CAP service delivery program is a time-consuming endeavor. When one takes into account the time investment necessary to guide the CAP screening team, review data collected during the screening process, engage in comprehensive assessment procedures, make recommendations for management, meet with teachers, parents, and other individuals to explain the recommendations made and ensure follow-through, and provide inservice training to all applicable persons, it can be seen that the audiologist may need to spend up to several hours per child. This is a daunting prospect for even the most energetic and enthusiastic of audiologists.

Add to this the fact that recent events in the federal government have virtually assured that educational funding will be cut drastically in the future, thus prohibiting the hiring of additional personnel, while, at the same time, more and more children are entering into the school system every day, and it is easy to see why many audiologists might approach the subject of CAP service delivery with a healthy degree of skepticism and trepidation.

Second, the audiologist may balk at the amount of training necessary for the appropriate interpretation of central auditory assessment tools and development of management plans. As discussed in this book, it is not enough simply to become familiar with the various test tools that can be utilized. Instead, a thorough understanding of the underlying processes, including anatomical and neurophysiological bases, is necessary. The typical educational audiologist has received little education in this area.

A primary reason for this lack of education is that **few educational programs for audiologists deal with the subject of CAPD in sufficient**

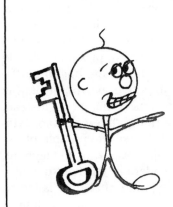

KEY CONCEPT

Familiarity with the administration of central auditory tests is not enough. In order to engage in comprehensive CAP service delivery, the clinician also must have the necessary background knowledge and competencies.

detail to allow for independent clinical application. In fact, we have encountered several audiology graduate programs that devote one day or less to the subject of CAPD and, when questioned, program administrators reply with one of the widely held myths surrounding the subject: "We can't really test it, and we can't do anything about it if we diagnose it. Therefore, there's nothing to teach." As a result, graduates entering the field of educational audiology carry similar misconceptions and lack of knowledge in the area and are surprised and unprepared when they are asked to address CAPD on a more and more frequent basis.

A second contributing factor to the insufficient education of audiologists regarding CAPD is the **lack of consensus regarding best practices in CAP service delivery**. It is generally acknowledged that, in recent years, debate has raged as to how CAPD should be viewed, assessed, and managed. In general, it appears that the debate has centered around finding the *one* best definition, the *one* best method of assessment, and the *one* best method of managing disorders of central auditory processing. During the 1994 CAPD consensus development conference in Albuquerque, New Mexico, it surprised some of us who attended as mere observers to hear the degree of emotional disagreement and debate. During the two-day run of the program, leaders in the field of CAPD held faithfully to their own, particular viewpoints on the subject and, in many cases, refused to acknowledge the input of others.

Debate raged over such subjects as whether CAPD is fundamentally a language-based disorder, whether electrophysiological tests should be utilized to diagnose CAPD, and if management approaches should focus on auditory, phonemic decoding, or language-based skills. Interestingly, when approached from an objective viewpoint, it was apparent that very little actual disagreement was taking place. Instead, each of the participants seemed to be describing different manifestations of this heterogeneous beast called CAPD. Like the parable of the four blind men who, while each is feeling a different part of an elephant, disagree over what the animal actually is, leaders in the field of CAPD seemed to hold so closely to their own viewpoints that they failed to recognize that each was describing a different part of the same animal.

When one accepts the extreme heterogeneity of the CAPD population, one recognizes that, in some cases, the disorder may be more language-based than in others. While management appropriate for one child may focus on language-related skills, management for another may be primarily auditory in nature. Electrophysiological measures may add valuable information in many, but not all, cases of CAPD.

Therefore, when looked at objectively, it appears that some degree of consensus regarding CAPD assessment and management has, indeed, been reached, and involves the recognition and acceptance of the fact that **the CAPD population is a heterogeneous one and, therefore, assessment and management should reflect this heterogeneity.** To this end, and as discussed throughout this book, assessment of CAPD should include the collection of information regarding educational, speech-language, cognitive, and other appropriate aspects of the child, as well as the evaluation of a wide variety of auditory processes using assessment tools that have demonstrated validity in the detection of disorders of the CANS. Management should be as deficit-specific as possible and should be directed toward the individual child's presenting type of disorder. Rather than adopting one limited view of CAPD, the clinician would do well to recognize that, depending on the individual child, any of the views espoused may be the correct one in any given instance. Therefore, **the clinician should strive to keep an open mind and to avoid the adoption of one, limited view of CAPD.**

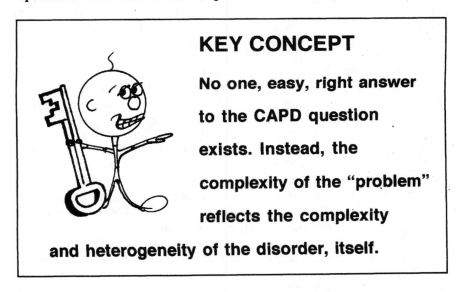

KEY CONCEPT

No one, easy, right answer to the CAPD question exists. Instead, the complexity of the "problem" reflects the complexity and heterogeneity of the disorder, itself.

All of this having been said, the audiologist would be correct in feeling that a great amount of education and training is involved in attaining the competencies necessary for CAP service delivery. This fact, combined with the lack of time to engage in training and service delivery activities, may result in reluctance on the part of many educational audiologists to become involved in the implementation of a CAP service delivery program, despite the evidence of need for such a program.

Educating the Audiologist

To obtain the support of the educational audiologist in the CAP service delivery program effort, it must first be acknowledged that the concerns raised by the audiologist are reasonable and valid. The provision of CAP services is, indeed, time consuming and requires specialized knowledge. On the other hand, the need for such services is undisputed. Therefore, efforts should be made to address the concerns of the audiologist in a realistic manner.

The issue of lack of time is a difficult one to resolve. However, it should be noted that **it may not be necessary for every educational audiologist to engage in comprehensive CAP service delivery.** Just as some physicians are better suited to certain specialties than are others, there may be some audiologists who, due to interest in the topic or other factors, may be more likely to become involved in the assessment and management of CAPD.

Later in this chapter, a model service delivery program will be presented that will provide for regional assessment centers to which all educational facilities in a given locale may refer for comprehensive central auditory assessment and recommendations for management. It may be possible, through interagency collaboration, for those audiologists who exhibit the desire and competence necessary to be primarily responsible for the delivery of comprehensive CAP services in a given location, thus eliminating the need for all audiologists to become involved in providing full-scale CAP services. In this manner, the responsibility for CAP service provision may be shared among several different educational agencies, and the waste of valuable time and resources that occurs with replication of services may be avoided.

Which brings us to the subject of training: It has been emphasized again and again throughout this book that **the provision of CAP services requires a working knowledge of the subject that can be obtained only through specialized education and training in the field.** Therefore, efforts to provide inservice and workshop education for audiologists should focus on the scientific and theoretical underpinnings of central auditory processing, as well as methods of practical application of scientific theory. In addition, it would behoove any clinician in the field to network with other professionals throughout the nation who, likewise, are involved in the provision of full-scale CAP services. Finally, we encourage educational institutions to include in the graduate education of fledgling audiologists courses specifically designed to build the competencies necessary for the independent provision of comprehensive central auditory processing services.

In conclusion, as the professional to whom the task of organizing a comprehensive CAP service delivery effort will fall, the audiologist is likely to raise understandable concerns regarding time available for such activities, as well as the necessary specialized training. Therefore, through interagency collaboration and networking, efforts should be made to allow for sufficient clinical time and educational opportunities so that the audiologists involved may have available the resources and support necessary for the provision of quality CAP services.

The Speech-Language Pathologist

The speech-language pathologist is the professional who will probably be most involved in the implementation of management suggestions, particularly if recommendations involve direct therapeutic techniques that can best be handled in an individual therapy situation, or if the child in question exhibits a language-based CAPD that requires more traditional language intervention. In addition, information from the speech-language pathologist concerning the individual child's speech and language capabilities is necessary for the CAP screening process. Therefore, the speech-language pathologist, like the audiologist, is likely to raise concerns that revolve around the time available for CAP-related activities.

Second, the speech-language pathologist historically has been intimately involved in the central auditory assessment process. As mentioned in Chapter 4, many of the speech-language tools on the market contain subtests that purport to assess auditory perceptuals abilities. These professionals may require justification for the fact that these tools, which have to date been utilized for diagnostic central auditory purposes, should actually be considered as screening tools only.

Educating the Speech-Language Pathologist

The speech-language pathologist is a key member of the CAP service delivery team. Therefore, it is necessary to obtain the cooperation and support from speech-language pathologists throughout the educational arena. In order to do this, the speech-language pathologist must first be educated regarding the nature of CAPD and the validity and reliability of assessment tools. It must be shown that, while the speech-language pathologist has much to offer in the CAP screening and management processes, **assessment tools that have documented validity in the detection of disorders of the CANS must be utilized for the actual diagnosis and delineation of central auditory processing disorders**.

Secondly, and perhaps more importantly, the nature of CAPD management should be of issue in any educational program directed toward the speech-language pathologist. Because it is the speech-language pathologist who likely will carry out many of the management suggestions made following comprehensive central auditory assessment, it is necessary that the speech-language pathologist attain a working knowledge of categories of CAPD, types of underlying processes that may be dysfunctional, purposes and goals of each management technique described, and methods of carrying out management recommendations. In addition, the contribution of auditory processing to speech perception, speech production, language, and learning should be addressed in any educational program for speech-language pathologists.

Finally, in cases of children who may already be on the speech-language pathologist's caseload, suggestions for infusing CAP therapeutic techniques into already existing therapy plans will be quite helpful, as will suggestions for home-based and resource-based therapy. In this way, the additional time investment on the part of the speech-language pathologist for CAPD management may be kept to a minimum.

The Educator

The classroom teacher has the responsibility of addressing the educational needs of all of the students in his or her classroom, and he or she may be responsible for 25 to 35 students in addition to the one child who exhibits CAPD. Although these educators may be extremely motivated to do whatever is necessary to help the child in need, it cannot be denied that little additional time is available for implementation of direct management suggestions in the classroom. Conversely, the educator may be unaware of the nature of CAPD and the unique needs such a child demonstrates and, instead, feel that the child in question is just "not trying hard enough" or "not paying attention."

The special education or resource teacher may be more aware of the difficulties exhibited by a given child; however, he or she may be unfamiliar with educationally based methods of management appropriate for use with various types of CAPD.

Educating the Educator

The key focus of educating the educator should be on the educational impact of CAPD and methods of classroom-based management. The educator is much less likely to be interested in the diagnostic process than in compensatory strategies, environmental modifications, and other educationally based methods of CAPD management. Also, the educator should receive information regarding the common indicators of CAPD for CAP screening purposes.

Therefore, activities directed toward education of the educator should center around developing an understanding of the characteristics of CAPD in general, the nature of a given child's CAPD, and the academic impact of such a disorder, as well as the rationale behind each management suggestion made. In addition, the regular education classroom teacher will benefit from guidance in how to implement classroom-based suggestions with the least amount of additional time investment.

The resource teacher may be in the position of implementing remediation techniques. For example, the child who exhibits an Auditory Decoding Deficit and is receiving remedial reading services may benefit greatly from the addition of Phonemic Decoding activities, including speech-to-print training, which can be added to the reading-based therapy program already in place.

Finally, educators should be familiarized with the various compensatory strategies that the child is being trained to use in the therapy situation so that the appropriate generalization and use of such strategies in the classroom can be monitored.

The Educational Psychologist

Like the speech-language pathologist, the educational psychologist has in his or her armament various test tools that have traditionally been utilized for diagnosis of CAPD. Indeed, in our experience, many of the children who come to school with a "CAPD label" often have been "diagnosed" by someone in the profession of psychology. Therefore, it should be recognized that a degree of territoriality may exist, and suggestions made regarding the appropriate methods of assessing CAPD may be met with some skepticism and distrust.

On the other hand, many children with CAPD may be under the care of the psychologist for associated symptoms of frustration and depression that may occur with continual academic and communicative struggles. Therefore, the psychologist is an important member of the CAP team in that he or she may be in the unique position to provide valuable information regarding the social-emotional impact of the disorder, as well as cognitive functioning and scatter of skills.

Educating the Psychologist

Through inservice education or other methods, all attempts should be made to educate the psychological profession regarding the neurophysiological bases of CAPD and the appropriate, valid measures of diagnosing the disorder. Once an understanding of the auditory nature of CAPD is fostered, the psychologist becomes much more likely to serve willingly as a key member of the CAP service delivery team.

In addition, the psychologist should become familiar with the CAP screening process and his or her contribution to CAP screening. The need for accurate measures of cognitive ability and other psychoeducational skills should be addressed. Finally, the potential impact of CAPD on a child's overall social and emotional well-being should not be overlooked, as the psychologist may be called upon to provide individual or family counseling services to those children in need of additional aid.

The Special Education Administrator

The administrator is responsible for providing the full range of special education services for all qualified children from a pool of ever-dwindling resources. As such, **the administrator is less likely to be interested in the theoretical underpinnings of auditory processing and its disorders and much more concerned with how CAP services can be provided with the least amount of drain upon current personnel and funding sources.**

A principle concern for administrators is the need for such a service delivery program. The administrator is likely to have questions regarding the numbers of children affected in his or her school or district, the purpose of each member's involvement in the program, and the time and equipment neecessary for implementing a comprehensive CAP program. If a regional assessment center approach is proposed, such as the one described later in this chapter, the administrater may have additional questions as to who will provide the direct diagnostic services for such a center, who will pay for assessment services, and how current caseloads will be affected by the additional duties required of those directly involved in the CAP endeavor.

Educating the Administrator

The key to obtaining administrative support for a CAP service delivery program is to foster an understanding of the rationale for comprehensive CAP services. The clinician should be prepared to address the estimated prevalence of CAPD, providing specific examples of children affected in a given school or district whenever possible; the academic, communicative, and emotional impact of such disorders; and current, state-of-the-art recommendations for service delivery. In addition, the clinician would do well to collect data regarding the number of CAP-related requests for information and assistance received in a given time period from professionals throughout the district or region. In this way, the clinician can help to foster an understanding of the need for CAP services, as well as the rationale behind the comprehensive program being proposed.

Regarding resources, although all attempts should be made to spread the responsibility for CAP service delivery among all involved professionals, it must be accepted that additional time or funding may be required for the implementation of such a program. If the presenting difficulties of a given child are deemed by the educational professionals working with the child to be needy of further investigation, it will ultimately fall to the educational system to provide the funding for such additional services. Therefore, along with the administrator, the clinician should be prepared to develop a plan for defining minimum referral criteria for CAP services and identifying methods of acquiring or allocating funds and personnel for the CAP service delivery endeavor.

Education of Other Appropriate Individuals

Medical professionals, private practice audiologists and psychologists, parents, and other individuals in a given region are appropriate targets for inservice and other educational activities concerning auditory processing disorders in the educational setting.

It is not uncommon to find professionals in the private practice setting becoming more and more involved with CAP service delivery. From neurologists and other medical professionals to audiologists, speech-language pathologists, and psychologists, interest in CAPD and its clinical manifestations is blossoming nationwide. Of primary concern to the clinician in the educational setting is the education of such professionals regarding appropriate methods of assessment and the educational impact of such disorders.

Due to lack of familiarity with the educational setting in general, **the private practitioner may be more likely to approach CAPD from a limited viewpoint, failing to take into account academic, cognitive, and communicative sequelae. As a result, the diagnostic and interpretive process may be limited in scope only to those skills that are auditory-based. Suggestions for management may fail to address the individualized academic and classroom-based needs of the child or, conversely, may address such needs in such a manner as to be impractical or inappropriate for the given child's educational setting.**

In addition, as federal funding for special education services undergoes further changes in the coming years, it is likely that many specialized services may be contracted out to private practitioners.

Therefore, the education of those in the private practice milieu is of utmost importance.

Through inservice education and networking, the need for these individuals to work closely with educational professionals must be emphasized. Private practitioners should be encouraged to consult with and involve the child's educators in all aspects of assessment and management. The whole child approach to diagnosis and management of CAPD should be advocated strongly, and open lines of communication between private practitioners and educational professionals should be made available at every step along the way. Through these efforts, the private practitioner becomes a member of the greater CAP team, and the likelihood of follow-through and success of management endeavors is greatly increased.

A final, critical component of the CAP team is the parent. Without understanding and support from the home environment, no CAP service delivery program can attain its full potential.

Parents of children with CAPD are likely to be in need of a great deal of information regarding the nature of the disorder, management suggestions, and prognosis for success. Even greater is the need for general, emotional support from clinicians and professionals in the educational arena. As discussed in Chapter 7, sufficient time should be made available during the diagnostic process to sit with the parents and explain the implications of assessment findings. Certain therapeutic techniques, such as Interhemispheric Exercises, may be particularly well suited for implementation in the home, and the rationale behind and methods of carrying out such activities should be delineated clearly. Parent support groups may be established to provide parents with a resource for emotional support and new information. The more the parents understand about their child's presenting disorder, the more likely appropriate follow-through will occur. Therefore, education of parents and other family members is of utmost importance for the success of any CAP service delivery program.

To conclude, education of key individuals is a primary step in the development of any CAP service delivery program. However, it must be recognized that each individual involved in CAP service delivery likely will have different educational needs depending on his or her specific discipline and degree of involvement. This section has attempted to identify some of the questions and concerns most likely to be raised by each member of the CAP team, and to suggest CAP-related topics most applicable for each discipline. Therefore, rather than approaching CAP education from a generic perspective, it is recommended that the clinician entering into the development and implementation of a CAP service delivery program make every attempt to establish methods of differentially addressing the concerns of each team member. The information presented in this section is summarized in Table 9–1.

Methods of Imparting Diagnostic Information

No matter how well organized and state-of-the-art any CAP service delivery program is, all efforts will be wasted unless the results of diagnostic assessment and recommendations for management are reported in a clear, understandable way to the referring party, parents, and other appropriate individuals. Therefore, this section will focus on ways of imparting information through report-writing, handouts, and use of the Child Study process.

Table 9–1
Summary of Educational Needs of Key Individuals

Team Member	Education Should Focus on
Audiologist	Training and knowledge base necessary for comprehensive CAP service delivery, theoretical underpinnings and methods of practical application of scientific theory, time management
Speech-Language Pathologist	Appropriate methods of diagnosing CAPD, CAPD management
Educator	Educational impact of CAPD, classroom management suggestions
Educational Psychologist	Neurophysiological bases of CAPD, appropriate methods of diagnosing CAPD, need for accurate measures of cognitive and psychoeducational abilities, emotional impact of CAPD
Administrator	Prevalence of CAPD, rationale for comprehensive CAPD services, current recommendations for service delivery, funding issues
Other Professionals	The nature and impact of CAPD, appropriate methods of diagnosing CAPD, and the need for private practitioners to work closely with educational professionals
Parents	The nature of CAPD, management suggestions, and prognosis for success

Writing Reports

When writing any report, it is important to make sure that the writing style is clear, that all salient points are covered, and that any potentially unfamiliar information or terminology is explained carefully. This is certainly the case with central auditory processing diagnostic reports, in which it may be assumed that the reader is unfamiliar with many of the tests utilized and the concepts presented therein.

In addition, when writing CAP reports, the clinician should avoid at all costs the inclusion of statements avowing that a CAPD is or is not present in a given child. Instead, steps should be taken to describe the assessment procedure, and interpretation should include a caveat to the reader that CAP testing is not without limitations and, therefore, interpretation of such tests should be undertaken with caution. **If the child demonstrates no apparent deficit in the areas tested, this should not be taken to mean that a CAPD is not present at all.** Rather, the clinician should state that the presence of a CAPD is not likely *in those areas specifically assessed.* In this manner, the reader is led to the understanding that difficulties or disorder may exist in processes or areas not addressed in the diagnostic evaluation.

This section will describe the major components that should be included in the CAP diagnostic report: a discussion of relevant background information, results of audiological evaluation, description and report of central auditory evaluation results, impression of results, and recommendations for management (Table 9–2). It should be noted that it is not our intent to suggest that this is the only manner in which diagnostic reports may be written. The suggestions offered here are intended merely as suggestions so that issues of importance are covered adequately in the report-writing process.

Background Information

The Background Information section of the CAP report should include relevant information collected during the screening and parent interview process related to primary referring concern; results of academic, cognitive, communicative, and other testing; medical and family history; and areas of difficulty in listening situations reported by the child and/or parents themselves. Emphasis for inclusion should be placed on those issues that led to the referral for comprehensive central auditory assessment; however, if a screening issue is "negative," that fact should be mentioned briefly (e.g., "Otologic history appears unremarkable" or "There does not appear to be a family history of learning problems") so that the reader understands that the issue was investigated.

Table 9-2

Components of the CAP Diagnostic Report

- Background Information
  - primary referring concern
  - results of academic, communicative, and other testing
  - medical and family history
  - areas of auditory difficulty
  - observations regarding the child's educational environment
- Results of Audiological Evaluation
- Central Auditory Assessment Results
  - description of test tools used
  - description of child's demeanor, attention, and behavior during testing
  - results of each test of central auditory processing
- Impressions
  - description of underlying process(es) indicated as dysfunctional by test results
  - description of CAPD subprofile suggested by test results
  - relationship of central auditory findings to information presented in Background Information section of report
- Recommendations
  - detailed description of any management suggestions made
  - recommendations for further testing, reevaluation, or medical follow-up, as needed

---

Also important for inclusion are any observations made regarding the child's educational environment. It has been our experience that, by including presenting symptomatology and other salient background information in the final diagnostic report, pieces of the puzzle that were not otherwise apparent often seem to fall into place. In addition, by leading the reader carefully through the history and presenting complaints of the child in question, findings on central auditory assessment and, particularly, recommendations for management often tend to make more sense, thus helping further to ensure appropriate cooperation and follow-through.

Results of Audiological Evaluation

If not mentioned during the Background Information section of the report, the results of any audiological testing performed should be delineated next. In this way, the reader is assured that the peripheral auditory system has been evaluated, and that the presence of peripheral hearing loss as a contributing factor to the reported symptoms can be ruled out.

Central Auditory Assessment Results

We recommend that this section begin with a brief description of each test utilized in the assessment process, including the task required from each test as well as the process or processes investigated. The primary reason for this is that, at the present time, many individuals are unfamiliar with tests of central auditory processing, and will require information regarding testing methodology. In addition, other clinicians who themselves are engaging in central auditory assessment will want to know not just the final results of testing, but the methods through which those results were obtained, as well. Therefore, the test protocol should be explained briefly, but with sufficient detail to foster an understanding of the methods through which the diagnostic impressions were derived.

Following the discussion of test protocol, the child's general demeanor, attention, and other behavioral factors during testing should be addressed, as well as the possible impact, if any, on reliability of the results. For example, if the child in question demonstrated inappropriate behavior during testing, or was easily distracted despite the carefully controlled environment, this finding should be mentioned, as should the fact that findings on test results may be confounded due to the observed behaviors. Conversely, if the child attended and cooperated well throughout the test session, such should be noted.

Finally, results of each test of central auditory processing should be reported. Rather than merely listing percentages or raw scores obtained, we recommend that each score be reported in terms of how it compares to normative values for the given age range, as raw score values rarely convey diagnostic significance when utilized alone. Significant differences between ears, or ear effects, should be noted whenever obtained. The purpose of this section of the report is not to interpret the test results, but to present them in a coherent fashion.

Impressions

In this section of the report, the conclusions drawn from the assessment findings are delineated. As stated previously, we recommend that this section begin with a caveat to the reader regarding the limitations of central tests and the need for caution when interpreting such tests. Then, the report should proceed to a discussion of the significance of the assessment findings.

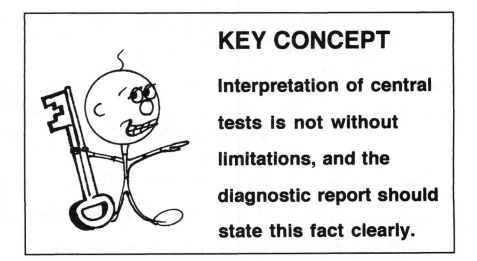

KEY CONCEPT

Interpretation of central tests is not without limitations, and the diagnostic report should state this fact clearly.

All attempts should be made to describe results in terms of the underlying process(es) found to be dysfunctional, and the likely behavioral, communicative, and academic impact of such dysfunction. Relating the findings to information presented in the Background Information section of the report is useful in helping the reader to understand the relative contribution of the given CAPD to the individual child's presenting history and complaints. If possible, the use of CAPD subprofiling, including a brief description of the appropriate profile(s), may also be useful in fostering reader understanding of the impact of the child's CAPD.

Recommendations

If the presenting history, test results, and impressions have been presented with sufficient detail and clarity, the recommendations made should, to the reader, appear to follow logically. In addition, it is helpful to separate recommendations for management into those that will occur in the classroom and those that will be addressed in a therapy situation.

In some cases, no therapeutic recommendations will be made, either because the assessment results do not suggest a need for therapy, or because the child is already receiving adequate services, as is frequently the case in language-based auditory processing disorders. In these situations, it is best to discuss *why* additional therapy suggestions are not being made, as well as the services currently in place that appear to be addressing the child's CAPD appropriately. Thus, the reader understands that intervention is, in fact, needed; however, the current program appears, at the present time, to be addressing the needs adequately. On the other hand, if the need for auditory processing intervention is not indicated by the results of central auditory evaluation, this should be discussed, as well.

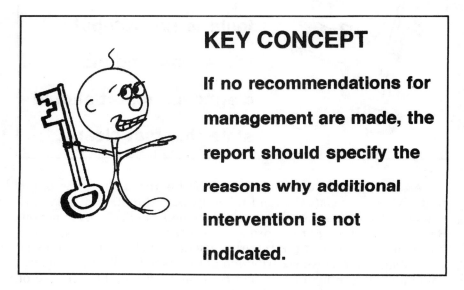

KEY CONCEPT

If no recommendations for management are made, the report should specify the reasons why additional intervention is not indicated.

Finally, it should be remembered that many of the intervention strategies discussed in Chapter 8 may not be familiar to many educational professionals. For this reason, recommendations for management should be described as clearly as possible. Remediation techniques should be supported with rationale, and examples should be given. In the next section, we will discuss the use of handouts to explain in detail the intervention methods that may be recommended. Handouts are an excellent way to guide the reader through management approaches, while reducing the report-writing and postevaluation counseling time investment on the part of the clinician providing comprehensive central auditory assessment services.

In conclusion, the diagnostic report is a key method of conveying information gleaned during the screening and assessment process. However, it is imperative that information contained in the report be written as clearly as possible, with sufficient detail so that the reader is able to understand the methodology used and the implications of the findings. When background history and screening information, test protocol, assessment results, and impressions of findings are explained in some detail, recommendations for management are more likely to seem part of a logical progression, and the chance of appropriate fol-low-through is enhanced.

Handouts

Handouts and other preprinted material can be invaluable resources for the busy clinician. In our clinic, each of the management techniques discussed in Chapter 8 is described in some detail, with step-by-step directions and examples of stimulus items. When a recommendation is made for a given type of remediation activity in the diagnostic report, the handout corresponding to the recommendation is attached. This practice not only saves valuable time, but also helps to ensure that remediation activities are conducted in a proper manner.

In addition, the clinician engaging in comprehensive CAP service delivery is likely to receive numerous requests for general information related to central auditory processing and its disorders. We have found it helpful to develop a general information packet that includes many of the key concepts presented in this book, from common indicators and definitions of CAPD to appropriate assessment methods. Of particular emphasis in our packet is the need for valid, reliable diagnostic procedures, as well as the heterogeneity of the CAPD population, which makes the presentation of general recommendations appropriate for every child with CAPD impossible.

To conclude, the use of preprinted handouts can be an excellent time-saving device for the clinician providing CAP services. However, caution should be exercised when developing these materials so that the reader clearly understands that the handouts are merely aids to understanding and do not take the place of valid diagnostic assessment and individualized management.

The Child Study Process

All special education programs have in place methods of bringing a variety of service providers together to discuss the educational concerns and needs of a particular child. This is done either before an Individual Educational Plan (IEP) staffing takes place, or at any time during the child's educational career when it is felt that additional concerns need to be addressed or the child's educational plan needs to be changed. These meetings usually involve the educators and service providers working with a given child, as well as the parents and, in some instances, the children themselves. The name by which these meetings are called varies from region to region but, for our purposes, we will call them *Child Studies*.

The Child Study process is an appropriate vehicle for disseminating information regarding auditory processing. It may be used before diagnostic assessment to discuss and delineate auditory-related concerns, as well as after central auditory evaluation to convey findings and recommendations for management. Through the use of the Child Study process, time is saved by addressing all appropriate individuals simultaneously, and questions can be answered promptly and within earshot of all involved. Finally, understanding of the disorder and management recommendations is fostered more easily when all persons involved in the education of the child are brought together.

We recommend that the clinician providing comprehensive CAP services set aside time to attend such meetings. In this manner, everyone involved with the given child can approach the issue from the same perspective, questions and misunderstandings can be clarified from the outset, and valuable time can be saved that may otherwise have been spent on individualized consultation with each service provider involved.

This section has discussed methods of imparting salient information to involved professionals and parents. Included have been suggestions for clear, concise report-writing, the use of handouts and other preprinted material, and the use of the Child Study process as a means of meeting face-to-face with service providers. The clinician should make use of these and other devices that will allow for better dissemination of information, while saving valuable time for everyone involved.

Comprehensive Central Auditory Processing Service Delivery

Throughout this text, we have discussed various aspects of central auditory processing, from neuroanatomy and neurophysiology to screening methods, assessment tools, and approaches to CAPD management. Because of the complexity of the subject, any service program designed to address central auditory processing will, likewise, be complex. This section will discuss those components necessary for developing and implementing a comprehensive CAP service delivery program. Also included will be the presentation of a model service delivery program which, through the use of regional assessment centers, may help to save time and money investment for each individual school or district, while still providing for quality service delivery.

Components of a Comprehensive CAP Service Delivery Program

Several components must be in place in order for a CAP service delivery program to be successful. These components are outlined in Table 9–3, and are reviewed in this section. Methods of funding a program such as that described in this book will differ depending upon regional characteristics. Therefore, beyond the general suggestions that have been made herein, funding will not be addressed. Each clinician involved in the development and implementation of CAP services should discuss funding-related issues with his or her respective administrator(s).

Training and Education

The first step necessary for the development and implementation of any CAP service delivery program is training and education of involved professionals. The level of training will vary depending on the degree of involvement. As discussed earlier in this chapter, the educational needs of educators and associated professionals will be different from those of the primary clinician providing comprehensive CAP services.

The CAP team leader, by necessity the audiologist, will need to receive training in all aspects of central auditory processing. Training in the scientific bases of CAP, screening and assessment methods, interpretation of central auditory assessment results, and management approaches is essential for any clinician entering into this complex field. **It is our opinion that it is more harmful to provide these services with poor or inadequate training in all aspects of CAP than it would be not to provide any CAP services at all.** The need for

Table 9-3
Necessary Components of Any Comprehensive CAP Service Delivery Program

Training and education of key individuals
Screening procedures
Resources for carrying out comprehensive central auditory assessment
Resources for implementing management suggestions
Methods of data collection and research to document program efficacy

appropriate training of any individual entering into the greater CAP arena cannot be overemphasized. The clinician desiring to provide comprehensive CAP services should seek out sources of the training needed, using the suggestions provided earlier in this chapter.

In addition to the need for training for the audiologist providing the bulk of the services, educational inservice opportunities must be provided for all professionals involved in the CAP effort. In many cases, the CAP team leader will provide such inservice training. The educational needs of each of the disciplines involved were presented in some detail earlier in this chapter.

Finally, the need for keeping up with new trends and information in the field of CAP cannot be overlooked. Therefore, in addition to initial training and inservice education, a system of continuing education must be in place for professionals involved in any CAP service delivery program.

Screening

The topic of CAP screening was dealt with in detail in Chapter 4. Therefore, we will not reiterate here what has already been covered. The reader should be aware, however, that a screening program for CAPD is an integral part of any comprehensive CAP service delivery program. It should also be remembered that the screening program should be based on a multidisciplinary team approach, allow for appropriate referral for comprehensive assessment when indicated, and include methods of data collection for monitoring program efficacy.

Comprehensive Central Auditory Assessment

The next integral component is the CAP diagnostic program itself. Once a child has been identified through the screening process as needing further central auditory assessment, there must be in place a means of performing diagnostic testing. This component includes the actual assessment procedures and methods of reporting the results to the referring party, as well as making recommendations for management.

The comprehensive assessment portion of the CAP service delivery program need not be available at the school, or even the district, level. Instead, a school or district may choose to refer to a regional assessment center for such services. **What is critical is that comprehensive CAP assessment services are available in a given region and that access to such services is ensured as part of the overall CAP program.**

Management

A critical component of any CAP service delivery program is the implementation of management suggestions. Methods of providing therapeutic intervention must be in place for children who are in need of such services, as well as classroom-based modifications and other management strategies. The decision regarding who should oversee the management effort and/or be primarily responsible for implementing therapy suggestions (e.g., speech-language pathologist, audiologist, resource teacher) will depend on the personnal constraints of the given school or district as well as the intervention needs of the individual child.

Regardless of which professional is primarily responsible for implementing management suggestions, it is imperative that the lines of communication among diagnostician, educators, therapists, and others involved in the CAP effort be kept open for ongoing monitoring of treatment efficacy.

Data Collection and Research

In addition to the provision of clinical services, we feel that it is important that the CAP service delivery program also be equipped for collecting of data and generating research. At the very least, the clinician providing diagnostic services must be knowledgeable regarding the collection of normative data and development of clinic-specific norms for each test tool in use. Also necessary is data collection related to screening program efficacy, as mentioned previously.

Although the above-mentioned data collection activities are generally considered to be integral parts of the CAP service delivery program, we recommend also that the clinician become familiar with scientific methodology and, as practitioners, take on the responsibility of contributing to the growing body of CAPD literature. Mentioned frequently throughout this book has been the need for further research, particularly in the areas of treatment efficacy and assessment methodology. **No one is better suited for generating treatment-related data than those practitioners engaged on a regular basis in providing CAP management services, and it is our opinion that a large portion of the much-needed data regarding treatment efficacy ultimately will come from these same practitioners.**

Therefore, we encourage clinicians engaged in CAP service delivery to commit themselves to the journey from practice back to science, and to engage in research-related activities that will further our knowledge of this complex field. General principles of scientific methodology and data collection will be discussed in the final chapter of this book.

In conclusion, the necessary components of the CAP service delivery program consist of education and training, screening, comprehensive diagnostic assessment, management, and data collection for the purposes of development of normative values, program monitoring, and future research needs.

A Regional Assessment Center Model Service Delivery Program

What follows is a description of a model CAP service delivery program currently in use in portions of the state of Colorado with good success. This program allows for the inclusion of all of the above-mentioned components, as well as reduces the time load on the part of individual audiologists and other educational professionals. We have found it to be particularly useful for the provision of CAP services in large geographical regions with smaller student populations. However, this program can also be utilized in smaller, more populated, regions. The program is outlined in Figure 9–1.

In our program, regional assessment centers, headed by trained audiologists, are established. The audiologist at the regional assessment center carries the responsibility of heading screening efforts and reviewing screening data, providing diagnostic evaluations, and making recommendations for management for all of the schools and/or districts in his or her region. Depending on population and geographical distance, each assessment center may be responsible for one or more school districts.

CAP screening is carried out at the school or district level. Educational personnel are provided with inservice training in order to delineate screening activities and other salient information necessary for screening and follow-through. When screening data suggest that further diagnostic evaluation is indicated, the child is referred to the regional assessment center for comprehensive central auditory testing. Upon completion of such testing, results of assessment and recommendations for management (if any) are conveyed to the referring school through the methods discussed in this chapter. The responsibility for implementing management suggestions is then taken up by the appropriate personnel at the school level.

Currently, we are investigating means of interdistrict funding in which districts participating in the regional assessment center program will cooperatively subsidize the effort. Although more data need

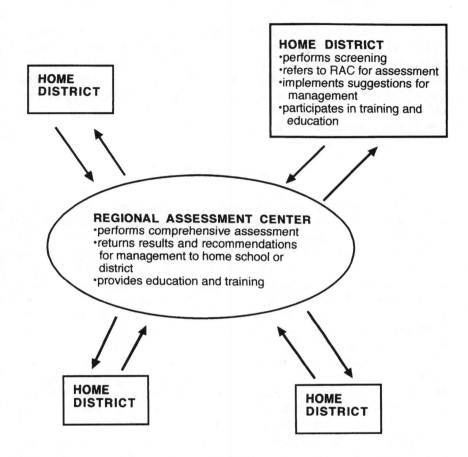

Figure 9-1. Regional assessment center model CAP service delivery program.

to be collected on the efficacy of a program such as that described here, our activities to date suggest that this method is a useful way of ensuring quality CAP services for all children in a given region while, at the sime time, lessening the time investment requirements on many of the professionals involved. An additional advantage to the program is that only those audiologists with the interest and energy to devote to training in the area of auditory processing need commit to the provision of comprehensive CAP services. **Those audiologists without the time, interest, or other means to invest in such pursuits are provided with the option of referring out for those CAP services for which they are not trained.**

The program described here represents just one example of how a CAP service delivery program can be established to address the needs of the given population. What is most important is an understanding of the necessary components of any CAP service delivery program. Once that understanding is attained, we urge the clinician to be creative and to take advantage of all available resources when developing ways of implementing CAP services.

Summary

This chapter has discussed a variety of considerations in CAP service delivery, including the need for education for all individuals involved, methods of conveying salient information to appropriate persons, and components necessary for inclusion in any CAP service delivery program.

The development and implementation of a CAP service delivery is a complex, time-consuming endeavor requiring input and cooperation from a variety of professionals and other individuals. However, it must be emphasized that each of the components described in this chapter, from education and training to screening, assessment, and management, must be included for any program to demonstrate effectiveness and overall success. It is our opinion that a CAP service delivery program that employs poorly trained individuals, is poorly planned, poorly executed, and lacks one or more of the necessary components discussed in this chapter is no better, and may actually be worse, than no CAP service delivery program at all.

Finally, the clinician must remain aware at all times of the ever-changing nature of central auditory assessment and management and make every effort to adapt and incorporate such changes into his or her comprehensive CAP service delivery program.

Review Questions

1. What purpose(s) does education of individuals involved in the delivery of CAP services serve?
2. Identify key topics important in the education of the following persons:

Audiologist	Speech-Language Pathologist
Educator	Psychologist
Parent	Private Practitioner

3. What components should be included in a central auditory diagnostic report?

4. How should the lack of significant findings upon diagnostic testing be addressed in the written CAP report?
5. How can the use of handouts aid the clinician in imparting CAP-related information?
6. What is a Child Study and how can it be used in the dissemination of CAP-related information?
7. What are the primary components of any CAP service delivery program?
8. Why is knowledge of data collection and scientific methodology important in CAP service delivery?
9. For your own setting, identify obstacles that are most likely to surface in the development and implementation of a comprehensive CAP service delivery program, and design a plan for addressing each of these obstacles.

CHAPTER

Back to Science

The preceding chapters of this book have focused on the practical application of scientific theory regarding central auditory processing. The purpose of this chapter is to provide the reader with a brief introduction to scientific methodology in the hopes of generating interest in the fascinating journey from practice back to science. In addition, it is the intent of this chapter to assist in developing an understanding and appreciation of the need for research-based activities on the part of clinicians engaged in central auditory processing service delivery. Discussed in this chapter will be the need for clinicians to perform as scientists in their daily settings; fundamentals of the scientific method, including terminology and basic concepts of research design; a brief overview of commonly used statistical formulas; and areas of need for further study within the field of central auditory processing and its disorders.

257

Learning Objectives

After studying this chapter, the reader should be able to

1. Discuss the justification underlying the need for clinicians to engage in research-based activities in their daily settings
2. Identify and discuss key concepts related to scientific methodology
3. Define common terms related to research design
4. Identify the purpose of several commonly used statistical procedures
5. Delineate several areas of need for future research in central auditory processing.

Why Should the Clinician Engage in Research?

Although the word *research* strikes fear in the hearts of many audiologists and speech-language pathologists in the trenches, **it should be recognized that what many of us do on a daily basis is essentially scientific study.** For example, when a patient enters the clinic for a standard audiological examination, the audiologist must first identify a clear objective of the clinical session (e.g., to identify whether a hearing loss is present and, if so, what type and to what degree?). Then, data collection activities must be performed in order to gather information that will, hopefully, meet the objective (e.g., obtaining pure-tone air- and bone-conduction thresholds, word recognition scores, immitance measures), while simultaneously assessing the reliability of the data being collected (e.g., determining the degree of agreement between pure-tone average and speech reception threshold, using a bracketing approach, and varying the rhythm of stimulus presentation to control for false responses). Finally, the data collected must be interpreted in light of what is known about auditory function in order to address the initial objective.

Likewise, (re)habilitative activities must follow the general principles of scientific research. The initial problem must be identified, baseline data collected, and a hypothesis must be formed regarding the effective treatment of the problem. Then, rehabilitative activities must be undertaken over a period of time, with repeated data collection occuring at regular intervals. Finally, the date must be interpreted in order to determine whether treatment has been effective, as well as to identify future directions for intervention.

In short, what each of us does every day in our respective settings is nothing short of scientific research. As Silverman (1977, p. 15) stated, **"There should be no difference, therefore, in the way you would go about answering clinically relevant questions or testing clinically relevant hypotheses for clinical and research purposes."**

Nevertheless, it appears that a general dichotomy exists to some extent between those engaged in clinical practice and those engaged in scientific research (Goldstein, 1972; Hamre, 1972; Jerger 1963). In other words, clinicians, although they are of necessity consumers of research, rarely engage in research-related activities for mass dissemination, whereas scientists spend their careers performing research-related activities for use by clinicians in the practical setting. This separation of the researcher from the clinician fails to acknowledge the interdependency of the two activities and results in a paucity of clinically relevant research for use in daily practice.

Silverman (1977) listed several benefits that a clinician may realize from functioning in the dual role of practitioner and scientist, including an increase in job satisfaction and stimulation; improvement in one's effectiveness as a clinician; and the provision of much-needed data regarding clinical diagnostic and treatment methods (Table 10–1). For example, because the daily clinical activities required of the audiologist and speech-language pathologist are so closely tied to research methodology, engaging in research activities would serve to improve clinical skills by helping to develop a more scientific approach to clinical decision making. Instead of asking whether a particular treatment approach has been effective, for instance, the clinician would learn to phrase clinical questions in a manner such that answers can be more specific and measurable (e.g., did therapy result in certain desired behaviors?). In addition, familiarity with the scientific method would aid clinicians in the collection of normative data for

---

Table 10–1

Ways in Which Engaging in Research Can Be of Benefit to the Clinician

Engaging in Research Activities Can
- Increase job satisfaction and stimulation, and reduce boredom
- Improve clinical skills by developing a scientific approach to clinical decision making
- Provide answers to clinic-related research questions regarding diagnostic methods and treatment efficacy

nonstandardized and new diagnostic procedures, as well as in the development of new diagnostic and treatment procedures.

Data generated by clinicians also can help to provide much-needed answers to questions that are difficult to address outside of the clinical venue. Take, for example, an issue mentioned repeatedly throughout this text, that of CAP treatment efficacy. Who better to engage in research and generate data regarding CAP treatment efficacy than those clinicians actively engaged in such pursuits in their daily practice? **Because of the nature of treatment efficacy research, which must be gathered over a period of time and is best generalized when obtained from situations most resembling the "real-life" treatment environment, clinicians may be in the best position to generate such data.** Additionally, clinicians may not only have access to the patients, opportunity, and setting that are needed for research of this type, but also may have a better idea of what questions are clinically relevant than would scientists not actively engaged in clinical practice.

Before concluding, it should be acknowledged that clinicians may be hesitant to engage in clinical research because of the feeling that such activities require more time than is available. However, as stated previously, the types of activities required of the clinical researcher are the same as those required for daily clinical practice. Naturally, although some additional time and support would be required for the analysis and presentation of data, the clinician should realize that the sources of such data may well lie within his or her current caseload. **By incorporating the scientific method into daily practice, all activities performed in the daily routine can be used for data collection purposes, and the clinician would be in a better position to judge the efficiency and effectiveness of his or her clinical activities.**

In conclusion, by engaging in research-based activities, the clinician can not only help to improve his or her own efficiency as a service provider, but also can help to answer important research questions that may best be addressed by those who are in the clinical setting. For these reasons, we encourage clinicians entering into the CAP arena to become familiar with scientific methodology and to perform their own CAP-related duties with an eye toward generating data that will help to clarify those areas that remain largely untested and untried, but critical to the overall big picture of CAPD assessment and management.

Fundamentals of the Scientific Method

When one sets out to incorporate the scientific method into daily clinical practice, one must become familiar with certain concepts and terms implicit in research methodology. This section will focus on critical elements of the scientific method and will introduce to the reader selected terminology, concepts, and types of research designs. Hopefully, these concepts will not be new to experienced clinicians; however, a review may help to remove some of the rust if they have not been used for awhile.

Terminology

When discussing research, various terms are used to describe a variety of facets of the scientific method. Many of these terms are frequently encountered when reading journal articles or materials such as this book, and the reader may be somewhat familiar with their meanings. The purpose of this section is to clarify for the reader some of the more commonly used terms in research.

Data

The term *data* refers to those attributes or events that are observed (or collected) during research activities. Data may be quantitative, or numerical (e.g., scores on a test, ages, percentile ranks, response time) or they may be qualitative, or descriptive (e.g., race, hair color, attention). What is critical when considering what data to collect during a research activity is that the attributes be measurable in some way, and that a clear plan for assigning values or coding the data is established prior to data collection.

To illustrate, if an investigator wishes to look at attention during testing as an attribute critical to a study, he or she must make sure that *attention* is defined in such a way as to be measurable. It may be decided that the percent of time spent on task will be an indicator of *attention*. On the other hand, *attention* may be assigned a value on a continuum from good to poor. In any case, the attribute or event being observed must be defined in a manner that allows it to be measured and coded as data.

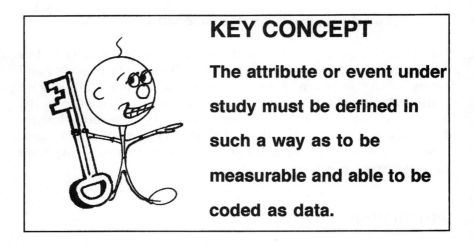

KEY CONCEPT

The attribute or event under study must be defined in such a way as to be measurable and able to be coded as data.

Variables

A variable is an outcome that can take on more than one value. For example, response time is a variable that can take on several numerical values. Likewise, race is a variable that can take on values such as Caucasian, African-American, Hispanic, and Asian.

To take our discussion of variables one step further, a *dependent variable* is a variable that measures the outcome of a research study. Conversely, an *independent variable* is a condition that is controlled by the researcher in order to test its effect on the outcome. For example, if one is studying the effect of age on performance on a test of central auditory processing, then age would be the independent variable, and the actual scored performance on the test would be the dependent variable.

When engaging in research activities, one must be aware of and control for additional confounding variables that may affect the ultimate outcome of the study. For example, in the above illustration, while age certainly has an effect upon central auditory test performance, so might variables such as cognitive capacity, history of otitis or other otologic or neurologic disorder, family history of learning disabilities, and so on. Therefore, in this example, one would want to choose a sample of children who exhibit normal cognitive capacity and no significant medical or family history in order to isolate, as much as possible, the effect of age alone on the test being studied.

Sample

Because it would be virtually impossible to include every person in the world in a given research study, we must select a sample that is as representative as possible of the population being studied. The more representative the chosen sample is of the target population, the more likely it will be that the findings of the study can be *generalized*, or applied, to the population as a whole. This process of inferring the results from a sample to a population is the basis for the *inferential method*, a method upon which many of the studies discussed in this book are based.

To provide a simplified illustration, if the clinician is collecting data for the purpose of developing clinic-specific normative values for a selected test of central auditory processing, the clinician will want to make sure that the sample that is chosen is representative of the population as a whole. In order to do this, the clinician will want to select children from different classrooms in a given school or region while simultaneously controlling for independent variables that may have a detrimental effect on test performance. In other words, all children within the desired age ranges who exhibit normal cognitive capacity and negative medical and family history should have equal chances of being selected for the normative study. The reader should be aware that those variables mentioned above may not be the only ones that might be considered when choosing a representative sample from a given population, but, rather, are intended here for illustrative purposes only.

A final consideration when discussing samples is that of sample size. As a general rule of thumb, the larger the sample size, the smaller the chance for error. However, due to constraints upon time and resources, it usually will be desirable to limit the sample size to a workable number that will still yield the desired results and minimize the chance for error. We recommend that, in multisubject studies designed for the purpose of developing representative data for a population (e.g., development of normative values for specific age groups), the sample size (N) be at least 30 within each group. As the study becomes more complex in terms of number of independent and dependent variables, as well as estimated variability within the population, then the size of the sample might need to be increased in order to minimize error. Likewise, if the target population is quite homogeneous, and the desired outcome is likely to demonstrate very little variability, then the sample size may be smaller and still yield reliable results that can be generalized to the target population as a whole.

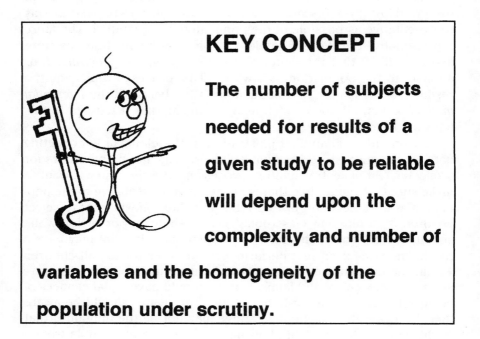

KEY CONCEPT

The number of subjects needed for results of a given study to be reliable will depend upon the complexity and number of variables and the homogeneity of the population under scrutiny.

Variability

Variability refers to the degree of spread that characterizes a group of scores within a sample or a population. In other words, scores that are closer together demonstrate a lesser degree of variability than do those that are farther apart. Measures of variability are those statistical procedures that determine the degree of heterogeneity of a selected characteristic of a sample. Specific measures of variability will be discussed in the section on statistical analysis.

Significance

Statistically speaking, *significance* refers to a finding that two experimental groups are different. The degree of significance is expressed in terms of *probability (p)*. For example, $p < .05$ can be interpreted to mean that there is less than a 5% chance that the differences observed in an experiment were due to chance or error or, conversely, that there is a 95% chance that the differences observed were real and not merely an artifact. Tests of significance are utilized in research in order to determine the level of confidence that can be placed in the findings. The two most commonly used confidence levels in clinical research are .05 and .01.

The concept of *statistical significance* should be distinguished from that of *clinical significance*. Suppose, for example, that the performance of a very large number of boys on a test of central auditory processing were compared to the performance of the same number of girls, and the results indicated that the girls performed 1% better on the test than did the boys. Even if a statistical test of significance indicated that the probability of the finding was less than .01, indicating that the finding was statistically significant, a difference in performance of a mere 1% on a central auditory test is likely to be so negligible as to be clinically insignificant. **Therefore, it should not be assumed that results of a study are clinically relevant simply because the findings are statistically significant.** Instead, the degree to which the findings can be utilized in the real-life, clinical setting will determine the degree of clinical significance a given study exhibits. Some common tests of statistical significance will be discussed later in this chapter.

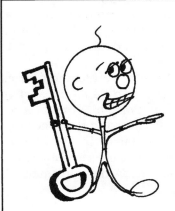

KEY CONCEPT

Statistical significance does not necessarily imply clinical significance. In order for findings of a study to be clinically significant, they must be applicable to the clinical setting.

Correlation

A correlation is a relationship between two or more variables. For example, the finding that the Right Ear Advantage (REA) decreases with increasing age indicates that the two variables—REA and age—have something in common, or are correlated. The higher the degree of relatedness among two or more variables, the higher the correlation is said to be.

Statistical tests for correlation can indicate whether the variables are *negatively* or *positively correlated*. A negative correlation is one in which an inverse relationship exists, or the value of one variable increases as the other decreases. The example provided above, in which the REA decreases as a function of increasing age, would be an example of a negative correlation.

Conversely, two variables are said to be positively correlated when they change in the same direction. For example, the percentage of total correct responses on the Frequency Patterns Test increases with increasing age. This would be an example of a positive correlation.

Correlations are expressed in values referred to as *correlation coefficients*. Correlation coefficients range in value from −1.00 to +1.00. The size of the number is an indicator of the strength of the correlation, regardless of whether the number is negative or positive. **Therefore, a correlation coefficient of −.78 indicates a stronger relationship between variables than does a correlation coefficient of +.50.** Likewise, a correlation coefficient of −0.90 indicates that two variables are strongly negatively correlated, whereas a correlation coefficient of +0.90 indicates that two or more variables are strongly positively correlated.

This section has introduced some of the more common terms used in research and is by no means intended to be an exhaustive overview of research-related terminology. Additional important terms, such as reliability and validity, have been discussed in the preceding chapters. It is hoped that, by becoming familiar with these terms, readers will be better able to understand technical terms utilized in the literature, as well as begin to gain the knowledge fundamentals for engaging in research activities, themselves.

Types of Research

Research can take on many forms, and the form chosen for a given study will depend upon the question being asked. **Scientific research serves a variety of functions, including identifying the causative fac-**

tors that lead to a given event, describing characteristics of a population or phenomenon, determining the nature of events that have
occurred in the past, and identifying the relationship between two
or more variables. A discussion of the types of research designs that
perform these functions, as well as considerations for engaging in
each type, follows.

Experimental Research

The primary goal of *experimental research* is to determine the effect of
a given variable on the outcome variable. In order to do this, subjects
are assigned by the investigator to different groups, with each group
receiving a different possible treatment in order to assess the differential effects of the treatment on the outcome. For example, if one wishes to compare the effect of daily phoneme training on performance on
Low-Pass Filtered Speech Tasks to the effect of no training whatsoever
over the same time period, one would assign matched subjects to the
two groups. Group One, no therapy, would be considered the *control
group*, while Group Two, the group receiving daily therapy, would be
considered the *experimental group*. Baseline data, in the form of Low-
Pass Filtered Speech scores, could be obtained from both groups
before the experiment, with repeated data collection at various times
throughout the allotted time period. The improvement in scores, if
any, that occurs in Group One could be compared to those obtained
from Group Two using selected tests of significance, which will be discussed later in this chapter.

Advantages to the experimental method include a high level of
control over subject variables, group assignments, and treatment variables. However, it may not always be possible or ethical to assign subjects to groups and manipulate the treatment each group receives in
order to determine relative effects. For example, if one wishes to study
the effect of early otitis media on central auditory processing abilities,
it would not be possible or ethical to assign children to two experimental groups, and then induce otitis in the members of one of the
groups in order to assess its effect on auditory skills. In these situations, rather than conducting a true experimental research study, the
investigator would need to utilize the type of research known as
causative-comparative research (Salkind, 1991).

In causative-comparative research, the investigator has no control
over the assignment of subjects to a particular group. Instead, subjects are assigned to groups based upon some characteristic that they
bring to the investigation (e.g., history of early chronic otitis media).
Although other factors, such as socioeconomic status, cognitive func-

tioning, age, and academic achievement, can be controlled for, the actual variable of interest—history of otitis—is already established and cannot be manipulated by the investigator. Data collection would then occur "after the fact," and tests for significant differences between groups would be conducted as in experimental research.

Much of the research completed in the area of central auditory processing is of the causative-comparative type of research design. Studies of lesion effects on various tests of central auditory function, for example, would be an example of this type. Conversely, much of the research that occurs in the area of treatment efficacy is likely to fall into the experimental research design category, because the treatment variable can be manipulated during the investigation process in order to determine cause and effect.

Descriptive Research

The goal of *descriptive research* is to describe the characteristics of a selected phenomenon (Salkind, 1991). For example, the collection of data for purposes of establishing normative values on tests of central auditory function could be considered descriptive research. In this type of study, the investigator is merely collecting information (in the form of performance on selected tests) from a group of subjects, and then describing the characteristics of the group's performance, without comparing the results to the findings from another group. Statistical formulas used in descriptive research design, including the mean and standard deviation, will be discussed later in this chapter.

Correlational Research

Correlational research helps to determine if and how two or more variables are related to one another, without implying cause and effect. In addition, correlational research is useful in making predictions based upon relationships among variables. For example, a study may be undertaken to determine the relationship between articulatory disorders (as measured by performance on a standardized test of articulation) and auditory closure deficits (as measured by performance on a monaural low-redundancy speech task). Results may show that, indeed, articulation disorders and auditory closure deficits are positively correlated. However, it should not be assumed that one factor (e.g., a deficit in auditory closure) causes the other (e.g., articulation disorder).

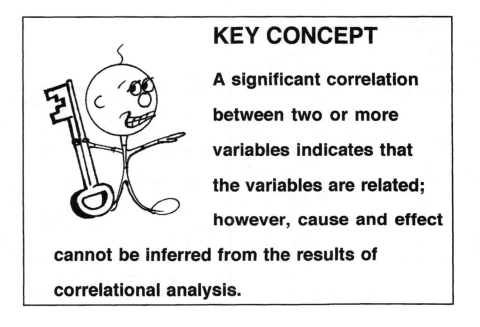

KEY CONCEPT

A significant correlation between two or more variables indicates that the variables are related; however, cause and effect cannot be inferred from the results of correlational analysis.

Instead, this information can be used only to document an association between the two variables and not to determine cause and effect.

Historical Research

Historical research is primarily concerned with describing the nature of events that have occurred in the past for the purpose of examining trends in data. To perform historical research, the investigator can use historical documents, journal articles, and personal interviews, among other tools, in order to perform data collection activities. For example, an investigator may wish to determine the effectiveness of a screening program for CAPD that has been in place over the past year. He or she might review the records of the past year to determine the number of children who, after having "failed" the screening and been referred on for comprehensive central auditory assessment, actually exhibited a central auditory processing disorder. The information obtained might be used to modify the screening protocol so that the number of inappropriate referrals is decreased, or it might serve to confirm that the majority of children referred did, indeed, exhibit a CAPD.

The types of research discussed in this section are summarized in Table 10–2.

Table 10–2
Overview of Types of Research

Type	Description
Experimental	Goal: to determine the effect of a given variable on the outcome variable. Clinician has control over the treatment variable and the assignment of subjects to groups.
Causal-Comparative	Goal: same as experimental; however, clinician has no control over the treatment variable and the assignment of subjects to groups.
Descriptive	Goal: to describe the characteristics of a selected phenomenon.
Correlational	Goal: to determine if and how two or more variables are related. Cause and effect cannot be inferred from the results of correlational research.
Historical	Goal: to describe the nature of events that have occurred in the past for the purpose of examining trends in data.

Final Considerations Regarding the Scientific Method

To summarize, the scientific method is a system of asking and answering questions. The question itself will determine the ultimate form the research design takes. By undertaking studies in which variables are carefully controlled and questions are asked in ways that allow for measurable data to be collected and analyzed, information regarding cause and effect, relationships among variables, characteristics of a phenomenon, and past trends can be obtained.

It should be emphasized, however, that answers obtained through the use of the scientific method should be considered tentative, and the reliability of findings depends upon such factors as control of extraneous variables, how representative the chosen sample is of the target population, and the methods chosen to investigate the topic. Even in cases of exceptional research design and variable control, results of any research study should be regarded as subject to change if new information becomes available that suggests the necessity of such a change. **The investigator should avoid at all times the tendency to consider the results of any study or series of studies as absolute fact and should be willing to modify his or her own**

hypotheses if subsequent evidence should cast doubt upon them. Finally, rather than expecting an unequivocal answer to research questions, the investigator should realize that the ultimate result of scientific inquiry is the generation of new questions and new directions for further research.

Basic Statistical Procedures

Once data are collected, they must then be organized and analyzed. It is the topic of statistical analysis, and the unavoidable mathematical formulas that go along with statistics, that turn many would-be scientists away from the fascinating realm of research. However, armed with a little understanding and a calculator or computer, many of the most commonly used statistical procedures can be performed with very little effort.

This section will describe several common statistical procedures used to analyze data for the purpose of answering research questions. It should be noted that there exist a variety of computer programs that will perform the statistical procedures discussed here with a mere click of the mouse. Formulas will be provided for the first two categories of statistical procedures, measures of central tendency and measures of variability, as these procedures are likely to be used frequently in clinical practice and can be performed with very little effort on the part of the clinician. Other statistical procedures that will be discussed in this section include tests of significance and measures of association.

Measures of Central Tendency

Measures of central tendency are designed to indicate the individual value that is in some way representative of the group of scores or values obtained. There are three measures of central tendency:

(a) the *mean*, which is the sum of the scores divided by the total number of scores. The mean is commonly referred to as the average, and can be computed using the following formula:

$$\overline{X} = \frac{\Sigma X}{n}$$

where $\overline{X}$ = mean

Σ = sum

X = individual score

n = number of scores in the sample

(b) the *median*, which is the score in a distribution above which half of the scores lie. In other words, the median represents the midpoint in a group of scores. The median can be computed simply by ordering the scores from lowest to highest value, counting the number of scores, and choosing that score which occurs at the midpoint or, in the case of an even number of scores, the average of the two middle scores. For example, for the following scores, the median value would be 14 since 3 of the scores occur below 14 and 3 occur above 14.

3   10   12   (14)   16   25   90

(c) the *mode*, which is the score that occurs most frequently in a distribution. In order to compute the mode, simply look at the values and determine which score occurs more often than the others. For example, for the following distribution, the mode would be 10 since it occurs 3 times.

3   8   (10)   11   5   (10)   4   5   (10)   9   6

For purposes of descriptive statistics, it is the median, or average, that will likely be the most common measure of central tendency used.

Measures of Variability

As previously mentioned in this chapter, variability refers to the spread or dispersion of scores in a sample. It can also be thought of as the degree to which the scores differ from a measure of central tendency, usually the mean. The two most commonly used measures of variability for our purposes are the range and the standard deviation.

The *range* is simply the difference between the highest and lowest scores in the distribution. Therefore, in the following example, the range would be 10 - 4, or 6.

4   5   7   9   10

The *standard deviation* represents the average amount that each individual score differs from the mean. The larger the standard deviation, the more variability exists in the sample. The standard deviation can be computed using the following formula:

$$SD = \sqrt{\frac{\Sigma(X-\overline{X})}{n-1}}$$

where SD = standard deviation

Σ = sum

$\overline{X}$ = mean

X = individual score

n = number of scores in the sample

The standard deviation is particularly important in the development of normative values. **For most tests of central auditory processing, performance is considered to be within normal limits if it falls within one to two standard deviations of the mean.** The decision regarding which value to use is based on the overall variability of the sample. If the choice of one standard deviation for the determination of "normal cutoff" means that several of the scores obtained from the normative sample would "fail" the test, then it would be more prudent to use two standard deviations for interpretive purposes. On the other hand, if the scores in the sample for a given test are very close together, one standard deviation may be sufficient for determining the normal cut-off.

The procedure for establishing normative values for a given test of central auditory processing is outlined in Table 10–3, and involves choosing an appropriate sample (controlling for age and other variables as discussed previously in this chapter), administering the test and obtaining individual scores, computing the standard deviation, and determining the minimum value necessary for performance on the test to be considered "within normal limits."

Tests of Significance

The concept of significance was discussed earlier in this chapter, and involves determining the probability of whether a given finding can be attributed to chance. There are numerous tests of significance that

Table 10–3
Procedure for Establishing Clinic-Specific Normative Values for a Test

Step One
   Choose appropriate subjects, making sure to match for age and controlling for confounding variables. Number of subjects should be no less than 30.
Step Two
   Administer test, making sure to keep test conditions uniform across subjects.
Step Three
   Score test using the appropriate scoring methods for the given assessment tool.
Step Four
   Calculate mean and standard deviation of scores from the sample.
Step Five
   Determine normal cut-off value. For example, if 2 standard deviations below the mean is determined to be the appropriate cut-off value, use the following formula:

$$\text{Cut-off} = \text{Mean} - (\text{Standard Deviation} \times 2)$$

can be used; however, the most common are the *t* test and analysis of variance.

The *t* test is designed to determine whether scores for two groups are significantly different. For example, in the example previously provided in this chapter in which the effect of phoneme training on Low-Pass Filtered Speech performance was being compared to the effect of no training on the same task, the scores obtained from Group A (therapy) could be compared to Group B (no therapy), and the probability of the presence of a significant difference between the groups could be determined using a *t* test for statistical significance.

Analysis of variance (ANOVA) (or *F* test) is similar to the *t* test, except that it is designed for use with more than two groups. The use of ANOVA in statistical analysis can determine whether significant differences exist overall in the means of three or more different groups.

Suppose that an investigation were designed to investigate the effects of three different types of therapeutic activities for a given disorder. In this example, there would be three experimental groups, one for each type of therapy. To determine if a difference exists among posttherapy scores obtained from the three groups, ANOVA could be utilized. A word of caution is warranted here: A finding of significance on analysis of variance indicates only that a significant difference exists *somewhere* in the groups, but does not suggest that all three groups are significantly different from each other. In order to determine relative differences, the data must be more closely scrutinized using additional analysis procedures.

Again, it should be emphasized that the two tests of significance discussed herein are offered merely as representative samples. A variety of significance tests can be used to analyze limitless combinations of data.

Measures of Association

Measures of association are intended to determine relationships, or correlation, among variables. As discussed previously, measures of association result in a correlation coefficient, or an indicator of the strength and direction of a relationship between two variables. Probably the most commonly utilized index of association, or correlation, in the field of communication disorders is the Pearson product-moment correlation coefficient (Pearson r), which is an indicator of relationship between two continuous variables. For example, in order to determine the relationship between a sample's performance on a test of auditory closure and a test of articulation, the Pearson r may be the statistical procedure of choice.

This section has provided the reader with methods of computing measures of central tendency and variability, and has briefly reviewed tests of significance and measures of association in an attempt to dispel some of the mystery and confusion that surround the entire topic of statistical analysis. For further information regarding specific tests of significance and association, as well as the myriad of other statistical procedures that can be utilized for data analysis, the reader is referred to Phillips (1996), or to the neighborhood bookstore, where large numbers of statistical manuals can be found. The information presented in this section is summarized in Table 10–4.

Meeting the Research Challenge

The arena of CAPD holds unlimited opportunities for clinicians wishing to contribute to the general bank of knowledge by engaging in research activities. Further study is needed in virtually all CAP-related areas, from identification to management and everything in between, and many of these topics lend themselves particularly well to studies conducted in the clinical setting. In this text, we have mentioned the need for research into treatment efficacy, an area plagued by a paucity of empirical data. Perhaps no other topic in the field of CAPD is in

Table 10-4
Overview of Basic Statistical Procedures

Procedure	Description
Measures of Central Tendency	Designed to indicate a value that is, in some way, representative of a group of scores. Includes the mean (average), median (the score above which half of the scores lie), and the mode (the score that occurs most frequently).
Measures of Variability	Indicates spread or dispersion of scores in a sample. Includes the range(difference between highest and lowest scores), and the standard deviation (the average amount that each score differs from the mean).
Tests of Significance	Determines the probability of whether a given finding was due to chance. Includes the t test (determines whether scores for 2 groups are significantly different) and ANOVA (designed for use with more than 2 groups).
Measures of Association	Indicates relationships or correlation among variables.

greater need of clinician involvement in research design and data collection than the study of the efficacy of methods of CAPD management and treatment.

But treatment efficacy is not the only research area in which clinician involvement could contribute significantly to the understanding of CAPD. In Chapter 7, we discussed several subprofiles of CAPD. It should be remembered that the validity and reliability of these profiles await confirmation. Clinicians in the educational setting can be instrumental in helping to define subprofiles of CAPD further, as well as in correlating performance on tests of central auditory function with academic, cognitive, social, emotional, and communicative sequelae (Ferre, 1994).

Causative factors contributing to the development of CAPD in children is an area of need for further study. When a child is diagnosed as exhibiting CAPD, the next question is invariably, "Why?" The possible contribution of various pre- and postnatal conditions, maternal and/or paternal drug or alcohol use, and a variety of other factors that contribute to the incidence of CAPD in children needs to be examined closely.

And, speaking of incidence, it was mentioned in Chapter 4 that the actual incidence of CAPD in the school-age population is currently unknown. Studies need to be undertaken to determine the incidence of CAPD in the regular educational population as well as in the learning disabled population, studies that will require large numbers of children available only to those investigators with access to the schools.

Regarding assessment, further research needs to be conducted into the development of assessment tools for very young children, and valid, reliable screening procedures for all ages. Predictors of future CAPD problems in the very young child need to be identified, and methods of assessment for the hearing impaired and other hard-to-test populations need to be investigated and developed.

Further research needs to be done in the area of CAP assessment, as well. Comparisons of performance on central auditory tests need to be compared to performance on similar tests within other modalities in order to determine the modality-specificity of the tests currently in use (McFarland & Cacace, 1995). Reliability of several of the test tools discussed in this book needs to be investigated in the school-age population.

These are only a few of the CAP-related areas in which further research is indicated, and in which the clinician in the educational setting can and should become involved. For, when considering assessment and management of CAPD in the educational setting, it is the clinician in that very setting who ultimately must generate the data that remain at present so badly needed within the area of central auditory processing and its disorders.

Summary

This chapter has attempted to provide the reader with a brief introduction to various facets of scientific research, including terminology, types of research designs, and basic statistical procedures. In addition, the need for clinician involvement into CAP-related research has been emphasized. It is our strongly held view that, unless and until clinicians within the educational setting become involved in asking and answering questions related to CAPD, the area of CAPD in children will remain as much a mystery as it is today.

It is our hope that this chapter, while barely touching upon the research-related topics selected for inclusion, has at least served the function of whetting the appetites of clinicians in the educational setting for confronting the challenges of the unknown and embarking on the journey toward knowledge. In this great, uncharted frontier of CAPD, it is the clinician who quests for enlightenment and patterns his or her activities accordingly who has the opportunity to map the territory and light the way for the rest of us.

Review Questions

1. What are some benefits that the clinician may enjoy by functioning in the dual role of scientist and practitioner?
2. How does the scientific method apply to everyday clinical activities?
3. Define the following terms:

data	variable
independent variable	dependent variable
sample	inferential method
variability	significance
correlation	

4. With regard to samples, what factor(s) helps to determine the degree to which the results of a study can be generalized to the population as a whole?
5. Contrast the concept of statistical significance with that of clinical significance.
6. What is the fundamental difference between negative and positive correlations?
7. List and define the four types of research discussed in this chapter.
8. How do experimental and causative-comparative research differ?
9. Using the following fictitious scores, compute the mean of the sample:

95	74	83	85	89	99
68	93	92	88	82	87
99	86	88	99	65	77
76	74	89	75	99	92
94	95	89	90	90	92

10. What is the median of the above sample? What is the mode?
11. What is the purpose of tests of significance?
12. How do t tests and ANOVA (F tests) differ from one another?
13. What is the primary purpose of measures of association or correlation?

References

Abel, S., Bert, B., & McLean, J. (1978). Sound localization: Value in localizing lesions of the auditory pathway. *Journal of Otolaryngology, 7*, 132–140.

Ackerman, S. (1992). *Discovering the Brain.* Washington, DC: National Academy Press.

Aiello, I., Sotgiu, S., Sau, G. F., Manca, S., Conti, M., & Rosati, G. (1995). Long latency evoked potentials in a case of corpus callosum agenesia. Italian *Journal of Neurological Sciences, 15,* 497–505.

Aoki, C., & Siekevitz, P. (1988). Plasticity in brain development. *Scientific American, 259,* 56–64.

American Speech-Language-Hearing Association (1990). Audiological assessment of central auditory processing: an annotated bibliography. *Asha, 32* (Suppl. 1), 13–30.

American Speech-Language-Hearing Association (1995). *Central auditory processing: current status of research and implications for clinical practice. A report from the ASHA task force on central auditory processing.* Rockville, MD: Author.

Arnst, D. J. (1982) SSW test results with peripheral hearing loss. In D. Arnst & J. Katz (Eds.), *The SSW test: Development and clinical use* (pp. 287–293). San Diego, CA: College-Hill Press.

Ashmead, D., Davis, D., Whalen, T., & Odom, R. (1991). Sound localization and sensitivity to interaural time differences in human infants. *Child Development, 61,* 1211–1226.

Baran, J. A., & Musiek, F. E. (1991). Behavioral assessment of the central auditory nervous system. In W. Rintelmann (Ed.), *Hearing assessment* (2nd ed., pp. 549–602). Austin, TX: PRO-ED.

Baran, J. A., Musiek, F. E., & Reeves, A. G. (1986). Central auditory function following anterior sectioning of the corpus callosum. *Ear and Hearing, 7,* 359–362.

Baran, J. A., Verkest, S., Gollegly, K., Kibbe-Michal, K., Rintelmann, W. F., & Musiek, F. E. (1985). Use of compressed speech in the assessment of central nervous system disorder. *Journal of the Acoustical Society of America, 78* (Suppl. 1), S41.

Beasley, D. S., Forman, B., & Rintelmann, W. F. (1972). Intelligibility of time-compressed CNC monosyllables by normal listeners. *Journal of Auditory Research, 12,* 71–75.

Beasley, D. S., Schwimmer, S., & Rintelmann, W. F. (1972). Intelligibility of time-compressed monosyllables. *Journal of Speech and Hearing Research, 15,* 340–350.

Bellis, T. J., & Ferre, J. M. (in press). Assessment and management of CAPD in children. *Educational Audiology Association Monograph.*

Belmont, I., & Handler, A. (1971). Delayed information processing and judgement of temporal order following cerebral damage. *Journal of Nervous and Mental Disease, 152,* 353–361.

Bergman, M. (1957). Binaural hearing. *Archives of Otolaryngology, 66,* 572–588.

Berlin, C. I., Cullen, J. K., Hughes, L. F., Berlin, J. L., Lowe-Bell, S. S., & Thompson, C. L. (1975). Dichotic processing of speech: Acoustic and phonetic variables. In M.D. Sullivan (Ed.), *Central auditory processing disorders* (pp. 36–46). Proceedings of a conference at the University of Nebraska Medical Center, Omaha.

Berlin, C., Hughes, L., Lowe-Bell, S., & Berlin, H. (1973). Dichotic right ear advantage in children 5 to 13. *Cortex, 9,* 393–401.

Berlin, C. I., Lowe-Bell, S. S., Jannetta, P. J., & Kline, D. G. (1972). Central auditory deficits after temporal lobectomy. *Archives of Otolaryngology, 96,* 4–10.

Bhatnagar, S. C., & Andy, O. J. (1995). *Neuroscience for the study of communicative disorders.* Baltimore: Williams & Wilkins.

Blaettner, U., Scherg, M., & Von Cramon, D. (1989). Diagnosis of unilateral telencephalic hearing disorders: Evaluation of a simple psychoacoustic pattern discrimination test. *Brain, 112,* 177–195.

Bliss, T., & Lomo, T. (1973). Long-lasting potentiation of synaptic transmission in the dentate area of the anaesthetized rabbit following stimulation of the perforant path. *Journal of Physiology, 232,* 331–356.

Bocca, E., Calearo, C., & Cassinari, V. (1954). A new method for testing hearing in temporal lobe tumors. *Acta Otolaryngologica (Stockholm), 44,* 219–221.

Bornstein, S. P. (1994). Time compression and release from masking in adults and children. *Journal of the American Academy of Audiology, 5,* 89–98.

Bornstein, S. P., Wilson, R. H., & Cambron, N. K. (1994). Low- and high-pass filtered Northwestern University Auditory Test No. 6 for monaural and binaural evaluation. *Journal of the American Academy of Audiology, 5,* 259–264.

Brazelton, T. B. (1973). *Neonatal behavioral assessment scale.* London: Spastics International Medical Publications.

Broadbent, D. E. (1954). The role of auditory localization in attention and memory span. *Journal of Experimental Psychology, 47*, 191–196.

Bryden, M. (1963). Ear preference in auditory perception. *Journal of Experimental Psychology, 16*, 359–360.

Buchwald, J. S., Hinman, C., Norman, R. S., Huang, C. M., & Brown, K. A. (1981). Middle and long-latency auditory evoked potentials recorded from the vertex of normal and chronically lesioned cats. *Brain Research, 205*, 91–109.

Butterworth, G., & Castillo, M. (1976). Coordination of auditory visual space in newborn human infants. *Perception, 5*, 155–160.

Caird, D. M., & Klinke, R. (1987). The effect of inferior colliculus lesions on auditory evoked potentials. *Electroencephalography and Clinical Neurophysiology, 68*, 237–240.

Carmon, A., & Nachshon, I. (1971). Effect of unilateral brain damage on perception of temporal order. *Cortex, 7*, 410–418.

Carrow-Woolfolk, E. (1981). *Carrow auditory-visual abilities test.* Hingham, MA: Teaching Resources Corp.

Cervette, M. J. (1984). Auditory brainstem response testing in the intensive care unit. *Seminars in Hearing, 5*, 57–68.

Chermak, G. D. (1992, February). Central auditory processing disorders (CAPD): Key concepts and clinical considerations. Paper presented at the American Speech-Language-Hearing Association Workshop on Central Auditory Processing, Orlando, FL.

Chermak, G. D., & Musiek, F. E. (1995, July). Managing central auditory processing disorders in children and youth. *American Journal of Audiology,* 61–65.

Chermak, G. D., Vonhof, M. R., & Bendel, R. B. (1989) Word identification performance in the presence of competing speech and noise in learning disabled adults. *Ear and Hearing, 10*, 90–93.

Chiappa, K. H. (1980). Brainstem auditory evoked potentials in 200 patients with multiple sclerosis. *Annals of Neurology, 7*, 135–143.

Chiappa, K. H., (1983.) *Evoked potentials in clinical medicine.* New York: Raven Press.

Clarkson, M., Clifton, R., & Morongiello, B. (1985). The effects of sound duration on newborns' head orientation. *Journal of Experimental Child Psychology, 39*, 20–36.

Clarkson, M., Clifton, R., Swain, I., & Perris, E. (1989). Stimulus duration and repetition rate influence newborns' head orientation toward sound. *Developmental Psychobiology, 22*, 683–705.

Clopton, B., & Silverman, M. (1978). Changes in latency and duration of neural responding following developmental auditory deprivation. *Experimental Brain Research, 32*, 39–47.

Colavita, F. B., Szeligo, F. V., & Zimmer, S. D. (1974). Temporal pattern discrimination in cats with insular-temporal lesions. *Brain Research, 79*, 153–156.

Courchesne, E., (1978). Neurophysiological correlates of cognitive development: Changes in long-latency event-related potentials from childhood to adulthood. *Electroencephalography and Clinical Neurophysiology, 45*, 468–482.

Cox, L. C. (1985). Infant assessment: Developmental and age related considerations. In Jacobsen, J. (Ed.) *The auditory brainstem response* (pp. 298–316). San Diego, CA: College-Hill Press.

Cranford, J. L. (1984). Brief tone detection and discrimination tests in clinical audiology with emphasis on their use in central nervous system lesions. *Seminars in Hearing, 5*, 263–275.

Cranford, J. L., Stream, R. W., Rye, C. V., & Slade, T. L. (1982). Detection versus discrimination of brief-duration tones: Findings in patients with temporal lobe damage. *Archives of Otolaryngology, 108*, 350–356.

Damasio, H., & Damasio, A. (1979). "Paradoxic" ear extinction in dichotic listening: Possible anatomic significance. *Neurology, 29*, 644–653.

Davis, H., & Onishi, S. (1969). Maturation of auditory evoked potentials. *International Audiology, 8*, 24–33.

Davis, P. A. (1939). Effects of acoustic stimuli on the waking human brain. *Journal of Neurophysiology, 2*, 494–499.

Dayal, V. S., Tarantino, L., & Swisher, L. P. (1966). Neuro-otologic studies in multiple sclerosis. *Laryngoscope, 76*, 1798–1809.

Despland, P. A. & Galambos, R. (1980). The auditory brainstem response (ABR) is a useful tool in the intensive care nursery. *Pediatric Research, 14*, 154–158.

Dirks, D. (1964). Perception of dichotic and monaural verbal material and cerebral dominance for speech. *Acta Oto-laryngology, 58*, 78–80.

Dirks, D., & Wilson, R. (1969). binaural hearing of speech for aided and unaided conditions. *Journal of Speech and Hearing Research, 12*, 650–664.

DiSimoni, F. (1978). *The Token Test for Children*. Hingham, MA: Teaching Resources Corp.

Disterhoft, J. F., & Stuart, D. K. (1976). Trial sequence of changed unit activity in auditory system of alert rat during conditioned response acquisition and extinction. *Journal of Neurophysiology, 39*, 266–281.

Drulovic, B., Ribaric-Jankes, K., Kostic, V., & Sternic, N. (1994). Multiple sclerosis as the cause of sudden "pontine" deafness. *Audiology, 33*, 195–201.

Durlach, N. I., Thompson, C. L., & Colburn, H. S. (1981). Binaural interaction in impaired listeners: A review of past research. *Audiology, 20*, 181–211.

Efron, R. (1963). Temporal perception, aphasia and deja vu. *Brain, 86*, 403–424.

Efron, R. (1985). The central auditory system and issues related to hemispheric specialization. In M.L. Pinheiro & F.E. Musiek (Eds.), *Assessment of central auditory dysfunction: Foundations and clinical correlates* (pp. 143–154). Baltimore: Williams & Wilkins.

Efron, R., & Crandall, P. H. (1983). Central auditory processing: Effects of anterior temporal lobectomy. *Brain and Language, 19*, 237–253.

Efron, R., Crandall, P. H., Koss, D., Divenyi, P. L., & Yund, E. W. (1983). Central auditory processing. III. The "Cocktail Party" effect and anterior temporal lobectomy. *Brain and Language, 19*, 254–263.

Efron, R., Dennis, M., & Yund, E. W. (1977). The perception of dichotic chords by hemispherectomized subjects. *Brain and Language, 4*, 537–549.

Efron, R., Yund, E. W., Nichols, D., & Crandall, P. H. (1977). An ear asymmetry for gap detection following anterior temporal lobectomy. *Neuropsychologia, 23*, 43–50.

Fairbanks, G., Everitt, W., & Jaeger, R. (1954). Methods for time or frequency compression-expansion of speech. *Trans IRE-PGA, AU-2*, 7–12.

Ferre, J. (1987). Pediatric central auditory processing disorder: Considerations for diagnosis, interpretation, and remediation. *Journal of the Academy of Rehabilitative Audiology, 20,* 73–81.

Ferre, J. (1992, November). CATfiles: Improving the clinical utility of central auditory function tests. Paper presented at the American Speech-Language-Hearing Association Annual Convention, San Antonio, TX.

Ferre, J. (1994, March). The clinical utility of the concept of central auditory processing - a commentary. Paper presented at the American Speech-Language-Hearing Association Task Force on Central Auditory Processing Consensus Development Conference, Albuquerque, NM.

Field, J., Muir, D., Pilon, R., Sinclair, M., & Dodwell, P. (1980). Infants' orientation to lateral sounds from birth to 3 months. *Child Development, 51,* 295–298.

Fifer, R., Jerger, J., Berlin, C., Tobey, E., & Campbell, J. (1983). Development of a dichotic sentence identification test for hearing impaired adults. *Ear and Hearing, 4,* 300–305.

Fischer, C., Bognar, L., Turjman, F., & Lapras, C. (1995). Auditory evoked potentials in a patient with a unilateral lesion of the inferior colliculus and medial geniculate body. *Electroencephalography and Clinical Neurophysiology, 96,* 261–267.

Flowers, A., Costello, M., & Small, V. (1973). *Flowers-Costello Tests of Central Auditory Abilities.* Dearborn, MI: Perceptual Learning Systems.

Franzen, M. D. (1989). *Reliability and validity in neuropsychological assessment.* New York: Plenum Press.

Galambos, R., Wilson, M. J., & Silva, P. D. (1994). Identifying hearing loss in the intensive care nursery: A 20-year summary. *Journal of the American Academy of Audiology, 5,* 151–162.

Gardner, M. F., (1985). *Test of auditory-perceptual skills.* Burlingame, CA: Psychological and Educational Publications.

Gatehouse, R. (1976). Further research in localization of sound by completely monaural subjects. *Journal of Auditory Research, 16,* 265–273.

Geisler, C., Frishkopf, L., & Rosenblith, W. (1958). Extracranial responses to acoustic clicks in man. *Science, 128,* 1210–1211.

Geschwind, N., & Levitsky, W. (1968). Human brain: left-right asymmetries in temporal speech region. *Science, 161,* 186–187.

Goldstein, R. (1972). Presidential address: 1971 national convention. *Asha, 14,* 58–62.

Goodin, D., Squires, K., Henderson, B, & Starr, A. (1978). Age related variations in evoked potentials to auditory stimuli in normal human subjects. *Electroencephalography and Clinical Neurophysiology, 44,* 447–458.

Green, D. M. (1966). Interaural phase effects in the masking of signals of different durations. *Journal of the Acoustical Society of America, 39,* 720–724.

Greene, T. (1929). The ability to localize sound. *Archives of Surgery: Chicagy, 6,* 1825–1841.

Grose, J. H., Hall, J. W., & Gibbs, C. (1993). Temporal analysis in children. *Journal of Speech and Hearing Research, 36,* 351–356.

Grote, C. L., Pierre-Louis, S. J., Smith, M. C., Roberts, R. H., & Varney, N. R. (1995). Significance of unilateral ear extinction on the dichotic listening test. *Journal of Clinical and Experimental Neuropsychology, 17*, 108.

Gustafsson, B., & Wigstrom, H. (1988). Physiological mechanisms underlying long-term potentiation. *Trends in Neuroscience, 11*, 156–162.

Haggard, M. P., & Hughes, E. A. (1991). Screening children's hearing: A review of the literature and implications of otitis media. *London: HMSO.*

Hall, J. W., & Derlacki, E. D. (1986). Binaural hearing after middle ear surgery. *Journal of Otology Rhinology and Laryngology, 95*, 118–124.

Hall, J. W., & Derlacki, E. D. (1988). Binaural hearing after middle ear surgery: MLD for interaural time and level cues. *Audiology, 27*, 89–98.

Hall, J. W., & Grose, J. H. (1990). The masking-level difference in children. *Journal of the American Academy of Audiology, 1*, 81–88.

Hall, J. W., & Grose, J. H. (1993). The effect of otitis media with effusion on the masking-level difference and the auditory brainstem response. *Journal of Speech and Hearing Research, 36*, 210–217.

Hall, J. W., & Grose, J. H. (1994). Development of temporal resolution in children as measured by the temporal modulation transfer function. *Journal of the Acoustical Society of America, 96*, 150–154.

Hall, J. W., Grose, J. H., & Pillsbury, H. C. (1990.) Predicting binaural hearing after stapedectomy from pre-surgery results. *Archives of Otolaryngology, Head and Neck Surgery, 116*, 946–950.

Hall, J. W., Grose, J. H., & Pillsbury, H. C. (1995). Long-term effects of chronic otitis media on binaural hearing in children. *Archives of Otolaryngology, 121*, 857–862.

Hall, J. W., Tyler, R. S., & Fernandez, M. A. (1984). Factors influencing the masking level difference in cochlear hearing-impaired and normal-hearing listeners. *Journal of Speech and Hearing Research, 27*, 145–154.

Hamre, C. E. (1972). Research and clinical practice: A unifying model. *Asha, 14*, 542–545.

Harris, J. D. (1960). Combinations of distortions in speech: The twenty-five per cent safety factor by multiple-cueing. *Archives of Otolaryngology, 72, 227–232.*

Hashimoto, I., Ishiyama, Y., Yoshimoto, T., & Nemoto, S. (1981). Brainstem auditory-evoked potentials recorded directly from the human brainstem and thalamus. *Brain, 104*, 841–859.

Hausler, R., Colburn, H. S., & Marr, E. (1983). Sound localization in subjects with impaired hearing. *Acta Oto-laryngology* (Suppl. 400), Monograph.

Hausler, R., & Levine, R. A. (1980). Brainstem auditory evoked potentials are related to interaural time discrimination in patients with multiple sclerosis. *Brain Research, 191*, 589–594.

Hebb, D. O. (1949). *The organization of behavior.* New York: John Wiley & Sons.

Heffner, H. E., & Heffner, R. S. (1986). Effect of unilateral and bilateral auditory cortex lesions on the discrimination of vocalizations by Japanese macaques. *Journal of Neurophysiology, 35*, 683–701.

Heilman, K. M., Hammer, L. C., & Wilder, B. J. (1973). An audiometric defect in temporal lobe dysfunction. *Neurology (NY), 3*, 384–386.

Heise, D. R. (1969). Separating reliability and stability in test-retest correlation. *American Sociological Review, 34,* 93–104.

Helfer, K. S., & Wilber, L. A. (1990). Hearing loss, aging, and speech perception in reverberation and noise. *Journal of Speech and Hearing Research, 33,* 149–155.

Hendler, T., Squires, N. K., & Emmerich, D. S. (1990). Psychophysical measures of central auditory dysfunction in multiple sclerosis: Neurophysiological and neuroanatomical correlates. *Ear and Hearing, 11,* 403–415.

Hirsh, I. J. (1948). The influence of interaural phase on interaural summation and inhibition. *Journal of the Acoustical Society of America, 20,* 536–544.

Hirsh, I. J. (1959). Auditory perception of temporal order. *Journal of the Acoustical Society of America, 31,* 759–767.

Hirsh, I. J., & Sherrick, Jr., C. E. (1961). Perceived order in different sense modalities. *Journal of Experimental Psychology, 62,* 423–432.

Hughes, J. W. (1946). The threshold of audition for short periods of stimulation. *Procedures of the Research Society of London, 133B,* 486–490.

Hurley, R., & Singer, J. (April, 1989). The effectiveness of selected auditory processing tests as screening tests with children. Paper presented at the American Academy of Audiology Annual Conference, Kiawah, S.C.

Irvine, D. R. F., Rajan, R., Wize, L. Z., & Heil, P. (1991). Reorganization in auditory cortex of adult cats with unilateral restricted cochlear lesions. *Society for Neuroscience, 17* (Abstract), 1485.

Irwin, R. J., Ball, A. K., Kay, N., Stillman, J. A., & Bosser, J. (1985). The development of auditory temporal acuity in children. *Child Development, 56,* 614–620.

Ivey, R. G. (1969). Tests of CNS auditory function. Unpublished Master's Thesis. Ft. Collins, CO: Colorado State University.

Jacobson, J. (Ed.) (1985). *The auditory brainstem response.* San Diego, CA: College-Hill Press.

Jacobson, J. T., Deppe, U., & Murray, T. J. (1983). Dichotic paradigms in multiple sclerosis. *Ear and Hearing, 3,* 311–317.

Jensen, J. K., Neff, D. L., & Callaghan, B. P. (1987). Frequency, intensity, and duration discrimination in young children. *Asha, 29,* 88.

Jerger, J. (1963). Viewpoint. *Journal of Speech and Hearing Research, 6,* 203–206.

Jerger, J., Brown, D., & Smith, S. (1984). Effect of peripheral hearing loss on the MLD. *Archives of Otolaryngology, 110,* 290–296.

Jerger, J., & Jerger, S. W. (1974). Auditory findings in brainstem disorders. *Archives of Otolaryngology, 99,* 342–349.

Jerger, J., & Jerger, S. (1975). Clinical validity of central auditory tests. *Scandinavian Audiology, 4,* 147–163.

Jerger, S., Jerger, J., Alford, B. R., & Abrams, S. (1983). Development of speech intelligibility in children with recurrent otitis media. *Ear and Hearing, 4,* 138–145.

Jerger, J., Lovering, L., & Wertz, M. (1972). Auditory disorder following bilateral temporal lobe insult: Report of a case. *Journal of Speech and Hearing Disorders, 37,* 524–535.

Jewitt, D., & Williston, J. (1971). Auditory-evoked far fields averaged from the scalp of humans. *Brain, 94,* 618–696.

Jirsa, R. E. (1992). The clinical utility of the P3 AERP in children with auditory processing disorders. *Journal of Speech and Hearing Research, 35*, 903–912.

Jongkees, L., & Van der Veer, R. (1957). Directional hearing capacity in hearing disorders. *Acta Oto-laryngology, 48*, 465–474.

Kalil, R. E. (1989, December). Synapse formation in the developing brain. *Scientific American*, 76–85.

Kalil, R. E., Dubin, M. W., Scott, G., & Stark, L. A. (1986). Elimination of action potentials blocks the structural development of retinogeniculate synapses. *Nature, 323*, 156–158.

Karaseva, T. A. (1972). The role of the temporal lobe in human auditory perception. *Neuropsychologia, 10*, 227–231.

Katz, J. (1962). The use of staggered spondaic words for assessing the integrity of the central auditory nervous system. *Journal of Auditory Research, 2*, 327–337.

Katz, J. (1968). The SSW test: An interim report. *Journal of Speech and Hearing Disorders, 33*, 132–146.

Katz, J. (1977). The staggered spondaic word test. In R.W. Keith (Ed.), *Central auditory dysfunction* (pp. 103–121). New York: Grune & Stratton.

Katz, J. (1986). *SSW Test User's Manual.* Vancouver, WA: Precision Acoustics.

Katz, J. (1992). Classification of auditory processing disorders. In J. Katz, N. Stecker, & D. Henderson (Eds.), *Central auditory processing: A transdisciplinary view* (pp. 81–91). St. Louis, MO: Mosby Year Book.

Katz, J. (1994). *Handbook of clinical audiology* (4th ed.). Baltimore: Williams & Wilkins.

Katz., J., Stecker, N., & Masters, M. G. (1994, March). Central auditory processing: A coherent approach. Paper presented at the American Speech-Language-Hearing Association Task Force on Central Auditory Processing Consensus Development Conference, Albuquerque, NM.

Keith, R. (1977). Synthetic sentence identification test. In R.W. Keith (Ed.), *Central auditory dysfunction* (pp. 73–102). New York: Grune & Stratton.

Keith, R. (1984). Dichotic listening in children. In D. Beasley (Ed.), *Audition in childhood: Methods of study* (pp. 1–23). San Diego, CA: College Hill Press.

Keith, R. (1986). *SCAN: A screening test for auditory processing disorders.* San Antonio,TX: The Psychological Corporation.

Keith, R. (1994a). *ACPT: Auditory continuous performance test.* San Antonio,TX: The Psychological Corporation.

Keith, R. (1994b). *SCAN-A: A test for auditory processing disorders in adolescents and adults.* TX: The Psychological Corporation, Harcourt Brace Jovanovich, Inc.

Kelly, J. (1986). The development of sound localization of auditory processing in mammals. In R.N. Aslin (Ed.), *Advances in neural and behavioral development: Vol. 2* (pp. 202–234). Norwood, NJ: Ablex.

Kiang, N. Y. S. (1975). Stimulus representation in the discharge patterns of auditory neurons. In D.B. Tower (Ed.), *The nervous system. Volume 3: Human communication and its disorders* (pp. 81–96). New York: Raven Press.

Kileny, P., Paccioretti, D., & Wilson, A. F. (1987). Effects of cortical lesions on middle-latency auditory evoked responses (MLR). *Electroencephalography and Clinical Neurophysiology, 66*, 108–120.

Kimura, D. (1961a). Some effects of temporal-lobe damage on auditory perception. *Canadian Journal of Psychology, 15*, 156–165.

Kimura, D. (1961b). Cerebral dominance and the perception of verbal stimuli. *Canadian Journal of Psychology, 15*, 166–171.

Kitzes, L. M., Farley, G. R., & Starr, A. (1978). Modulation of auditory cortex unit activity during the performance of a conditioned response. *Experimental Neurology, 62*, 678–697.

Knudsen, E. J. (1983). Early auditory experience aligns the auditory map of space in the optic tectum of the barn owl. *Science, 222*, 939–942.

Knudsen, E. J. (1987). Early auditory experience shapes auditory localization behavior and the spatial tuning of auditory units in the barn owl. In J. Rauschecker & P. Marler (Eds.), *Imprinting and cortical plasticity* (pp. 7–23). New York: John Wiley & Sons.

Knudsen, E. J., Esterly, S. D., & Knudsen, P. F. (1984). Monaural occlusion alters sound localization during a sensitive period in the barn owl. *Journal of Neuroscience, 4*, 1001–1011.

Knudsen, E., & Knudsen, P, (1985). Vision guides the adjustment of auditory localization in young barn owls. *Science, 230*, 545–548.

Kolata, G. (1984). Studying learning in the womb: Behavioral scientists are using established experimental methods to show that fetuses can and do learn. *Science, 20*, 302–303.

Kraus, N., McGee, T., Carrell, T. D., & Sharma, A (1995). Neurophysiologic bases of speech discrimination. *Ear and Hearing, 16*, 19–37.

Kraus, N., McGee, T., Micco, A., Sharma, A., Carrell, T., & Nicol, T. (1993). Mismatch negativity in school-age children to speech stimuli that are just perceptibly different. *Electroencephalography and Clinical Neurophysiology, 88*, 123–130.

Kraus, N., Ozdamar, O., Hier, D., & Stein, L. (1982). Auditory middle latency responses in patients with cortical lesions. *Electroencephalography and Clinical Neurophysiology, 54*, 247–287.

Kraus, N. Smith, D., Reed, N., Stein, L., & Cartee, C. (1985). Auditory middle latency responses in children: Effects of age and diagnostic category. *Electroencephalography and Clinical Neurophysiology, 62*, 343–351.

Kurdziel, S. A., Noffsinger, P. D., & Olsen, W. (1976). Performance by cortical lesion patients on 40 and 60 percent time-compressed materials. *Journal of the Americal Audiological Society, 2*, 3–7.

Lackner, J. R., & Teuber, H. L. (1973). Alterations in auditory fusion thresholds after cerebral injury in man. *Neuropsychologia, 11*, 409–415.

Lecours, A. R. (1975). Myelogenetic correlates of development of speech and language. In E. H. Lenneberg and E. Lenneberg (Eds), *Foundation of language development, Vol. 1* (pp. 121–135). New York: Academic Press.

Lenneberg, E. H. (1967). *Biological foundations of language.* New York: John Wiley & Sons.

Lessler, K. (1972, February). Health and educational screening of school-age children: Definition and objectives. *American Journal of Public Health, 62*, 191–198.

Levine, R. A., Gardner, J. C., Stufflebeam, S. M., Fullterton, B. C., Carlisle, E. W., Furst, M., Rosen, B. R., & Kiang, N. Y. S. (1993a). Binaural auditory processing in multiple sclerosis subjects. *Hearing Research, 68*, 59–72.

Levine, R. A., Gardner, J. C., Stufflebeam, S. M., Fullterton, B. C., Carlisle, E. W., Furst, M., Rosen, B. R., & Kiang, N. Y. S. (1993b). Effects of multiple sclerosis brainstem lesions on sound lateralization and brainstem auditory evoked potentials. *Hearing Research, 68*, 73–88.

Lewis, M. (1986). *Learning disabilities and prenatal risks.* Urbana, IL: University of Illinois Press.

Licklider, J. C. R. (1948). The influence of interaural phase relations upon the masking of speech by white noise. *Journal of the Acoustical Society of America, 20*, 150–159.

Lindamood, C., & Lindamood, P. (1971). *The Lindamood Auditory Test of Cenceptualization (LAC).* Boston: Teaching Resources Corp.

Litovsky, R. (1991). *Developmental changes in sound localization precision under conditions of the precedence effect.* Unpublished doctoral dissertation, University of Massachusetts, Amherst. As reported in Clifton, R. K. (1992). The development of spatial hearing in infants. In L. A. Werner & E. W. Rubel (Eds.), *Developmental psychoacoustics* (pp. 135–157). Washington, DC: American Psychological Association.

Luria, A. (1973). *The working brain: An introduction to neuropsychology.* New York: Basic Books.

Lynn, G. E., & Gilroy, J. (1972). Neuro-audiological abnormalities in patients with temporal lobe tumors. *Journal of Neurological Sciences, 17*, 167–184.

Lynn, G. E., & Gilroy, J. (1975). Effects of brain lesions on the perception of monotic and dichotic speech stimuli. In M. D. Sullivan (Ed.), *Central auditory processing disorders* (pp. 47–83). Proceedings of a conference at the University of Nebraska Medical Center, Omaha.

Lynn, G. E., & Gilroy, J. (1977). Effects of brain lesions on the perception of monotic and dichotic speech stimuli. In M. D. Sullivan (Ed.), *Central auditory processing disorders* (pp. 47–83). Proceedings of a conference at the University of Nebraska Medical Center, Omaha.

Lynn, G. E., Gilroy, J., Taylor, P. C., & Leiser, R. P. (1981). Binaural masking-level differences in neurological disorders. *Archives of Otolaryngology, 107*, 357–362.

Massaro, D. W. (1972). Preperceptual images, processing time, and perceptual units in auditory perception. *Psychological Review, 79*, 124–145.

Matzker, J. (1959). Two new methods for the assessment of central auditory functions in cases of brain disease. *Annals of Otology, Rhinology and Laryngology, 68*, 1155–1197.

Maue-Dickson, W. (1981). The auditory nerve and central auditory pathways: Prenatal development. In Martin, F. N. (Ed.), *Medical Audiology. Disorders of Hearing* (pp. 371–392). Englewood Cliffs, NJ: Prentice-Hall.

McFarland, D. J., & Cacace, A. T. (1995). Modality specificity as a criterion for diagnosing central auditory processing disorders. *American Journal of Audiology, 4*, 36–48.

McGee, T., Kraus, N., Comperatore, C., & Nicol, T. (1991). Subcortical and cortical components of the MLR generating system. *Brain Research, 544,* 211–220.

McGurk, H., Turnure, C., & Creighton, S. (1977). Auditory-visual coordination in neonates. *Child Development, 48,* 138–143.

Merzenich, M. M., & Haas, J. H. (1982, December). Reorganization of mammalian somatosensory cortex following peripheral nerve injury. *Trends in Neuroscience,* 434–436.

Merzenich, M. M., Rencanzone, G., Jenkins, W. M., Allard, T. T., & Nudo, R. J. (1988). Cortical representational plasticity. In P. Rakic & W. Singer (Eds.), *Neurobiology of neocortex* (pp. 41–67.) New York: John Wiley & Sons.

Miller, G. A., & Gildea, P. M. (1987). How children learn words. *Scientific American, 257,* 94–99.

Milner, B., Taylor, S., & Sperry, R. (1968). Lateralized suppression of dichotically presented digits after commissural section in man. *Science, 161,* 184–185.

Moller, A. R., Jannetta, P. J., & Moller, M. B. (1981). Neural generators of brainstem evoked potentials. Results from human intracranial recordings. *Annals of Otology, 90,* 591–596.

Moore, D. R., Hutchings, M. E., King, A. J., & Kowalchuk, N. E. (1989). Auditory brainstem of the ferret: Some effects of rearing with unilateral ear plug on the cochlea, cochlear nucleus, and projections to the inferior colliculus. *Journal of Neuroscience, 9,* 1213–1222.

Moore, D. R., & Irvine, D. R. F. (1981). Plasticity of binaural interaction in the cat inferior colliculus. *Brain Research, 208,* 198–202.

Morales-Garcia, C., & Poole, J. O. (1972). Masked speech audiometry in central deafness. *Acta Otolaryngologica (Stockholm), 74,* 307–316.

Morongiello, B., & Clifton, R. (1984). Effects of sound frequency on behavioral and cardiac orienting in newborn and five-month-infants. *Journal of Experimental Child Psychology, 38,* 429–446.

Morrongiello, B. A., & Trehub, S. E. (1987). Age-related changes in auditory temporal perception. *Journal of Experimental Child Psychology, 44,* 413–426.

Mueller, H. G., Beck, W. G., & Sedge, R. K. (1987). Comparison of the efficiency of cortical level speech tests. *Seminars in Hearing, 8,* 279–298.

Mueller, H. G., & Bright, K. E. (1994). Monosyllabic procedures in central testing. In J. Katz (Ed.), *Handbook of clinical audiology,* (4th ed., pp. 222–238). Baltimore: Williams & Wilkins.

Muir, D., Abraham, W., Forbes, B., & Harris, L. (1979) The ontogenesis of an auditory localization response from birth to 4 months of age. *Canadian Journal of Psychology, 43,* 199–216.

Muir, D., & Clifton, R. (1985). Infants' orientation to the localization of sound sources. In G. Gottlieb & N. Krasnegor (Eds.), *The measurement of audition and vision during the first year of postnatal life: A methodological overview* (pp. 171–194). Norwood, NJ: Ablex.

Musiek, F. E. (1983a). Assessment of central auditory dysfunction: The Dichotic Digits Test revisited. *Ear and Hearing, 4,* 79–83.

Musiek, F. E. (1983b). Assessment of three dichotic speech tests on subjects with intracranial lesions. *Ear and Hearing, 4,* 318–323.

Musiek, F. E. (1983c). The evaluation of brainstem disorders using ABR and central auditory tests. *Monographs in Contemporary Audiology, 4,* 1–24.

Musiek, F. E. (1986). Neuroanatomy, neurophysiology, and central auditory assessment. Part III: Corpus callosum and efferent pathways. *Ear and Hearing, 7,* 349–358.

Musiek, F. E. (1994). Frequency (pitch) and duration pattern tests. *Journal of the American Academy of Audiology, 5,* 265–268.

Musiek, F. E., Baran, J. A., & Pinheiro, M. L. (1990). Duration pattern recognition in normal subjects and patients with cerebral and cochlear lesions. *Audiology, 29,* 304–313.

Musiek, F. E., & Chermak, G. D. (1994). Three commonly asked questions about central auditory processing disorders: Assessment. *American Journal of Audiology, 3,* 23–27.

Musiek, F. E., & Chermak, G. D. (1995). Three commonly asked questions about central auditory processing disorders: Managment. *American Journal of Audiology, 4,* 15–18.

Musiek, F. E., Gollegly, K. M., & Baran, J. A. (1984.) Myelination of the corpus callosum and auditory processing problems in children: Theoretical and clinical correlates. *Seminars in Hearing, 5,* 231–241.

Musiek, F., Gollegly, K., Kibbe, K., & Reeves, A. (1985). Electrophysiologic and behavioral auditory findings in multiple sclerosis. *American Journal of Otology, 10,* 343–350.

Musiek, F. E., Gollegly, K. M., Kibbe, K. S., & Verkest-Lenz, S. B. (1991). Proposed screening test for central auditory disorders: Follow-up on the Dichotic Digits Test. *American Journal of Otology, 12,* 109–113.

Musiek, F. E., Gollegly, K. M., Lamb, L. E., & Lamb, P. (1990). Selected issues in screening for central auditory processing dysfunction. *Seminars in Hearing, 11,* 372–384.

Musiek, F., Gollegly, K., & Ross, M. (1985). Profiles of types of auditory processing disorders in children with learning disabilities. *Journal of Children with Communication Disorders, 9,* 43.

Musiek, F., & Guerkink, N. (1982). Auditory brainstem response and central auditory test findings for patients with brainstem lesions. *Laryngoscope, 92,* 891–900.

Musiek, F. E., & Hoffman, D. W. (1990). An introduction to the functional neurochemistry of the auditory system. *Ear and Hearing, 11,* 395–402.

Musiek, F. E., Kibbe, K., & Baran, J. A. (1984). Neuroaudiological results from split-brain patients. *Seminars in Hearing, 5,* 219–229.

Musiek, F. E., Kurdziel-Schwan, S., Kibbe, K. S., Gollegly, K. M., Baran, J. A., & Rintelmann, W. F. (1989). The dichotic rhyme task: Results in split-brain patients. *Ear and Hearing, 10,* 33–39.

Musiek, F. E., & Lamb, L. (1994). Central auditory assessment: An overview. In J. Katz (Ed.), *Handbook of clinical audiology,* (4th ed., pp. 197–211). Baltimore: Williams & Wilkins.

Musiek, F. E., & Pinheiro, M. L. (1987). Frequency patterns in cochlear, brainstem, and cerebral lesions. *Audiology, 26*, 79–88.

Musiek, F. E., Pinheiro, M. L., & Wilson, D. H. (1980). Auditory pattern perception in "split-brain" patients. *Archives of Otolaryngology, 106*, 610–612.

Musiek, F. E., & Reeves, A. G. (1990). Asymmetries of the auditory areas of the cerebrum. *Journal of the American Academy of Audiology, 1*, 240–245.

Musiek, F. E., Reeves, A. G., & Baran, J. A. (1985). Release from central auditory competition in the split-brain patient. *Neurology, 35*, 983–987.

Musiek, F. E., Verkest, S. B., & Gollegly, K. M. (1988). Effects of neuro-maturation on auditory-evoked potentials. *Seminars in Hearing, 9*, 1–13.

Musiek, F. E., Weider, D. J., & Mueller, R. (1982). Audiological findings in Charcot-Marie-Tooth syndrome. *Archives of Otolaryngology, 109*, 595–599.

Myklebust, H. (1954). *Auditory disorders in children.* New York: Grune & Stratton.

Naatanen, R., & Gaillard, A. W. K. (1983). The N2 deflection of ERP and the orienting reflex. In A. W. K. Gaillard & W. Ritter (Eds.), *EEG correlates of information processing: Theoretical issues* (pp. 119–141). Amsterdam: North Holland.

Naatanen, R., Gaillard, A. W. K., & Montysalo, S. (1978). Early selective-attention effect on evoked potential reinterpreted. *Acta Psychologica, 42*, 313–329.

Naatanen, R., & Kraus, N. (Eds.) (1995). Special issue: Mismatch negativity as an index of central auditory function. *Ear and Hearing, 16*, 1–146.

Niccum, N., Rubens, A., & Speaks, C. (1981). Effects of stimulus material on the dichotic listening performance of aphasic patients. *Journal of Speech and Hearing Research, 24*, 526–534.

Niccum, N., Speaks, C., Katsuki-Nakamura, J., & Van Tassell, D. (1987). Effects of simulated conductive hearing loss on dichotic listening performance for digits. *Journal of Speech and Hearing Disorders, 52*, 313–318.

Noback, C. R., (1985). Neuroanatomical correlates of central auditory function. In M. L. Pinheiro and F. E. Musiek (Eds.), *Assessment of central auditory dysfunction: Foundations and clinical correlates* (pp. 7–21). Baltimore: Williams & Wilkins.

Noffsinger, D., Martinez, C., & Schaefer, A. (1982). Auditory brainstem responses and masking level differences from persons with brainstem lesions. *Scandinavian Audiology, 15*, 81–93.

Noffsinger, D., Martinez, C. D., & Wilson, R. H. (1994). Dichotic listening to speech. Background and preliminary data for digits, sentences, and nonsense syllables. *Journal of the American Academy of Audiology, 5*, 248–254.

Noffsinger, D., Olsen, W. O., Carhart, R., Hart, C. W., & Sahgal, V. (1972). Auditory and vestibular aberrations in multiple sclerosis. *Acta Oto-Laryngology* (Suppl. 303), 1–63.

Noffsinger, D., Schaefer, A. B., & Martinez, C. D. (1984). Behavioral and objective estimates of auditory brainstem integrity. *Seminars in Hearing, 5*, 337–349.

Noffsinger, D., Wilson, W. H., & Musiek, F. E. (1994). Department of Veterans Affairs compact disc recording for auditory perceptual assessment: Background and introduction. *Journal of the American Academy of Audiology, 5*, 231–235.

Nordlund, B. (1964). Directional audiometry. *Acta Oto-Laryngology, 57,* 1–18.

Nordlund, B., & Fritzel, B. (1963). The influence of azimuth on speech signals. *Acta Oto-Laryngology, 56,* 632–642.

Nozza, R. J. (1987). The binaural masking level difference in infants and adults: Developmental change in binaural hearing. *Infant Behavior Development, 10,* 105–110.

Nozza, R. J., Wagner, E. F., & Crandall, M. A. (1988). Binaural release from masking for a speech sound in infants, preschoolers, and adults. *Journal of Speech and Hearing Research, 31,* 212–218.

Olds, J., Disterhoft, J. F., Segal, M., Kornblith, C. L., & Hirsh, R. (1972). Learning centers of rat brain mapped by measuring latencies of conditioned unit responses. *Journal of Neurophysiology, 35,* 202–219.

Olsen, W. O. (1983). Dichotic test results for normal subjects and for temporal lobectomy patients. *Ear and Hearing, 4,* 324–330.

Olsen, W., & Noffsinger, D. (1976). Masking level differences for cochlear and brainstem lesions. *Annals of Otology, 85,* 820–825.

Olsen, W. O., Noffsinger, D., & Carhart, R. (1976). Masking level differences encountered in clinical populations. *Audiology, 15,* 287–301.

Olsen, W. O., Noffsinger, P. D., & Kurdziel, S. A. (1975). Speech discrimination in quiet and in white noise by patients with peripheral and central lesions. *Acta Otolaryngologica (Stockholm), 80,* 375–382.

Osterhammel, P. A., Shallop, J. K., & Terkildsen, K. (1987). The effect of sleep on the auditory brainstem response (ABR) and the middle latency response (MLR). *Scandinavian Audiology, 14,* 47–50.

Ozdamar, O., & Kraus, N. (1983). Auditory middle latency responses in humans. *Audiology, 22,* 34–49.

Papsin, B. C., & Abel, S. M. (1988). Temporal summation in hearing-impaired listeners. *Journal of Otolaryngology, 17,* 93–100.

Perrault, N., & Picton, T. W. (1984). Event-related potentials recorded from the scalp and nasopharyns. I. N1 and P2. *Electroencephalography and Clinical Neurophysiology, 47,* 637–647.

Phillips. J. L. (1996). *How to think about statistics.* New York: W. H. Freeman and Company.

Pickles, J. O. (1985). Physiology of the cerebral auditory system. In M. L. Pinheiro & F. E. Musiek (Eds.), *Assessment of central auditory dysfunction: Foundations and clinical correlates* (pp. 67–86). Baltimore: Williams & Wilkins.

Picton, T., Woods, D., Baribeau-Braun, J., & Healey, T. (1977). Evoked potential audiometry. *Journal of Otolaryngology, 6,* 90–119.

Pillsbury, H. C., Grose, J. H., & Hall, J. W. (1991.) Otitis media with effusion in children. *Archives of Otolaryngology, Head and Neck Surgery, 117,* 718–723.

Pinheiro, M. L. (1976). Auditory pattern perception in patients with right and left hemisphere lesions. *Ohio Journal of Speech and Hearing, 2,* 9–20.

Pinheiro, M. L., & Musiek, F. E. (1985). Sequencing and temporal ordering in the auditory system. In M. L. Pinheiro & F. E. Musiek (Eds.), *Assessment of central auditory dysfunction: Foundations and clinical correlates* (pp. 219–238). Baltimore: Williams & Wilkins.

Pinheiro, M. L., & Ptacek, P. H. (1971). Reversals in the perception of noise and tone patterns. *Journal of the Acoustical Society of America, 49*, 1778–1782.

Pinheiro, M. L., & Tobin, H. (1969). Interaural intensity difference for intracranial localization. *Journal of the Acoustical Society of America, 46*, 1482–1487.

Pinheiro, M. L., & Tobin, H. (1971). The interaural intensity difference as a diagnostic indicator. *Acta Oto–Laryngology, 71*, 326–328.

Polich, J., Howard, L., & Starr, A. (1985). Effects of age on the P-300 component of the event related potential from auditory stimuli: Peak definition, variation, and measurement. *Journal of Gerontology, 40,* 721–726.

Porter, R., & Berlin, C. (1975). On interpreting developmental change in the dichotic right ear advantage. *Brain and Language, 2,* 186–200.

Ptacek, P. H., & Pinheiro, M. L. (1971). Pattern reversal in auditory perception. *Journal of the Acoustical Society of America, 49*, 493–498.

Quaranta, A., & Cervellera, G. (1974). Masking level differences in normal and pathological ears. *Audiology, 13*, 428–431.

Quine, D. B., Regan, D., & Murray, T. J. (1983). Delayed auditory tone perception in multiple sclerosis. *Canadian Journal of Neurological Sciences, 10*, 183–186.

Rauschecker, J. P., & Marler, P. (1987). Cortical plasticity and imprinting: Behavioral and physiological contrasts and parallels. In J. P. Rauschecker & P. Marler (Eds.), *Imprinting and cortical plasticity* (pp. 349–366). New York: John Wiley & Sons.

Rencanzone, G. H., Schreiner, C. E., & Merzenich, M. M. (1993.) Plasticity in the frequency representation of primary auditory cortex following discrimination training in adult owl monkeys. *Journal of Neuroscience, 13*, 87–103.

Restak, R. M. (1986). *The Infant Mind.* Garden City, NY: Doubleday & Company.

Reynolds, W. M. (1987). *Auditory Discrimination Test* (2nd ed.). Los Angeles: Western Psychological Services.

Rintelmann, W. F. (1985). Monaural speech tests in the detection of central auditory disorders. In M. L. Pinheiro & F. E. Musiek (Eds.), *Assessment of central auditory dysfunction: Foundations and clinical correlates* (pp. 173–200). Baltimore: Williams & Wilkins.

Ritter, W., Simson, R., Vaughan, H. G., & Macht, M. (1982). Manipulation of event-related potential manifestations of information processing stages. *Science, 218,* 909–911.

Robertson, D., & Irvine, D. R. F. (1989). Plasticity of frequency organization in auditory cortex of guinea pigs with partial unilateral deafness. *Journal of Comparative Neurology, 282*, 456–471.

Roeser, R. J., Johns, D. F., & Price, L. L. (1976). Dichotic listening in adults with sensorineural hearing loss. *Journal of the American Audiology Society, 2,* 19–25.

Roeser, R. J., Millay, K. K., & Morrow, J. M. (1983). Dichotic Consonant-Vowel (CV) perception in normal and learning-impaired children. *Ear and Hearing, 4,* 293–299.

Romand, R. (Ed.), (1983). *Development of auditory and vestibular systems.* New York: Academic Press.

Roser, D. (1966). Directional hearing in persons with hearing disorders. *Journal of Laryngology and Rhinology, 45,* 423–440.

Roush, J., & Tait, C. A., (1984). Binaural fusion, masking level differences, and auditory brainstem responses in children with language-learning disabilities. *Ear and Hearing, 5*, 37–41.

Rubens, A. B., Froehling, B., Slater, G., & Anderson, D. (1985). Left ear suppression on verbal dichotic tests in patients with multiple sclerosis. *Annals of Neurology, 18*, 459–463.

Rugg, M. D. (1984a). Event-related potentials and the phonological processing of words and non-words. *Neuropsychologia, 22*, 435–443.

Rugg, M. D., (1984b). Event-related potentials in phonological matching tasks. *Brain and Language, 23*, 225–240.

Ryugo, D. K., & Weinberger, N. M. (1978). Differencial plasticity of morphologically distinct populations in the medial geniculate body of the cat during classical conditioning. *Behavioral Biology, 22*, 275–301.

Sahley, T. L., Kalish, R. B., Musiek, F. E., & Hoffman, D. W. (1991). Effects of opioid drugs on auditory evoked potentials suggest a role of lateral olivocochlear dynorphins in auditory function. *Hearing Research, 55*, 133–142.

Salamy, A. (1978). Commissural transmission: Maturational changes in humans. *Science, 200*, 1409–1410.

Salamy, A. (1984). Maturation of the auditory brainstem response from birth through early childhood. *Journal of Clinical Neurophysiology, 1*, 293–329.

Salamy, A., Mendelson, T., Tooley, W., & Chaplin, E. (1980). Differential development of brainstem potentials in healthy and high-risk infants. *Science, 210*, 553–555.

Salkind, N. J. (1991). *Exploring research*. New York: Macmillan.

Sanchez-Longo, L., & Forster, F. (1958). Clinical significance of impairments in sound localizations. *Neurology, 8*, 119–125.

Sanchez-Longo, F., Forster, F., & Auth, T. (1957). A clinical test for sound localization and its applications. *Neurology, 7*, 655–663.

Satz, K., Achenback, E., Pattishall, E., & Fennell, E. (1965). Order of report, ear asymmetry and handedness in dichotic listening. *Cortex, 1*, 377–395.

Scherg, M., Vasjar, J., & Picton, T. (1989). A source analysis of the late human auditory evoked potentials. *Journal of Cognitive Neuroscience, 1*, 336–355.

Schneider, B. A., Trehub, S. E., Morrongiello, B. A., & Thorpe, L. A. (1989). Developmental changes in masked thresholds. *Journal of the Acoustical Society of America, 86*, 1733–1741.

Schoeny, Z. G., & Carhart, R. (1971). Effects of unilateral Meniere's disease on masking-level differences. *Journal of the Acoustical Society of America, 50*, 1143–1150.

Semel, E., Wiig, E. H., & Secord, W. (1987). *Clinical Evaluation of Language Fundamentals—Revised: Examiner's manual*. San Antonio, TX: The Psychological Corporation.

Sidtis, J. (1982). Predicting brain organization from dichotic listening performance: Cortical and subcortical functional asymmetries contribute to perceptual asymmetries. *Brain and Language, 17*, 287–300.

Silverman, F. H. (1977). *Research design in speech pathology and audiology*. Englewood Cliffs, NJ: Prentice-Hall.

Sinha, S. O. (1959). *The role of the temporal lobe in hearing*. Unpublished master's thesis, Montreal, Quebec, Canada: McGill University.

Sloan, C. (1995). *Treating auditory processing difficulties in children*. San Diego, CA: Singular Publishing Group.

Smith, B. B., & Resnick, D. M. (1972). An auditory test for assessing brain stem integrity: Preliminary report. *Laryngoscope, 82*, 414–424.

Sparks, R., & Geschwind, N. (1968). Dichotic listening in man after section of neocortical commissures. *Cortex, 4*, 3–16.

Sparks, R., Goodglass, H., & Nickel, B. (1970). Ipsilateral versus contralateral extinction in dichotic listening resulting from hemispheric lesions. *Cortex, 6*, 249–260.

Speaks, C., Gray, T., Miller, J., & Rubens, A. (1975). Central auditory deficits and temporal-lobe lesions. *Journal of Speech and Hearing Disorders, 40*, 192–205.

Speaks, C., Niccum, N., & Van Tasell, D. (1985). Effects of stimulus material on the dichotic listening performance of patients with sensorineural hearing loss. *Journal of Speech and Hearing Research, 28*, 16–25.

Squires, K., & Hecox, K. (1983). Electrophysiological evaluation of higher level auditory processing. *Seminars in Hearing, 4*, 415–432.

Staffel, J. G., Hall, J. W., Grose, J. H., & Pillsbury, H. C. (1990). NøSø and NøSπ detection as a function of masker bandwidth in normal-hearing and cochlear-impaired listeners. *Journal of the Acoustical Society of America, 87*, 1720–1727.

Starr, A., Amlie, R. N., Martin, W. H., & Sanders, S. (1977). Development of auditory function in newborn infants revealed by auditory brainstem potentials. *Pediatrics, 60*, 831–839.

Streeter, G. L. (1906). On the development of the membranous labyrinth and the acoustic and facial nerves in the human embryo. *American Journal of Anatomy, 6*, 139–165.

Stryker, M. P., & Harris, W. A. (1986). Binocular impulse blockade prevents the formation of ocular dominance columns in cat visual cortex. *Journal of Neuroscience, 6*, 2117–2133.

Sugishita, M., Otomo, K., Yamazaki, K., Shimizu, H., Yoshioka, M., & Shinohars, A. (1995). Dichotic listening in patients with partial section of the corpus callosum. *Brain, 118*, 417–427.

Sutton, S., Braren, M., Zubin, J., & John, E. R. (1965.) Evoked-potential correlates of stimulus uncertainty. *Science, 150*, 1187–1188.

Suzuki, T., Hirabayashi, M., & Kobayashi, K. (1983). Auditory middle responses in young children. *British Journal of Audiology, 17*, 5–9.

Sweetow, R. W., & Reddell, R. C. (1978). The use of masking level differences in the identification of children with perceptual learning problems. *Journal of the American Auditory Society, 4*, 52–56.

Swisher, L., & Hirsh, I. J. (1972). Brain damage and the ordering of two temporally successive stimuli. *Neuropsychologia, 10*, 137–152.

Thompson, M. E., & Abel, S. M. (1992a). Indices of hearing in patients with central auditory pathology. I: Detection and discrimination. *Scandinavian Audiology, 21* (Suppl. 35), 3–15.

Thompson, M. E., & Abel, S. M. (1992b). Indices of hearing in patients with central auditory pathology. II: Choice response time. *Scandinavian Audiology, 21* (Suppl. 35), 17–22.

Tobin, H. (1985). Binaural interaction tasks. In M. L. Pinheiro & F. E. Musiek (Eds.), *Assessment of central auditory dysfunction: Foundations and clinical correlates* (pp. 155–172). Baltimore: Williams & Wilkins.

Tonal and speech materials for auditory perceptual assessment (1992). Long Beach, CA: Research and Development Service, Veterans' Administration Central Office.

Tonning, F. (1971). Directional audiometry. II. The influence of azimuth on the perception of speech. *Acta Oto-Laryngology, 72,* 352–357.Tonning, F. (1973). Directional audiometry. VIII. The influence of hearing aids on the localization of white noise. *Acta Oto-Laryngology, 76,* 114–120.

Tonning, F. (1975). Auditory localization and its clinical applications. *Audiology, 14,* 368–380.

Townsend, T. H., & Goldstein, D. P. (1972). Supra-threshold binaural unmasking. *Journal of the Acoustical Society of America, 51,* 621–624.

Turner, R. G., & Nielsen, D. W. (1984). Application of clinical decision analysis to audiological tests. *Ear and Hearing, 5,* 125–133.

Vaughan Jr., H. G., & Ritter, W. (1970). The sources of auditory evoked responses recorded from the human scalp. *Electroencephalography and Clinical Neurophysiology, 28,* 360–367.

Viehweg, R., & Campbell, R. (1960). Localization difficulty in monaurally impaired listeners. *Annals of Otology, Rhinology and Laryngology, 69,* 622–634.

Walsh, E. (1957). An investigation of sound localization in patients with neurological abnormalities. *Brain, 80,* 222–250.

Wedenberg, E. (1965). Prenatal Test of Hearing. *Acta Otolaryngology, Suppl. 206,* 27–32.

Weiss, M., Zelazo, P., & Swain, I. (1988). Newborn response to auditory stimulus discrepancy. *Child Development, 59,* 1530–1541.

Welsh, L. W., Welsh, J. J., & Healy, M. (1980). Central auditory testing and dyslexia. *Laryngoscope, 90,* 972–984.

Welsh, L. W., Welsh, J. J., Healy, M., & Cooper, B. (1982). Cortical, subcortical, and brainstem dysfunction: A correlation in dyslexic children. *Annals of Otology, Rhinology and Laryngology, 91,* 310–315.

Wepman, J. M., & Morency, A. (1973). *Auditory sequential memory test.* Los Angeles: Western Psychological Services.

Werner, L. A., Marean, G. C., Halpin, C. F., Spetner, N. B., & Gillenwater, J. M. (1992). Infant auditory temporal acuity: Gap detection. *Child Development, 63,* 260–272.

Wertheimer, M. (1961). Psychomotor coordination of auditory and visual space at birth. *Science, 134,* 1692.

Wexler, B., & Hawles, T. (1983). Increasing the power of dichotic methods: The fused rhymed words test. *Neuropsychologia, 21,* 59–66.

White, E. J. (1977). Children's performance on the SSW test and Willeford battery: Interim clinical data. In R. W. Keith (Ed.), *Central auditory dysfunction* (pp. 319–340). New York: Grune & Stratton.

Wightman, F., Allen, P., Dolan, T., Kistler, D., & Jamieson, D. (1989). Temporal resolution in children. *Child Development, 60*, 611–624.

Willeford, J. (1976). Differential diagnosis of central auditory dysfunction. In L. Bradford (Ed.), *Audiology: An audio journal for continuing education* (Vol. 2). New York: Grune & Stratton.

Willeford, J. (1977). Assessing central auditory behavior in children: A test battery approach. In R. W. Keith (Ed.), *Central auditory dysfunction* (pp. 43–72). New York: Grune & Stratton.

Willeford, J. A., & Bilger, J. M. (1978). Auditory perception in children with learning disabilities. In J. Katz (Ed.), *Handbook of clinical audiology (2nd ed.)* (pp. 410–425). Baltimore: Williams & Wilkins.

Willeford, J. A., & Burleigh, J. M. (1985). *Handbook of central auditory processing disorders in children.* New York: Grune & Stratton.

Willeford, J. A., & Burleigh, J. M. (1994). Sentence procedures in central testing. In J. Katz (Ed.), *Handbook of clinical audiology, fourth edition* (pp. 256–268). Baltimore: Williams & Wilkins.

Wilson, L., & Mueller, H. G. (1984). Performance of normal hearing individuals on Auditec filtered speech tests. *Asha, 27*, 189.

Wilson, R. H. (1994). Word recognition with segmented-alternated CVC words: Compact disc trials. *Journal of the American Academy of Audiology, 5*, 255–258.

Wilson, R. H., Arcos, J. T., & Jones, H. C. (1984). Word recognition with segmented-alternated CVC words: A preliminary report on listeners with normal hearing. *Journal of Speech and Hearing Disorders, 47*, 111–112.

Wilson, R. H., Preece, J. P., Salamon, D. L., Sperry, J. L., & Bornstein, S. P. (1994). Effects of time compression and time compression plus reverberation on the intelligibility of the Northwestern University Auditory Test No. 6. *Journal of the American Academy of Audiology, 5*, 269–277.

Wilson, R. H., Zizz, C. A., & Sperry, J. L. (1994). Masking-level difference for spondaic words in 2000-msec bursts of broadband noise. *Journal of the American Academy of Audiology, 5*, 236–242.

Woodcock, R. (1976). *Goldman-Fristoe-Woodcock Auditory Skills Test Battery— Technical manual.* Circle Pines, MN: American Guidance Service.

Woodcock, R. (1977). *Woodcock-Johnson Psycho-educational Test Battery: Technical report.* Allen, TX: DLM Teaching Resources.

Yakovlev, P. I., & Lecours, A. R. (1967). The myelogenetic cycles of regional maturation of the brain. In A. Minkowski (Ed.), *Regional development of the brain in early life* (pp. 3–70). Oxford, England: Blackwell.

Appendix

Answers to
Review Questions

Chapter One

1. *sagittal:* A cut in which the brain is divided into right and left sides.

   coronal: A cut dividing the brain into front and back sections.

   horizontal: A cut which divides the brain into upper and lower portions.

   transverse: A cut which is diagonal to the horizontal plane.

anterior: Towards the front.

posterior: Towards the back.

rostral: Towards the head and away from the tail.

caudal: Towards the tail and away from the head.

lateral: Away from the midline.

medial: Towards the midline.

2.   **a.** *central sulcus:* This is the fissure or valley that separates the frontal and parietal lobes.

     b. *frontal lobe:* This lobe lies posterior to the central sulcus and anterior to the occipital lobe. The primary motor cortex is located along the posterior portion of the frontal lobe.

     c. *lateral (Sylvian) fissure:* This sulcus marks the superior boundary of the temporal lobe.

     d. *occipital lobe:* The occipital lobe makes up the posterior-most portion of each cerebral hemisphere. The primary and secondary visual cortices are located here.

     e. *temporal lobe:* This lobe is located inferior to the frontal and parietal lobes and anterior to the occipital lobe. It contains the primary auditory cortex, portions of the auditory association areas, and portions of the language association areas.

     f. *parietal lobe:* This lobe lies posterior to the central sulcus and anterior to the occipital lobe. Its primary functions include perception of somatic sensation and integration for multimodality information.

     g. *longitudinal fissure:* This is the sulcus or valley that separates the right and left hemispheres.

3. *limbic system:* The limbic system is responsible for providing emotional drive for various functions necessary for survival.

   ventricles: These cavities within the brain function in the production and circulation of cerebrospinal fluid.

   meninges: The meninges are three fibrous tissue layers which form a protective covering for the brain and central nervous system.

4.   **a.** putamen

     b. external capsule

     c. caudate

    d. internal capsule
    e. claustrum
    f. globus padillus

5. Excitatory transmitters lower a postsynaptic neuron's membrane potential, allowing the cell to fire and transmit an impulse. Conversely, inhibitory neurotransmitters elevate the membrane potential of a neuron and make it less likely to fire.

6. The three main divisions of the brainstem are the midbrain, pons, and medulla oblongata.

7. The *cochlear nuclei* preserve the tonotopic organization initiated in the cochlea and pass auditory information on to higher brainstem structures.

The *superior olivary complex* contains "binaural cells" that receive information from both ipsilateral and contralateral cochlear nuclei and which are sensitive to timing and intensity differences between the ears. This makes the superior olivary complex important in binaural interaction.

The *lateral lemniscus* receives crossed and uncrossed projections from more caudal brainstem structures, continuing the bilateral representation of auditory input.

The *inferior colliculus* is important for localization and other binaural processes. Some projections from the inferior colliculus travel to the superior colliculus, reticular formation, and cerebellum for reflexive localization movements.

The *medial geniculate* body acts as a relay station for auditory information. Projections from the medial geniculate body travel to the auditory cortices via the internal capsule, external capsule, and insula.

8. *supratemporal plane:* This is the upper surface of the temporal lobe. It is on the posterior portion of this area that Heschl's gyrus is located.
Heschl's gyrus: This is the primary auditory cortex, which is responsible for auditory sensation and perception.
planum temporal: This is the portion of the temporal lobe extending from Heschl's gyrus to the end of the lateral fissure. Some axonal connections between Heschl's gyrus and Wernicke's area travel along the planum temporal.

supramarginal gyrus: This gyrus curves around the posterior limit of the lateral fissure and makes up part of the auditory association cortex (Wernicke's area).

angular gyrus: Along with the supramarginal gyrus, which borders it posteriorly, the angular gyrus makes up part of the auditory association cortex (Wernicke's area).

insula: The insula, located medially to Heschl's gyrus, contains fibers responsive to acoustic stimuli. Some auditory nerve impulses arriving via the internal capsule are passed on to Heschl's gyrus by the insula.

arcuate fasciculus: This nerve fiber bundle provides communication between the auditory association cortex and Broca's area in the frontal lobe.

9. **a.** anterior commissure
    b. rostrum
    c. genu
    d. body
    e. splenium

10. The primary function of the corpus callosum is to transfer information between the cerebral hemispheres. Because each side of the brain is dominant for different functions involved in effective auditory processing, it is crucial that the corpus callosum be intact for auditory tasks such as dichotic listening.

11. The efferent auditory system is responsible for both excitatory and inhibitory activity in the CANS. It is possible that the efferent system assists in detection of signals in noise. In addition, the olivocochlear bundle, which is the most caudal structure in the efferent auditory system, plays a role in auditory attention.

12. *Intra-axial:* a lesion arising from within the brainstem. A pontine glioma is an example of an intra-axial lesion. *Extra-axial:* a lesion originating on the auditory nerve adjacent to the brainstem. The most common example of an extra-axial brainstem lesion is the acoustic schwannoma.

13. *VIIIth nerve:* A lesion here is likely to produce abnormal hearing acuity and/or difficulty understanding speech for the ear ipsilateral to the lesion.

    brainstem: Central auditory effects of brainstem lesions may be unilateral or bilateral depending on the size of the lesion and the location at which it occurs in the brainstem.

    right temporal lobe: A lesion of this lobe commonly results in left ear suppression on dichotic listening tests.

Impaired sound localization ability for stimuli located in the left (contralateral) auditory field also may occur.

left temporal lobe: A lesion of this lobe may result in bilateral suppression during dichotic listening, deficits in discrimination of acoustic stimuli, and impaired sound localization ability for stimulu located in the right (contralateral) auditory field.

both temporal lobes: Bilateral temporal lobe lesions are rare and may result in cortical or central deafness.

corpus callosum: Lesions of the posterior portion of the corpus callosum result in a bilateral deficit on any auditory task that requires interhemispheric transfer of auditory information, as well as a left ear deficit on dichotic speech tasks.

efferent auditory system: Because this system is hypothesized to serve inhibitory functions, a lesion of the efferent system may result in difficulty hearing in noise or in auditory attention.

Chapter Two

1. Central auditory processes are the auditory system mechanisms and processes responsible for phenomena such as localization/lateralization, auditory discrimination, auditory pattern recognition, temporal aspects of audition, and auditory performance decrements with competing or degraded acoustic signals.
2. *Dichotic* refers to a condition in which different stimuli are presented to each ear simultaneously. *Diotic* refers to a situation in which identical stimuli are presented to both ears at the same time.
3. Kimura theorized that the contralateral pathways from the ear to the auditory cortex are stronger and more numerous than the ipsilateral pathways. For monotic stimuli, either type of pathway suffices for transmission of the signal. However, for dichotic stimuli, the contralateral pathways dominate and suppress the ipsilateral pathways. Consequently, a lesion in one hemisphere manifests itself as a deficit in the contralateral ear during dichotic listening.
4. The REA is the phenomenon in which performance for the right ear is better than that for the left ear among

normal right-handed listeners during dichotic listening tasks. The REA is presumed to indicate a preexisting ear asymmetry, and provides evidence of left hemisphere dominance for speech perception.

5. *right temporal lobe:* Lesions result in left ear suppression or extinction.

    left temporal lobe: Lesions result in contralateral or bilateral suppression or extinction.

    corpus callosum: If only the anterior portion of the corpus callosum is lesioned, there will be no effect seen on dichotic listening performance. If the posterior portion is lesioned, however, left ear extinction likely will occur during dichotic stimulation. Further, scores for the right ear may be enhanced due to a release from competition normally routed through the right hemisphere.

    cochlea: Sensorineural hearing loss may affect the size and direction of the ear advantage.

    middle ear: Conductive hearing loss does not appear to affect performance on dichotic listening tasks as long as the stimuli are presented at a sufficient intensity level.

6. Temporal processing refers to the way in which the CANS deals with the time-related aspects of the acoustic signal.

7. Tasks that rely on temporal processing include perception of the order of musical notes to determine if the pitch is rising or falling and recognition of subtle cues such as voice onset time and order of phonemes for speech perception.

8. *temporal lobe:* Lesions result in a contralateral deficit on two-tone ordering or gap detection tasks, and a bilateral deficit on temporal patterning tasks involving 2 or more successive stimuli.

    corpus callosum: Lesions result in a bilateral deficit on temporal patterning tasks involving 2 or more successive stimuli.

    brainstem: The effect of brainstem pathology on temporal processing is variable and depends upon the site of lesion and the type of task.

    cochlea: Lesions of the cochlea do not appear to affect temporal patterning tasks when the stimulus is of sufficient intensity. Cochlear site-of-lesion may, however, result in a temporal integration function that is less steep than normal.

middle ear: Middle ear pathology resulting in conductive hearing loss has little or no impact on temporal processing.

9.   Binaural interaction refers to the way in which the ears work together. This process depends primarily on the integrity of the brainstem auditory structures.

10.   Auditory functions that rely on binaural interaction include localization and lateralization of auditory stimuli, binaural release from masking, detection of signals in noise, and binaural fusion.

11.   The MLD is the difference in binaural masked thresholds for a signal between homophasic and antiphasic conditions. In the homophasic condition, both signal and noise are binaural and in phase, or binaural and out of phase. Consequently, both are perceived either at midline (in phase) or at the ear (out of phase). However, if one of the types of stimuli is in phase and the other is out of phase (antiphasic condition), they are perceived at different places, and the masked threshold improves. This improvement in masked threshold is the masking-level difference that occurs as a result of binaural release from masking.

SπNπ: both signal and noise are binaural and out of phase.

S$\emptyset$N$\emptyset$: both signal and noise are binaural and in phase.

SπN$\emptyset$: signal is binaural and out of phase; noise is binaural and in phase.

S$\emptyset$Nπ: signal is binaural and in phase; noise is binaural and out of phase.

12.   The antiphasic condition in which the signal delivered to the two ears is out of phase and the masking noise is in phase (SπN$\emptyset$) results in the largest MLDs. This occurs because the signal is perceived to be located at the ears while the noise is perceived to be located at midline.

13.   *temporal lobe:*   Lesions here may disrupt binaural perception, yet not directly affect binaural interaction.
midbrain and pons: Pathology in these structures could be expected to affect the reception and processing of binaural input. Lesions in the pontomedullary junction have been shown to be especially likely to result in abnormally small MLDs.

cochlea: MLDs are abnormally reduced in cases involving cochlear pathology. Localization and lateralization, on the other hand, are affected much less by cochlear pathology than by lesions occurring in other parts of the CANS. Indeed, even unilateral deafness does not necessarily destroy localization ability. There is, however, a great deal of variability in binaural interaction functions among listeners with cochlear lesions.

middle ear: Conductive hearing loss has been shown to degrade localization abilities, impair the ability to recognize speech-in-noise, and result in reduced MLDs. In cases of children with chronic otitis media, binaural interaction deficits may persist even after the conductive hearing loss is treated and hearing sensitivity returns to normal.

14. Multiple sclerosis causes focal lesions throughout the CANS. It slows neural transmission time, and may disrupt brainstem integration of binaural input. Individuals with multiple sclerosis may have difficulty processing interaural timing and intensity differences critical for localization of auditory stimuli, and with binaural fusion even in diotic listening conditions. Finally, individuals with multiple sclerosis are likely to exhibit reduced MLDs.

Chapter Three

1. The brain and spinal cord begin to develop during the 3rd week after conception, with the appearance of the neural plate.
2. The primary cerebral lobes are clearly formed by 28 weeks gestational age.
3. *ectoderm:* gives rise to the outer skin, the nervous system (including the CANS), and the inner and outer ear.
   mesoderm: gives rise to the skeleton, including the bony structures of the middle ear, the circulatory system, and the reproductive organs.
   endoderm: gives rise to the digestive and respiratory systems.
4. The inner ear is functional and adultlike in size and structure by the end of 20 weeks gestational age. The brainstem auditory pathways are structurally complete by 30 weeks after conception.

5. Myelination is the progressive development of myelin, a sheath that insulates and protects nerve fibers and enhances the speed and efficiency of neural transmission. Myelination proceeds in a caudal-to-rostral fashion, with brainstem structures complete before the first year of age, while myelination of cortical communication areas continues until adolescence and early adulthood.

6. Dendritic branching refers to the process in which dendrites—extensions of nerve cells that transmit neural impulses—grow and branch out in different directions. This process increases the surface area available for connections with other nerve cells, with the result that more information can readily be transferred through the nervous system.

7. *ABR*: The ABR is an electrical, far-field recording of synchronous activity in the auditory nerve and brainstem in response to auditory stimuli. The ABR waveform is characterized by five to seven distinct waves that occur in the 10 msec following presentation of click or tone pip stimuli. Wave latencies, interwave intervals, and wave amplitudes reach adult values by age 2 to 3 years.

   MLR: The MLR is recorded in the same manner as the ABR; however, the MLR represents neural activity in the 10 to 90 msec following stimulus presentation. The MLR waveform consists of three primary waves: Na, Pa, and Pb. Waves Na and Pa are present in nearly 100% of children by the age of 10 to 12 years.

   LEP: These are long latency, endogenous potentials which occur in response to internally generated processes related to attention to auditory stimuli. The auditory cortex is presumed to be the generator of this response. The three LEP waves, N1, P1, and P3, occur at 100, 200, and 300 msec, respectively, in adults. N1 and P2 reach adult values in adolescence. P3 latencies reach adult values in the early to mid teenage years.

8. Dichotic listening requires communication between the cerebral hemispheres via the corpus callosum, as well as proper functioning of both temporal lobes. In young children, a Right Ear Advantage (REA) often is observed on dichotic listening tasks due to incomplete myelination of the corpus callosum, which inhibits efficient interhemispheric transfer of information. The REA decreases as a function of increasing age.

9. When dichotic stimuli are less linguistically complex, the REA is less pronounced, even in the young child, and remains relatively constant with increasing age. When linguistically loaded stimuli such as sentences are utilized, however, young children exhibit a more pronounced REA which decreases with increasing age until 10 or 11 years of age.

10. Temporal processing abilities such as gap detection, temporal resolution, and temporal patterning improve as a function of increasing age until approximately 12 years of age. While the peripheral mechanism responsible for encoding temporal aspects of the acoustic signal appear to be well developed in young children, the ability of the CANS to extract and process temporal cues improves as a function of increasing age.

11. As with dichotic listening and temporal processing, binaural interaction abilities appear to improve with increasing age. Localizing behaviors become progressively more accurate from a few months of age until approximately 5 years of age. Integration and processing of binaural cues which occur in higher level brainstem pathways do not reach maximum efficiency until approximately age 6. Finally, MLDs generally show an improvement in performance from infancy until 6 years of age.

12. Performance on the majority of central auditory tests should reach adult values by age 11 or 12 years.

13. Abilities related to auditory processing change in a way that reflects the neuromaturation of the CANS from birth to age 12 years. Functioning that is normal for one stage of development or age group likely will be abnormal for a later stage or age. Therefore, age-appropriate normative data must be obtained in order to interpret performance on tests of central auditory processing accurately.

14. *Neuroplasticity* refers to the nervous system's ability to make organizational changes in response to internal and external changes. In essence, this term means that the CNS is able to form new connections as well as alter the functions that certain portions typically perform, in response to demands placed upon it.

15. Auditory deprivation may result in morphological changes within the CANS that impact auditory processing abilities. It has been shown that children with a

history of chronic otitis media with effusion exhibit reduced MLDs and difficulty hearing in noise even after PE tubes are in place and hearing sensitivity has returned to normal. These children also display abnormal ABR interwave intervals, suggesting dysfunction of structures in the brainstem. Similar results also have been seen in adults following otosclerosis-related auditory deprivation.

16. *Long-term potentiation* is the increase in synaptic activity and efficiency resulting from strong and repeated stimulation of a sensory system. It has been reported that long-term potentiation may involve an increase in nerve cell size and postsynaptic density.

17. If the nervous system has the ability to reorganize and acquire new skills and behaviors, and if long-term potentiation represents an ability to improve neural transmission in sensory systems, then it may be hypothesized that increased auditory stimulation of inefficient CANS pathways may result in structural changes as well as concomitant functional changes such as improved auditory processing abilities.

Chapter Four

1. The purpose of screening for CAPD is to identify those children in need of further, comprehensive central auditory assessment while, at the same time, reducing the number of inappropriate referrals for such costly services.

2. a. Prevalence of the disorder: 3–7% of school-aged children exhibit some form of learning disability. It is likely that the number of children with CAPD in this population is high. Children in this subgroup must be properly identified if effective management is to be initiated for them.

   b. CAPD screening may help identify children in need of medical follow-up that might otherwise go undetected.

   c. CAPD screening would decrease the number of overreferrals for comprehensive central auditory evaluations.

   d. Identification of CAPD will help reduce the shopping around and anxiety on the parts of parents and children that result from efforts to identify the underlying causes of learning and listening difficulties.

    e. Identification of CAPD will allow for insightful educational planning based on the individual child's auditory strengths and weaknesses.

    f. It is the audiologist's responsibility to evaluate all aspects of hearing.

3. A multidisciplinary team approach to CAPD screening provides more comprehensive information regarding the child's educational, social, communicative, cognitive, and medical characteristics than could easily be gathered by any one individual alone. This approach also reduces the time demand placed on any single individual and provides a more insightful answer to the question of whether additional testing is warranted.

4. *The Audiologist:* manages and coordinates the screening effort and performs standard audiological evaluations in order to rule out hearing loss as a contributing factor to a given child's listening and learning difficulties.

The Speech-Language Pathologist: defines the child's receptive and expressive langauge abilities as well as oral and written language skills. The speech-language pathologist also provides results of auditory perceptual subtests of speech-language test tools.

The Educator: provides descriptive information regarding the child's daily listening and learning behavior in the classroom environment. The educator also can illuminate areas of academic strengths and weaknesses for a given child.

The Psychologist: contributes information concerning the child's cognitive skills and capacity for learning, helps to identify attention-related disorders or emotional disturbances that may interfere with the learning process, and provides results of tests that tap auditory perceptual behaviors.

The Parent: provides information regarding family history of hearing or learning disorders, developmental milestones, auditory behaviors in the home environment, and medical history.

The Physician: rules out pathological conditions for which medical intervention may be indicated and which may be a contributing factor to learning difficulties.

5. Although these tests may have subtests that tap auditory perceptual abilities, they seldom provide information related to the specific nature of an auditory deficit. Most of these tests are confounded by language and other higher level neurocognitive variables, do not provide for sufficient acoustic control, and have no documented validity in the identification of disorders of the CANS.

6. Test of Auditory Perceptual Skills (TAPS)

   Goldman-Fristoe-Woodcock Auditory Skills Battery (GFWB)

   Lindamood Auditory Conceptualization Test (LAC)

   Auditory Discrimination Test (ADT)

   Carrow Auditory Visual Abilities Test

   Token Test for Children

   Flowers-Costello Test of Central Auditory Abilities

   Woodcock-Johnson Psychoeducational Battery—Revised

   Clinical Evaluation of Language Fundamentals—Revised (CELF-R)

7. First, that there is a reasonable likelihood that the child in question exhibits a CAPD must be established. Next, the results of a comprehensive central auditory evaluation must lead to recommendations for management that are not already being implemented. Finally, the child must have the capacity to participate in comprehensive central auditory assessment procedures.

8. The child with CAPD may behave as if he or she has a peripheral hearing loss even though hearing sensitivity is normal. In the classroom, these children are likely to perform more poorly in subjects requiring use of verbal language skills and may have difficulty with multistep directions. They may be distractible. Children with CAPD may refuse to participate in class dicussion or, conversely, may participate but respond in a manner that indicates a lack of understanding of discussion content. The child with CAPD may or may not exhibit a language disorder. It is not uncommon to see decreased performance in areas such as vocabulary, sequencing, and auditory discrimination/phonemic decoding among children with CAPD. Although IQ may be normal or above normal, verbal scores often are markedly lower than performance scores, leading to a classification of "learning disabled"

for many children with CAPD. Music skills may be poor, but art and drawing skills often are good in these children. Overall, children with CAPD tend to show a pattern in which skills and behaviors that rely on listening and verbal language are relatively depressed when compared to those which do not. Finally, many children with CAPD present with significant histories of chronic otitis media and/or family history of learning disorders.

9. If a child is suspected of exhibiting a CAPD, but comprehensive central auditory assessment cannot be performed, first it should be acknowledged that CAPD can neither be ruled in or out. Second, although a deficit-specific management plan cannot be developed, intervention strategies that address the child's most salient complaints should be initiated.

10. The success of a CAPD screening program necessitates the availability of resources for follow-through in the form of diagnostic assessment for those children for whom the need for further evaluation is indicated. The screening should not be considered the endpoint of the assessment process. In addition, it is important to monitor the outcome of the screening program in terms of the number of children referred for screening, the number referred for comprehensive evaluation, and the number finally identified as exhibiting CAPD, in order to evaluate program efficacy. Finally, the success of any CAPD screening program depends upon the cooperative interaction among all individuals involved.

Chapter Five

1. A test battery approach to central auditory assessment is necessary because no single test is sufficient in scope to address the complexity of the CANS. Therefore, a number of tests that assess different processes should be utilized. Second, the outcome of central auditory assessment should provide a description of the child's auditory strengths and weaknesses, rather than simply indicate the presence or absence of a disorder, in order to allow for more effective, deficit-specific management. Finally, the differentiation of site-of-dysfunction may influence

the recommendations made for management, particularly if medical referral is indicated. To identify the site of lesion accurately, it is critical that different tools that assess different levels of the central auditory system are used. Finally, it is the audiologist's responsibility to assess the central auditory system as part of overall hearing assessment, and a test battery approach to central auditory assessment represents the state-of-the-art in CAP evaluation.

2. *false positive:* Also called a false alarm, this is a positive finding on a test when the disorder is not, in fact, present.

    false negative: Also known as a miss, this is a negative finding in a subject who does, in fact, have the disorder.

    true positive: Also referred to as a hit, this is a positive result for a subject in whom the disorder does exist, or the correct identification of the presence of a disorder.

    true negative: Also called a correct rejection, this is a negative result for a subject who does not have the disorder in question, or the correct identification of the absence of a disorder.

    sensitivity: refers to the test's ability to identify correctly the presence of a disorder. It is calculated by dividing the number of true positives (hits) by the total of true positives plus false negatives (misses).

    specificity: refers to the test's ability to identify correctly the absence of a disorder. It is calculated by dividing the number of true negatives (correct rejections) by the total of false positives (false alarms) and true negatives.

    efficiency: refers to the test's overall ability to identify both the presence and absence of a particular disorder correctly, or the overall degree of both sensitivity and specificity.

3. Reliability refers to the repeatability of test results, or the degree to which the test will yield the same results within the test session or upon repeat testing. Procedural variables, or errors of measurement, that can affect reliability include calibration of equipment; practice effects, ceiling and floor effects, the use of too few items, and other factors directly related to the measurement being studied. Patient variables that can affect reliability include patient age; degree and stability of peripheral hearing loss; stability of the disorder itself; overall

health, attention, linguistic, and cognitive abilities; and the presence of additional, related disorders.

4. *Dichotic Digits Test:* Two digits from 1 to 10 (excluding 7) are presented to each ear simultaneously. The listener is instructed to repeat all four digits heard. This test is sensitive to lesions of the brainstem, cortex, and corpus callosum and is relatively unaffected by peripheral hearing loss.

Dichotic Consonant-Vowel Test: Stimuli consist of six CV segments. Different segments are presented to each ear simultaneously and the subjects must choose both segments heard from a printed list. This test is sensitive to cortical lesions but does not identify laterality of dysfunction.

Staggered Spondaic Word Test (SSW): This test involves the dichotic presentation of spondees in a manner such that the second syllable of the spondee presented to one ear overlaps the first syllable of the spondee presented to the other ear. The SSW is simple enough for use with a variety of ages and is relatively resistant to peripheral hearing loss. The SSW is sensitive to brainstem and cortical dysfunction.

Competing Sentence Test (CST): The CST involves the dichotic presentation of sentences. The listener is instructed to repeat the sentence heard in the target ear, while ignoring the sentence presented in the nontarget ear. This test has been suggested to be valuable in the investigation of neuromaturation and language processing abilities.

Synthetic Sentence Identification Test with Contralateral Competing Message (SSI-CCM): Stimuli consist of 10 third-order approximations of English sentences. These sentences are presented to the target ear while ongoing competition in the form of continuous discourse is presented to the nontarget ear. The listener chooses which of the target sentences he or she hears from a printed list. This test assesses the process of binaural separation and is helpful in distinguishing brainstem from cortical pathology.

Dichotic Sentence Identification Test (DSI): The DSI is similar to the SSI-CCM but is designed for use with hearing-impaired listeners. This test uses the SSI stimuli presented dichotically and requires the listener to choose from a printed list both sentences heard, thus tapping the process of binaural integration.

Dichotic Rhyme Test (DRT):   Stimuli for this test consist of rhyming CVC words beginning with one of the stop consonants. Pairs of words differing only in the initial consonant are presented dichotically. Due to the close acoustical alignment of the stimuli, the typical listener hears and reports only one word. This test taps the process of binaural integration and has been shown to be sensitive to dysfunction of the corpus callosum.

5. *Binaural separation:*   Competing Sentences, SSI-CCM.
   Binaural integration: Dichotic Digits, Dichotic CVs, SSW, DSI, DRT.

6. *Frequency Patterns Test, or Pitch Pattern Sequence Test:* This test consists of 120 pattern sequences, each made up of three tone bursts in varying patterns of high- and low-frequency. Thirty items are presented to each ear, and the listener is required to report the pattern heard verbally (e.g., high-high-low; low-high-low). This test is sensitive to disorders of the cerebral hemispheres and/or the corpus callosum.

   Duration Patterns Test: This test is similar to Frequency Patterns; however, the stimuli differ in terms of duration, rather than frequency. Again, the subject verbally describes the pattern heard (e.g., long-short-long; short-long-short). This test is sensitive to disorders of the cerebral hemispheres and/or corpus callosum and is relatively resistant to peripheral hearing loss.

   Psychoacoustic Pattern Discrimination Test (PPDT):   This test utilizes dichotically presented sequences of noise bursts or click trains. The listener must indicate discrimination of a monaural change in the pattern by pressing a button. The PPDT is sensitive to disorders of the cerebral hemispheres.

7. Both Frequency Patterns and Duration Patterns tap the processes of discrimination (frequency or duration, respectively), temporal ordering, and linguistic labeling of auditory stimuli. The PPDT assesses temporal patterning abilities and discrimination of temporal changes in acoustic stimuli.

8. Methods of reducing the redundancy of a speech signal include low-pass filtering, in which high-frequency com-

ponents of the word are filtered out; time compression, in which the temporal characteristics of a signal are altered without affecting the frequency characteristics; reverberation, which can be added to speech signals in order to reduce redundancy further; and the addition of background noise.

9. The lack of standardized test tools and material-specific normative data has resulted in conflicting findings for speech-in-noise tests. In addition, great variability is seen in speech-in-noise scores for both normal and lesioned subjects. Consequently, although speech-in-noise tests may be useful in describing auditory abilities, interpretation of results should be undertaken with caution.

10. Monaural low redundancy speech tasks assess the process of auditory closure.

11. *Rapidly Alternating Speech Perception (RASP):* In this test, speech is alternated quickly between the ears at periodic intervals. The sequential bursts fuse in the brainstem, and the target message is intelligible to the normal listener. Listeners with lesions of the low brainstem may have difficulty with this task; however, studies suggest that the RASP may not be sensitive to anything other than gross lesions.

    Binaural Fusion tests (BF): In these procedures, different portions of a signal are presented to each ear. The stimuli can be portioned via band-pass filtering with high-frequency information being delivered to one ear and low-frequency information being delivered to the other. Alternatively, CVC words can be used as stimuli, with the consonants presented to one ear and the vowels presented to the other. The test assesses the listener's ability to fuse the segmented stimuli into an intelligible whole. Research indicates that BF tasks have some limited utility in the identification of brainstem lesions.

    Interaural Difference Limen tasks: These procedures involve pairs of tonal stimuli that are presented to both ears simultaneously. Either the onset time or the intensity of the stimulus to one ear is manipulated relative to the other ear. The listener is required to indicate when he or she perceives the signal as lateralizing to one side or the other. This type of task appears to provide some measure of brainstem integrity; however, it requires precise control of the acoustic stimuli and, therefore, its clinical utility is limited at this time.

Masking Level Difference (MLD): This test involves the presentation of speech or tonal stimuli and noise while systematically varying the phase relationships between the ears. The MLD examines the difference in masked thresholds of speech or tones across different phase relationships. The MLD has been shown to be highly sensitive to brainstem lesions.

12. In general, and with the exception of the MLD, binaural interaction tests in use today demonstrate questionable sensitivity. In addition, some tests of binaural interaction, such as interaural difference limen tasks, are difficult to administer and require more precise acoustic control of stimuli than is provided by standard audiological equipment. Finally, with the exception of the MLD, binaural interaction tests provide no more information regarding brainstem integrity than is currently available through procedures such as ABR.

13. The Mismatched Negativity (MMN) response is a small, negative deflection superimposed on the P2 wave of the late evoked response following the presentation of an "oddball" stimulus embedded in a string of identical, standard stimuli. Conscious attention to the stimuli is not required to elicit the MMN. This response can be obtained with very small differences between the deviant and standard stimuli, and virtually any acoustic stimuli will suffice. Therefore, the MMN may provide a reliable, objective indicator of speech perception ability.

14. Electrophysiological testing can provide an objective supplement to behavioral procedures. In some cases, objective evidence of a processing disorder may be needed for legal or educational classification purposes, and electrophysiology may provide these objective data. In addition, behavioral data reflecting speech perception and other auditory processes may be provided by electrophysiological measures, particularly in hard-to-test populations. Finally, the ABR remains the most sensitive test of brainstem function in use today.

Chapter Six

1. Equipment needed for comprehensive behavioral central auditory assessment includes a two-channel audiometer,

a good quality tape player and/or compact disc player, and a sound booth.

2. The first step in the evaluation process should be an interview with the child and accompanying caregiver(s) to explain the evaluation procedure and to gather a thorough case history. The next step involves the actual adminstration of the selected test battery, during which the child should be monitored carefully for signs of fading attention or fatigue. Finally, the assessment results should be explained to the child and his or her caregiver(s) and preliminary recommendations for management made.

3. Because different tests of central auditory function assess different auditory processes, it is wise to include tests that tap each of these processes. The age and cognitive ability of the child also will influence the choice of tests that will be included in the test battery, as will the desired outcome of the assessment procedure. Finally, through ongoing interpretation of test results during the assessment itself, it may be determined that additional tests need to be added to the battery in order to provide further clarification of dysfunctional areas.

4. Dichotic Digits:
   Presentation Level: 50 dB SL (re: spondee threshold) or at MCL
   Instructions: The listener is informed that he or she will hear different numbers in each ear and should repeat all numbers heard.
   Scoring: Percent correct per ear
   Dichotic CVs:
   Presentation Level: 55 dBHL
   Instructions: The listener is instructed to indicate, using a printed list, which two CV segments were heard.
   Scoring: Percent correct per ear
   SSW:
   Presentation Level: 50 dB SL (re: PTA or spondee threshold) is recommended; however, intensities as low as 25 dB SL may be used.
   Instructions: The listener is instructed to repeat the words heard.
   Scoring: Raw SSW score indicates percentage of errors in each of four conditions (left and right competing and

noncompeting), percentage of errors by ear, and total percentage of errors.

Competing Sentences:

Presentation Level: Target: 35 dB SL (re: PTA), Competing: 50 dB SL

Instructions: The listener is instructed to repeat the sentence heard in the target ear, while ignoring the message in the competing ear.

Scoring: Percent correct per ear

SSI-CCM

Presentation Level: Primary message: 30 dB HL, Competing signal: varied from 30 to 50 dB HL

Instructions: The listener is instructed to ignore the competing signal and to identify the sentence heard in the target ear from a printed list of items.

Scoring: Percent correct per ear

DSI:

Presentation Level: 50 dB SL (re: PTA of 500, 1000, and 2000 Hz)

Instructions: The listener is to identify both sentences heard from a list of printed items.

Scoring: Percent correct per ear

Dichotic Rhyme Test:

Presentation Level: 50 dB SL (re: spondee threshold)

Instructions: The listener is instructed to repeat the word that is heard.

Scoring: Percent correct per ear

Frequency Patterns test:

Presentation Level: 50 dB SL (re: 1000 Hz threshold)

Instructions: The listener should be instructed that he or she will hear sets of three tones that will vary in pitch, and is to describe the pattern of the tones heard in terms of high and low. When initially instructing the listener, both visual and voiced pitch cues should be provided. Visual cues are then removed in order to ensure that the listener understands the task. In cases in which the listener performs poorly on the test, he or she can be instructed to hum or sing the patterns rather than label them verbally.

Scoring: Percent correct per ear

Duration Patterns test:

Presentation Level: 50 dB SL (re: 1000 Hz threshold)

Instructions: The instructions for this test are the same as for that of the Frequency Patterns test; however, the listener is instructed to label the patterns in terms of duration (e.g., long and short).

Scoring: Percent correct per ear

Low-Pass Filtered Speech:

Presentation Level: 50 to 70 dB HL

Instructions: The listener is instructed to repeat the words heard, and to guess if unsure.

Scoring: Percent correct per ear

Time-Compressed Speech:

Presentation Level: 50 to 70 dB HL

Instructions: The listener is instructed to repeat the words heard, and to guess if unsure.

Scoring: Percent correct per ear

SSI-ICM:

Presentation Level: Target: 30 dB HL, Competing signal: varied from 20 to 50 dB HL

Instructions: The listener is instructed to select the target sentence heard from a printed list.

Scoring: The score is calculated by taking the average of percentages correct at 0 dB S/N and 20 dB S/N

Binaural Fusion:

Presentation Level: 20 dB SL (re: thresholds at 500 and 2000 Hz) for adults, and 30 dB SL for children

Instructions: The listener is directed to repeat the words heard.

Scoring: Percent correct

Consonant-Vowel-Consonant (CVC) Fusion:

Presentation Level: 30 dB SL

Instructions: The listener is directed to repeat the words heard.

Scoring: Percent correct

Masking Level Difference (MLD):

Presentation Level: Stimuli are presented at 16 different signal to noise ratios in 2 dB increments from 0 dB S/N to −30 dB S/N

Instructions: The listener is asked to repeat the words heard.

Scoring: Thresholds are determined for both the SøNø and SπNø conditions. The MLD is calculated by determining the difference between the two thresholds.

5. The following tests may be suitable for use in cases of peripheral hearing loss: Dichotic Digits, SSW, DSI, Frequency Patterns, Duration Patterns, CVC Fusion

6. *Dichotic Digits, Dichotic CVs, SSW, DSI, DRT:* Binaural Integration

    Competing Sentences, SSI-CCM: Binaural Separation

    Frequency Patterns: Frequency Discrimination, Temporal Ordering, Linguistic Labeling

    Duration Patterns: Duration Discrimination, Temporal Ordering, Linguistic Labeling

    LPFS, Time Compressed Speech, SSI-CM: Auditory Closure

    Binaural Fusion, CVC Fusion, MLD: Binaural Interaction

Chapter Seven

1. The results of central auditory testing can help to answer questions related to the presence or absence of a disorder, the underlying processes affected, the site-of-dysfunction within the CANS, and the relationship of the CAPD to educational, cognitive, and communicative difficulties.

2. A lax criterion for identification of a disorder requires an abnormal finding on any single test in the battery. A strict approach demands abnormal findings on all tests utilized in order to identify the presence of a disorder positively.

3. The two components that should be present for finding the presence of a CAPD are an abnormal result on a test of central auditory processing and an indication of significant impact of the disorder upon learning or listening behavior.

4. Process-based interpretation refers to the assessment of a variety of specific auditory processes (i.e., auditory closure, binaural separation and integration, temporal patterning, binaural interaction, interhemispheric transfer of information) with the goal of identifying areas of auditory strengths and weaknesses. This type of interpretation allows for a detailed description of the child's underlying dysfunctional processes with an eye toward the development of a deficit-specific management program.

5. *Auditory Closure (Decoding):* The individual with a deficit in this process may have difficulty understanding

speech whenever the extrinsic redundancy of the message is reduced. He or she may have no problems understanding speech in a quiet environment; however, if the deficit is severe, even word recognition in quiet may be affected.

Binaural Separation and Integration: As in Auditory Closure, a deficit in the areas of Binaural Separation and/or Integration will manifest itself primarily in difficulty understanding speech-in-noise or when more than one person is talking at the same time. However, although the behavioral symptoms of Auditory Closure deficits and Binaural Separation/Integration deficits are similar, the underlying processes that are dysfunctional are very different, as will be the recommendations for management.

Temporal Patterning: Individuals with deficits in Temporal Patterning may have difficulty in the recognition and use of prosodic aspects of speech, including the identification of key words, and subtle differences of meaning indicated by changes in stress and intonational patterns. Expressively, they may exhibit monotonic speech, themselves. Finally, these individuals may have problems with sequencing critical elements, including sequencing individual sounds in words.

Binaural Interaction: The primary behavioral characteristic of a deficit in this process is difficulty in the detection of speech in a noisy background. Individuals with Binaural Interaction problems also may have impaired ability to localize auditory stimuli.

Interhemispheric Transfer: Persons with deficits in transfer of information between cerebral hemispheres may exhibit any combination of behavioral auditory characteristics.

6. *Auditory Closure (Decoding):* Poor performance on monaural low-redundancy speech tests and speech-in-noise tests. If the deficit is severe enough, even word recognition in quiet may be affected.

Binaural Separation and Integration: Poor performance on dichotic listening tasks. Individuals with Binaural Separation deficits also will perform poorly on tests of speech-in-noise.

Temporal Patterning: Poor performance on tests of temporal patterning (e.g., Frequency and Duration Patterns), in both the linguistic labeling and humming response conditions.

Binaural Interaction: Abnormally reduced MLDs, poor performance on speech-in-noise tests, and abnormal ABR results.

Interhemispheric Transfer: Left ear suppression on dichotic speech tasks combined with poor performance on tests of temporal patterning (e.g., Frequency and Duration Patterns) in the linguistic labeling response condition. However, performance on temporal patterning tasks will improve when the individual is asked to hum or sing the response.

7. *Auditory Closure (Decoding):* Environmental modifications to improve access to auditory information, activities designed to improve auditory closure from phonemic to sentence levels, preteaching of new concepts and vocabulary, and frequent repetition of key messages. In addition, consonant and vowel discrimination training may be indicated.

Binaural Separation and Integration: Environmental modifications to enhance auditory information while decreasing background noise; compensatory strategies focusing on direction of attention and selective listening.

Temporal Patterning: Prosody training and key word extraction. Reading aloud daily with particular emphasis on intonation, stress, and rhythm characteristics of speech may help develop awareness of prosodic aspects of speech.

Binaural Interaction: Environmental modifications to enhance access to auditory signals. Training in localization of auditory stimuli may be warranted. Additionally, the need for medical intervention should be ruled out.

Interhemispheric Transfer: Interhemispheric exercises to improve communication between the cerebral hemispheres. Additional management techniques should target the individual child's listening and educational difficulties.

8. When site-of-lesion has been determined through a comprehensive central auditory assessment, the clinician is better able to make informed decisions regarding the need for medical referral, and the management approach selection is likely to be more efficient. Finally, knowing the site of lesion or site of dysfunction facilitates monitoring the efficacy of rehabilitation in terms of tracking

changes in the effects of lesions. It should be noted, however, that site of lesion may not be identifiable with any degree of certainty in many cases.

9. *Brainstem:* Abnormal findings in the Synthetic Sentence Identification Test with Ipsilateral Competing Message, Masking-Level Difference, and Staggered Spondaic Words are indicative of lesions in this area. Also, Dichotic Digits, Competing Sentences, and Low-Pass Filtered Speech appear to be sensitive to brainstem dysfunction. Finally, brainstem dysfunction also can be identified through abnormalities in acoustic reflex testing, speech audiometry, and Auditory Brainstem Response testing.

Cerebral: For dichotic listening tasks and monaural low redundancy speech tasks, listeners with cerebral lesions tend to demonstrate abnormal performance in the ear contralateral to the involved hemisphere. Scores on Frequency and Duration Patterns tests likely will be depressed for both ears, regardless of site-of-lesion. Finally, listeners with temporal lobe lesions tend to demonstrate greater difficulty with consonant discrimination tasks and often require a longer response time than do normal listeners.

Interhemispheric: Findings in cases of corpus callosum lesions include left ear deficits on dichotic speech tasks and bilateral deficits on temporal patterning tasks when the listener is required to label verbally what was heard. However, performance on temporal patterning tasks tends to improve when the listener is asked to hum or sing the response. Performance on tests of monaural low-redundancy speech is generally normal with this type of lesion.

10. *Auditory Decoding Deficit:* Children characterized in this subprofile will experience difficulty understanding speech in noise. Sound blending, discrimination, and retention of phonemes often are poor. Reading, speech to print skills, vocabulary, syntax, and semantic skills may be weak. These children tend to perform poorly on tests of monaural low- redundancy speech, with right ear performance often worse than left ear performance.

Integration Deficit: Children in this subprofile may have difficulty with multimodality tasks that require interhemispheric cooperation. Use of prosodic cues in understanding speech may be impaired. Academically, these children tend to have difficulty with reading recognition, spelling, and writing due to an inability to recognize and use gestalt patterns adequately. On tests of central auditory function, Integration Deficit is characterized by left ear suppression on dichotic listening tasks, combined with bilateral deficits on tests of temporal patterning in the linguistic labeling condition.

Associative Deficit: Children in this category often exhibit receptive language deficits, and pragmatic and social communication skills may be poor. Although early academic achievement may be age-appropriate, increasing linguistic demands in the classroom by approximately the 3rd grade often precipitate general academic difficulties. Associative Deficit is characterized by the inability to apply the rules of language to incoming auditory stimuli. At its most severe, this dysfunction can result in the inability to attach linguistic meaning to phonemic units. On central auditory tests, children in this subprofile tend to exhibit bilateral deficits on dichotic listening tasks. Temporal patterning performance and speech sound discrimination usually are good; however, word recognition may be poor.

Output-Organization Deficit: This subprofile involves an impaired ability to sequence, plan, and organize responses. Children with Output-Organization Deficit may present with poor organizational skills, difficulty following directions, reversals, and poor word recall and retrieval abilities. Sequencing errors and sound blending difficulties also may be demonstrated. Children in this category may show good reading comprehension abilities, whereas writing and spelling skills may be poor due to the multi-element nature of these tasks. On central auditory testing, these children often have difficulty with any task that requires report of more than two critical elements. Therefore, performance on monaural low redundancy speech tests may be good; however, tests such as Frequency and Duration Patterns, Dichotic Digits, Competing Sentences, and Staggered Spondaic Words likely will indicate poor performance.

11. *Auditory Decoding Deficit:* An effective management approach for this deficit may resemble traditional aural rehabilitation, including consonant and vowel training, instruction in speech to print skills, vocabulary building

and other auditory closure activities, and environmental modifications designed to enhance access to auditory information. Finally, preteaching of new information and vocabulary will increase the extrinsic redundancy of the learning environment, and repetition of key information may be helpful, but only if the repetition is clearer acoustically than the original presentation of the message.

Integration Deficit: Management approaches aimed at improving interhemispheric transfer of information are likely to be beneficial for children in this subprofile. In addition, training in the use of prosodic aspects of speech typically is indicated. It is desirable to place children with Integration Deficit with a teacher who is dynamic and animated. The use of multimodality cues, unless appropriately implemented, may be contraindicated for individuals with Integration Deficit.

Associative Deficit: Management approaches for children with Associative Deficit should include elements of speech-language intervention. Metacognitive techniques aimed at strengthening the memory trace associated with item recall are helpful. Further, preteaching of new information and the imposition of external organization within the classroom are appropriate classroom-based strategies. Finally, frequent checks for understanding should be made by asking the child to paraphrase or demonstrate what is expected, rather than requesting simple repetition of instructions. It should be noted that repetition of key information is rarely effective for a child with Associative Deficit. Instead, information should be rephrased using simpler language and smaller linguistic units.

Output-Organization Deficit: As with Associative Deficit, children with Output-Organization Deficit likely will benefit from intervention designed to aid in the development of organizational skills. Speech-language intervention often is indicated for remediation of the expressive language component found in this subprofile. Finally, both repetition and rephrasing of key information may be useful for the child with Output-Organization Deficit, but only if the message and required response are broken down into linguistic units of no more than two critical elements.

Chapter Eight

1. The three main categories of CAPD management in the educational setting are (a) environmental modifications and classroom-based strategies designed to improve the child's access to auditory information; (b) remediation techniques designed to provide direct intervention for deficit areas; and (c) compensatory strategies designed to teach the child how to overcome residual dysfunction and maximize the use of auditory information.

2. The clinician should be cautious when asked to make "general recommendations" for all children with CAPD, as some suggestions will not be appropriate for children with certain types of auditory deficits. However, the following suggestions are helpful for all listeners in general: reduction in or elimination of adverse noise sources, education of significant individuals regarding listening and the nature of auditory disorders, and optimization of the learning environment based on the individual child's needs.

3. *Auditory Decoding Deficit:*   Appropriate classroom-based management strategies would include preferential seating, possible use of an FM auditory trainer to improve the signal-to-noise ratio in the classroom, repetition of key information, use of multimodality cues and hands-on demonstration, and frequent checks for understanding.

   Integration Deficit: Classroom-based management strategies appropriate for use with this profile might include provision of a notetaker, avoidance of use of multimodality cues (unless they are used correctly, as described in the text), and placement with an animated teacher.

   Associative Deficit: Appropriate classroom-based management strategies might include rephrasing of key information using smaller linguistic units, preteaching of new concepts, frequent checks for understanding by asking the child to rephrase or demonstrate what is expected, and imposition of external organization within the classroom.

   Output-Organization Deficit: Classroom-based suggestions that may be helpful are similar to those for Associative Deficit and include imposition of external organization within the classroom, frequent checks for understanding, repetition or rephrasing of critical information, and breaking down key information into linguistic units of no more than two critical elements.

4. *Auditory Closure Activities:* These are activities designed to assist the child in learning to fill in the missing components of an auditory message in order to perceive a meaningful whole. Activities such as these would be most useful with children who exhibit a deficit in the process of Auditory Closure, including children who fit into the Auditory Decoding Deficit subprofile.

    Vocabulary Building: These activities teach the child to utilize contextual derivation to determine word meaning. Like other Auditory Closure Activities, they are useful for children with deficits in Auditory Closure.

    Phoneme Training: The primary purpose of phoneme training is to help the child learn to develop accurate phonemic representation and to improve speech-to-print skills. This is accomplished through training of minimal contrast phoneme pair discrimination. These activities are particularly suited for use with children with Auditory Decoding Deficit.

    Prosody Training: Prosody training is designed to assist the child in learning to recognize and use prosodic aspects of speech such as rhythm, stress, and intonation. Activities include recognition of syllabic stress changes within words and changes in temporal cues within sentences. Prosody training is useful for children with deficits in the process of temporal patterning, such as is found in Integration Deficit.

    Temporal Patterning Training: The goal of temporal patterning training is for the child to discriminate differences in, analyze, and imitate rhythmic patterns of auditory stimuli. These activities are useful for children with deficits in temporal patterning, as in Integration Deficit, who are unable to perform the discriminations of subtle changes in stress and rhythm required for Prosody Training, or are unable to sequence information.

    Interhemispheric Exercises: Interhemispheric exercises are designed to improve efficiency of interhemispheric transfer of information and may include verbal and nonverbal activities. These exercises are designed for use with children with Integration Deficit, some cases of neuromaturational delay, or other deficits that include inadequate interhemispheric transfer of information.

5. Compensatory strategies useful for children with CAPD include metalinguistic, metacognitive, and linguistic strategies designed to aid the child in actively monitoring and self-regulating his or her own comprehension abilities and developing general problem-solving skills. Included are training in the rules of language; chunking, paraphrasing, and verbal rehearsal; the use of external organizational aids; and increasing internal motivation to succeed.

6. Children with CAPD tend to be passive rather than active listeners. Steps need to be taken to increase the child's internal motivation to implement compensatory strategies and other management suggestions, thus returning the locus of control back to the student. In this way, the child takes responsibility for his or her own listening behavior and is able to self-monitor and problem-solve in cases in which comprehension is troublesome. Only through the inclusion of the child as an active participant in his or her own management program will the success of that program be ensured.

7. Management approaches appropriate for the very young child could include virtually any activity used with older children. Phoneme training, reading aloud with selective listening goals, interhemispheric exercises, "guess the emotion" games to identify prosodic cues, and games designed to improve direction-following skills can all be fun and useful for very young children suspected of exhibiting CAPD.

8. Johnny appears to exhibit the characteristics of deficits in the areas of Binaural Separation and Integration, and Interhemispheric Transfer. His performance pattern suggests a neuromaturational delay, and he fits the description of the Integration Deficit subprofile. A management program appropriate for Johnny would include classroom-based modifications such as provision of a note taker and placement with an animated teacher; remediation activities such as Prosody Training and Interhemispheric Exercises; and compensatory strategies designed to aid in sequencing information, such as verbal rehearsal and chunking.

9. Mary exhibits a deficit in the process of Auditory Closure

and appears to fit the profile of Auditory Decoding Deficit. Management for Mary would include environmental modifications designed to improve acoustical clarity of the spoken message, while decreasing background noise, and use of an FM auditory trainer might be considered. Phoneme Training, including speech-to-print skills, would be appropriate in order to help Mary develop accurate phonemic representation, and Auditory Closure activities, including Vocabulary Building, may be indicated. Compensatory strategies appropriate for Mary would include methods of increasing internal motivation and self-monitoring of her own comprehension, as well as methods of identifying difficult listening situations and developing problem-solving strategies to overcome those difficulties.

10. Fred exhibits deficits in the areas of Binaural Separation and Integration of auditory stimuli. His academic and central test profile suggests the presence of an Associative Deficit. Fred would benefit from direct speech-language intervention to address his receptive language deficits. In addition, Fred's classroom teacher will need to be aware of the need for information to be broken down into smaller linguistic units, rather than repeated verbatim, making frequent checks for understanding, and imposing means of external organization, as opposed to independent work projects. Fred should be taught compensatory strategies designed to aid the memory trace, including chunking, verbal rehearsal, and paraphrasing of key information. Training in the rules of language likely will be indicated, as well.

11. Alex exhibits the characteristics of Output-Organization Deficit, which includes difficulty with any auditory task requiring report of two or more critical elements. As such, Alex will need to learn how to utilize organizational aids, such as notebooks and calendars, as well as metalinguistic and metacognitive strategies designed to strengthen the memory trace. His teachers will need to be aware of the need for key information to be pretaught, and to be broken into linguistic units of no more than two critical elements. Speech-language intervention likely will be indicated in order to address the expressive language component of Alex's disorder.

Chapter Nine

1. Education of key individuals involved in CAP service delivery will serve to inform them of the current issues surrounding the topic of CAPD in the educational setting, and to help ensure their cooperation in the service delivery effort. In addition, education of these individuals will delineate each person's role and expected contribution to the effort, and facilitate provision of quality identification and follow-through services.

2. *Audiologist:* Key topics important in the education of the audiologist include specific training in the scientific underpinnings of central auditory processing; practical application of scientific theory; identification, assessment, and management issues; and time management.

   Speech-Language Pathologist: The speech-language pathologist will benefit from education in the areas of appropriate methods of diagnosing CAPD, as well as implementation of CAPD management approaches.

   Educator: Classroom and special education teachers likely will be particularly interested in information regarding the educational impact of CAPD and methods of CAPD management, particularly classroom-based management techniques.

   Psychologist: The psychologist will require information regarding appropriate methods of diagnosing CAPD, as well as the need for his or her contribution of information regarding cognitive capacities and psychoeducational abilities of the child in question. In addition, a discussion of the neurophysiological bases of CAPD should be included in any educational program aimed at the psychologist.

   Parent: Parents of children with CAPD should be informed as to the general nature of CAPD, types of management approaches useful for children with CAPD, and prognosis for success.

   Private Practitioner: The private practitioner will need specific education regarding appropriate methods of diagnosing CAPD and the need for the diagnostician to work closely with educational personnel in the assessment and management process.

3. Components of any diagnostic CAP report should include Background Information, Results of Audiological Evaluation, Results of Central Auditory Assessment, Impressions, and Recommendations for management or follow-up.

4. If results of a central auditory assessment yield no significant findings, the clinician should state clearly in the diagnostic report that the presence of a CAPD is not likely in those areas specifically assessed. In this manner, the reader can be led to the understanding that auditory difficulties may exist in areas not specifically addressed by the evaluation process.

5. The use of handouts in imparting CAP-related information will allow the clinician to provide detailed information regarding management activities and other CAP-related topics, while saving valuable time that may otherwise be used in the repetitive relay of the same information to multiple sources.

6. A Child Study is a meeting in which all of the key service providers involved in the education of a given child are brought together to discuss educational options and methods of addressing the child's needs. This meeting can be a particularly useful forum for the clinician engaged in CAP service delivery to impart diagnostic information and suggestions for management in such a way as to ensure understanding and cooperation among persons involved, and to answer questions in a timely fashion.

7. The primary components of any CAP service delivery program include Education and Training, Screening, Comprehensive CAP Assessment, Management, and Follow-through, and a procedure for monitoring program efficacy through Data Collection and Research.

8. Knowledge of data collection and scientific methodology will serve to provide the clinician with a means of monitoring program efficacy, as well as answering pertinent questions regarding treatment efficacy and other timely topics.

9. This question should be addressed by each individual reader in his or her own way, paying particular attention to those areas cited in this chapter.

Chapter Ten

1. By functioning in the dual role of scientist and practitioner, the clinician will be able to approach clinical decision making from a scientific perspective, thus improving the effectiveness of his or her clinical skills. In addition, job satisfaction and stimulation will likely increase, and the clinician will be in a position to add important information to the body of CAP-related literature concerning diagnostic and remediation techniques.

2. The process of engaging in diagnostic activities, as well as in choosing therapy techniques and monitoring their effectiveness, relies upon the scientific method. Therefore, the activities that every clinician engages in on a daily basis involve the incorporation of scientific methodology into the clinical setting.

3. *data:* attributes or events observed during research activities.

   variable: an outcome that can take on more than one value. Variables can be independent or dependent.

   independent variable: a condition controlled by the researcher in order to test its effect upon the outcome.

   dependent variable: a variable that measures the outcome of a research study.

   sample: the group chosen from the general population for study in a given research project.

   inferential method: the process of inferring the results from a sample to a population.

   variability: the degree of spread or dispersion that characterizes a group of scores within a sample or a population.

   significance: a finding that two experimental groups are different. Significance is expressed in terms of probability that the findings were due to chance.

   correlation: a relationship between two or more variables. The finding that two or more variables are correlated does not imply cause and effect.

4. Factors that help to determine the degree to which the results of a study can be generalized to the population as a whole include the representativeness of the sample chosen, the sample size, and the significance of the findings.

5. Statistical significance refers to a finding that two experimental groups are different. The degree to which such findings will be clinically significant, however, depends on whether the findings can be utilized in the real-life, clinical setting.

6. A negative correlation is one in which the inverse relationship exists, or one in which the value of one variable increases as the value of another decreases. Conversely, a positive correlation indicates that changes in two or more related variables occurs in the same direction (e.g., as one increases, so does the other).

7. *Experimental Research:* This type of research is designed to determine the effect of a given variable on the outcome variable and involves manipulation of an independent, or "treatment," variable.
Descriptive Research: The goal of descriptive research is to describe the characteristics of a selected phenomenon and involves the collection of data without manipulation of variables.
Correlational Research: The purpose of this type of research is to determine if and how two or more variables are related to one another, without implying cause and effect.
Historical Research: Historical research is concerned primarily with describing the nature of events that have occurred in the past for the purpose of examining trends in data.

8. In experimental research design, the clinician has complete control over the assignment of subjects to sample groups and manipulation of the primary independent variable under study. In contrast, causative-comparative research is useful when the independent variable is already established and cannot be manipulated by the researcher. In this type of research, the assignment of subjects to sample groups is essentially out of the hands of the researcher.

9. Mean = 86.8

10. Median = 93.5; Mode = 99

11. Tests of significance determine whether two or more groups are different and, if so, the probability that the differences found are due to chance.

12. *t* tests are designed to determine whether scores for two groups are significantly different. ANOVA (*F* tests) serve the same function; however, these tests of significance are designed for use with more than two groups.

13. The primary purpose of measures of association or correlation is to determine whether a significant relationship exists between two or more variables.

Index